Comprehensive Care of the Patient with Chronic Illness

Editor

DOUGLAS S. PAAUW

MEDICAL CLINICS
OF NORTH AMERICA

www.medical.theclinics.com

Consulting Editors
DOUGLAS S. PAAUW
EDWARD R. BOLLARD

September 2015 • Volume 99 • Number 5

ELSEVIER

1600 John F. Kennedy Boulevard • Suite 1800 • Philadelphia, Pennsylvania, 19103-2899

http://www.theclinics.com

MEDICAL CLINICS OF NORTH AMERICA Volume 99, Number 5
September 2015 ISSN 0025-7125, ISBN-13: 978-0-323-39571-7

Editor: Jessica McCool
Developmental Editor: Alison Swety

Medical Clinics of North America (ISSN 0025-7125) is published bimonthly by Elsevier Inc., 360 Park Avenue South, New York, NY 10010-1710. Months of publication are January, March, May, July, September, and November. Business and editorial offices: 1600 John F. Kennedy Boulevard, Suite 1800, Philadelphia, PA 19103-2899. Periodicals postage paid at New York, NY, and additional mailing offices. Subscription prices are USD $255.00 per year (US individuals), $471.00 per year (US institutions), $125.00 per year (US Students), $320.00 per year (Canadian individuals), $612.00 per year (Canadian institutions), $200.00 per year (Canadian and foreign students), $390.00 per year (foreign individuals), and $612.00 per year (foreign institutions). To receive student/resident rate, orders must be accompanied by name of affiliated institution, date of term, and the signature of program/residency coordinator on institution letterhead. Orders will be billed at individual rate until proof of status is received. Foreign air speed delivery is included in all Clinics' subscription prices. All prices are subject to change without notice. **POSTMASTER:** Send address changes to *Medical Clinics of North America*, Elsevier Health Sciences Division, Subscription Customer Service, 3251 Riverport Lane, Maryland Heights, MO 63043. **Customer Service: Telephone: 1-800-654-2452** (U.S. and Canada); **1-314-447-8871** (outside U.S. and Canada). **Fax: 314-447-8029. E-mail: journalscustomerserviceusa@elsevier.com** (for print support); **journalsonlinesupport-usa@elsevier.com** (for online support).

Reprints. For copies of 100 or more of articles in this publication, please contact the Commercial Reprints Department, Elsevier Inc., 360 Park Avenue South, New York, NY 10010-1710. Tel.: 212-633-3874; Fax: 212-633-3820; E-mail: reprints@elsevier.com.

Medical Clinics of North America is also published in Spanish by McGraw-Hill Interamericana Editores S. A., P.O. Box 5-237, 06500 Mexico, D.F., Mexico.

Medical Clinics of North America is covered in *MEDLINE/PubMed (Index Medicus), Current Contents, ASCA, Excerpta Medica, Science Citation Index,* and *ISI/BIOMED.*

PROGRAM OBJECTIVE
The goal of the *Medical Clinics of North America* is to keep practicing physicians up to date with current clinical practice by providing timely articles reviewing the state of the art in patient care.

TARGET AUDIENCE
All practicing physicians and other healthcare professionals.

LEARNING OBJECTIVES
Upon completion of this activity, participants will be able to:
1. Review techniques in the management of patients with chronic diseases such as kidney and liver diseases, HIV, sarcoidosis, lung disease, and bowel disease.
2. Discuss ongoing issues in primary care for the childhood cancer survivor.
3. Recognize the unique considerations and methods of care necessary in the treatment of homeless and refugee patients.

ACCREDITATION
The Elsevier Office of Continuing Medical Education (EOCME) is accredited by the Accreditation Council for Continuing Medical Education (ACCME) to provide continuing medical education for physicians.

The EOCME designates this enduring material for a maximum of 15 *AMA PRA Category 1 Credit*(s)™. Physicians should claim only the credit commensurate with the extent of their participation in the activity.

All other health care professionals requesting continuing education credit for this enduring material will be issued a certificate of participation.

DISCLOSURE OF CONFLICTS OF INTEREST
The EOCME assesses conflict of interest with its instructors, faculty, planners, and other individuals who are in a position to control the content of CME activities. All relevant conflicts of interest that are identified are thoroughly vetted by EOCME for fair balance, scientific objectivity, and patient care recommendations. EOCME is committed to providing its learners with CME activities that promote improvements or quality in healthcare and not a specific proprietary business or a commercial interest.

The planning committee, staff, authors and editors listed below have identified no financial relationships or relationships to products or devices they or their spouse/life partner have with commercial interest related to the content of this CME activity:
Nicole Chow Ahrenholz, MD; Douglas Berger, MD, MLitt; Edward R. Bollard, MD, DDS, FACP; Fred R. Buckhold III, MD; Anjali Fortna; Mahri Z. Haider, MD, MPH; Jan Hirschmann, MD; Jocelyn James, MD; Meghan M. Kiefer, MD, MPH; Jared Wilson Klein, MD, MPH; Michael J. Lenaeus, MD, PhD; Iris W. Liou, MD; Jessica McCool; Douglas S. Paauw, MD, MACP; Jean R. Park, MD; Sheryl A. Pfeil, MD; Santha Priya; Simha Reddy, MD; Michael J. Ryan, MD; Justin Shinn, MD; Megan Suermann; Alison Swety; Genji Terasaki, MD; Anna Volerman, MD; Christopher J. Wong, MD.

The planning committee, staff, authors and editors listed below have identified financial relationships or relationships to products or devices they or their spouse/life partner have with commercial interest related to the content of this CME activity:
Katharine A. Bradley, MD, MPH has stock ownership in Johnson & Johnson Services, Inc.
Genevieve Pagalilauan, MD has an employment affiliation with *Hopkins Practical Review in Internal Medicine*, published by Oakstone Publishing, LLC.

UNAPPROVED/OFF-LABEL USE DISCLOSURE
The EOCME requires CME faculty to disclose to the participants:
1. When products or procedures being discussed are off-label, unlabelled, experimental, and/or investigational (not US Food and Drug Administration [FDA] approved); and
2. Any limitations on the information presented, such as data that are preliminary or that represent ongoing research, interim analyses, and/or unsupported opinions. Faculty may discuss information about pharmaceutical agents that is outside of FDA-approved labelling. This information is intended solely for CME and is not intended to promote off-label use of these medications. If you have any questions, contact the medical affairs department of the manufacturer for the most recent prescribing information.

TO ENROLL

To enroll in the *Medical Clinics of North America* Continuing Medical Education program, call customer service at 1-800-654-2452 or sign up online at http://www.theclinics.com/home/cme. The CME program is available to subscribers for an additional annual fee of USD $295.

METHOD OF PARTICIPATION

In order to claim credit, participants must complete the following:

1. Complete enrolment as indicated above.
2. Read the activity.
3. Complete the CME Test and Evaluation. Participants must achieve a score of 70% on the test. All CME Tests and Evaluations must be completed online.

CME INQUIRIES/SPECIAL NEEDS

For all CME inquiries or special needs, please contact elsevierCME@elsevier.com.

MEDICAL CLINICS OF NORTH AMERICA

Contributors

CONSULTING EDITORS

DOUGLAS S. PAAUW, MD, MACP
Professor of Medicine, Division of General Internal Medicine, Rathmann Family Foundation Endowed Chair for Patient-Centered Clinical Education; Medicine Student Programs, Professor of Medicine, University of Washington School of Medicine, Seattle, Washington

EDWARD R. BOLLARD, MD, DDS, FACP
Professor of Medicine, Associate Dean of Graduate Medical Education, Designated Institutional Official, Department of Medicine, Penn State-Hershey Medical Center/Penn State University College of Medicine, Hershey, Pennsylvania

EDITOR

DOUGLAS S. PAAUW, MD, MACP
Professor of Medicine, Division of General Internal Medicine, Rathmann Family Foundation Endowed Chair for Patient-Centered Clinical Education; Medicine Student Programs, Professor of Medicine, University of Washington School of Medicine, Seattle, Washington

AUTHORS

NICOLE CHOW AHRENHOLZ, MD
Clinical Instructor, Section of General Internal Medicine, Department of Medicine, Harborview Medical Center, University of Washington, Seattle, Washington

DOUGLAS BERGER, MD, MLitt
Acting Instructor, Department of Medicine, VA Puget Sound, University of Washington, Seattle, Washington

KATHARINE A. BRADLEY, MD, MPH
Senior Investigator, Group Health Research Institute; Affiliate Professor, Departments of Medicine and Health Services, University of Washington, Seattle, Washington

FRED R. BUCKHOLD III, MD
Assistant Professor, Division of General Internal Medicine; Program Director, Internal Medicine Residency Training Program, Department of Internal Medicine, Saint Louis University School of Medicine, Saint Louis, Missouri

MAHRI Z. HAIDER, MD, MPH
Clinical Instructor, Section of General Internal Medicine, Department of Medicine, Harborview Medical Center, University of Washington, Seattle, Washington

JAN HIRSCHMANN, MD
Professor, Department of General Internal Medicine, Puget Sound VA Medical Center, University of Washington School of Medicine, Seattle, Washington

JOCELYN JAMES, MD
Acting Instructor, Division of General Internal Medicine, Department of Medicine, Harborview Medical Center, University of Washington, Seattle, Washington

MEGHAN M. KIEFER, MD, MPH
Acting Assistant Professor, Division of General Internal Medicine, Department of Medicine, University of Washington School of Medicine, Seattle, Washington

JARED WILSON KLEIN, MD, MPH
Clinical Instructor, Division of General Internal Medicine, Department of Medicine, Harborview Medical Center, University of Washington, Seattle, Washington

MICHAEL J. LENAEUS, MD, PhD
Clinical Instructor, Department of General Internal Medicine, University of Washington Medical Center, Seattle, Washington

IRIS W. LIOU, MD
Assistant Professor, Division of Gastroenterology, Department of Medicine, University of Washington, Seattle, Washington

DOUGLAS S. PAAUW, MD, MACP
Professor of Medicine, Division of General Internal Medicine, Rathmann Family Foundation Endowed Chair for Patient-Centered Clinical Education; Medicine Student Programs, Professor of Medicine, University of Washington School of Medicine, Seattle, Washington ˙

GENEVIEVE PAGALILAUAN, MD
Associate Professor, Division of General Internal Medicine, Department of Medicine, University of Washington, Seattle, Washington

JEAN R. PARK, MD
Assistant Professor of Clinical Medicine, Division of Hospital Medicine, Department of Internal Medicine, The Ohio State University College of Medicine and Wexner Medical Center, Columbus, Ohio

SHERYL A. PFEIL, MD
Associate Professor of Clinical Medicine, Division of Gastroenterology, Hepatology, and Nutrition, Department of Internal Medicine, The Ohio State University College of Medicine and Wexner Medical Center, Columbus, Ohio

SIMHA REDDY, MD
Clinical Instructor, Division of General Internal Medicine, Department of Medicine, VA Puget Sound Health Care System, University of Washington, Seattle, Washington

MICHAEL J. RYAN, MD
Associate Professor, Division of Nephrology, Department of Medicine, University of Washington School of Medicine, Seattle, Washington

JUSTIN SHINN, MD
Department of Internal Medicine, University of Washington School of Medicine, Seattle, Washington

GENJI TERASAKI, MD
Assistant Professor, Section of General Internal Medicine, Department of Medicine, Harborview Medical Center, University of Washington, Seattle, Washington

ANNA VOLERMAN, MD
Assistant Professor, Department of Medicine and Pediatrics, University of Chicago, Chicago, Illinois

CHRISTOPHER J. WONG, MD
Assistant Professor, Division of General Internal Medicine, Department of Medicine, University of Washington, Seattle, Washington

Contents

> Chronic liver disease results from a wide range of conditions, for which individual management is beyond the scope of this article. General education, counseling, and harm reduction practices are important to the primary care of these patients, as are monitoring for cirrhosis and management of its complications. For patients with advanced liver disease, comprehensive care includes considering referral for liver transplantation, educating and empowering patients to prioritize goals of care, and optimizing symptom relief.

> Chronic kidney disease (CKD) is defined by reduced estimated glomerular filtration rate, increased proteinuria, or both. CKD affects more than 10% of US adults, or 20 million people, and the numbers are rising as the population ages. However, CKD remains underdiagnosed. Diabetes and hypertension are the most common causes of CKD. Although end-stage renal disease is a feared complication of CKD, patients with CKD have a much greater risk of dying of cardiovascular (CV) disease than progressing to kidney failure. Special effort should be made to address modifiable CV risk factors in patients with CKD.

> Obstructive lung disease includes asthma and chronic obstructive pulmonary disease (COPD). Because a previous issue of *Medical Clinics of North America* (2012;96[4]) was devoted to COPD, this article focuses on asthma in adults, and addresses some topics about COPD not addressed previously. Asthma is a heterogeneous disease marked by variable airflow obstruction and bronchial hyperreactivity. Onset is most common in early childhood, although many people develop asthma later in life. Adult-onset asthma presents a particular challenge in the primary care clinic because of incomplete understanding of the disorder, underreporting of symptoms, underdiagnosis, inadequate treatment, and high rate of comorbidity.

Inflammatory bowel disease (IBD) includes 2 major disorders, ulcerative colitis and Crohn's disease, both of which are due to inflammatory dysregulation in the gastrointestinal tract. Ulcerative colitis and Crohn's disease have many overlapping as well as distinguishing features in pathophysiology and management. This article highlights aspects of IBD that are most applicable to a primary care physician's practice. Also detailed are disease-related and treatment-related, and routine health maintenance practices for patients with IBD.

More than one in four American adults consume alcohol in quantities exceeding recommended limits. One in 12 have an alcohol use disorder marked by harmful consequences. Both types of alcohol misuse contribute to acute injury and chronic disease, making alcohol the third largest cause of preventable death in the United States. Alcohol misuse alters the management of common conditions from insomnia to anemia. Primary care providers should screen adult patients to identify the full spectrum of alcohol misuse. A range of effective treatments are available – from brief counselling interventions and mutual help groups to medications and behavioral therapies.

This article discusses the unique considerations when caring for patients who lack housing, one of the most essential human needs. Special attention is provided to diseases and conditions that are affected by homelessness as well as to particularly vulnerable populations of homeless patients.

 Video of 82-year-old man's description of how torture relates to chronic leg pain accompanies this article

Refugees share a common experience of displacement from their country of origin, migration, and resettlement in an unfamiliar country. More than 17 million people have fled their home countries due to war, generalized violence, and persecution. US primary care physicians must care for their immediate and long-term medical needs. Challenges include (1) language and cultural barriers, (2) high rates of mental health disorders, (3) higher prevalence of latent infections, and (4) different explanatory models for chronic diseases. This article discusses management strategies for common challenges that arise in the primary care of refugees.

Foreword

Comprehensive Care of the Patient with Chronic Illness

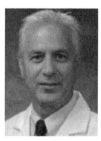

Edward R. Bollard, MD, DDS, FACP
Consulting Editor

The prevalence of one or more chronic medical conditions in patients presenting to the practicing general internist increases with age. In fact, in 2012, it was estimated that half of all adults—117 million people—had one or more chronic health conditions,[1] and that almost two-thirds of those over 65 years of age had multiple chronic medical conditions.[2] Historically, the care of the patient with chronic medical conditions has often been fragmented, leading to poor patient satisfaction and outcomes, as well as increased financial burden to our health care system. The comprehensive understanding of these chronic conditions and the ability to provide both longitudinal primary care as well as complex interdisciplinary care for these patients are essential.

In this issue of the *Medical Clinics of North America*, Dr Douglas S. Paauw and his expert colleagues present a comprehensive approach to the management of several chronic medical conditions. I believe the content will provide guidance to the practicing physician in what will result in more standardized, evidence-based, and patient-centered outcomes to our ongoing care of these patients.

Edward R. Bollard, MD, DDS, FACP
Department of Medicine
Penn State–Hershey Medical Center/
Penn State University College of Medicine
500 University Drive
PO Box 850 (Mail Code H039), Hershey, PA 17033-0850, USA

E-mail address:
ebollard@hmc.psu.edu

Med Clin N Am 99 (2015) xv–xvi
http://dx.doi.org/10.1016/j.mcna.2015.07.002
0025-7125/15/$ – see front matter © 2015 Published by Elsevier Inc.

REFERENCES

1. Ward BW, Schiller JS, Goodman RA. Multiple chronic conditions among US adults: a 2012 update. Prev Chronic Dis 2014;11:e62.
2. Partnership for Solutions. Chronic Conditions: Making the Case for Ongoing Care. Robert Wood Johnson Foundation; 2002.

Preface

Walking the Narrow Path— Managing the Patient with Chronic Medical Illnesses

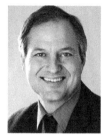

Douglas S. Paauw, MD, MACP
Editor

This issue of *Medical Clinics of North America* covers comprehensive care of patients with chronic medical illness. Primary care physicians frequently take care of patients who have long-term, ongoing chronic medical conditions that impact the way we interpret practice guidelines, dose drugs, manage symptoms, and set goals. There are nuances in the everyday management of patients with chronic organ system dysfunction. A good example of this is in our patients with chronic renal disease, where many commonly used drugs become ineffective (ie, thiazide diuretics) or more toxic and contraindicated (bisphosphonates).

The issue covers several themes that impact the approach to primary care delivery. Articles covering the primary care of patients with major organ system dysfunction (renal, pulmonary, and liver) are included. Two articles are dedicated to covering underlying diseases (HIV and sarcoid) that can present in many ways and be perplexing to physicians responsible for ongoing care. The remainder of the issue includes articles on patient populations that carry increased risk and complexity (solid organ transplant patients, childhood cancer survivors, homeless patients, refugees, and patients with chronic alcohol misuse).

I hope that this issue will bring together expert information from multiple sources that will help in the ongoing management of these complex patients. As primary care providers, we are expected to know the obvious as well as the hidden perils our patients face. Understanding and recognizing what makes up this complexity and how we need

Med Clin N Am 99 (2015) xvii–xviii
http://dx.doi.org/10.1016/j.mcna.2015.07.001
0025-7125/15/$ – see front matter © 2015 Published by Elsevier Inc.

medical.theclinics.com

to individualize our management plans to account for these different risks help us walk the narrow path to providing excellent care.

Douglas S. Paauw, MD, MACP
Division of General Internal Medicine
Department of Medicine
University of Washington School of Medicine
Seattle, WA 98195, USA

E-mail address:
DPaauw@medicine.washington.edu

Comprehensive Care of Patients with Chronic Liver Disease

Jocelyn James, MD[a],*, Iris W. Liou, MD[b]

KEYWORDS

- Chronic liver disease • Cirrhosis • Ascites • Varices
- Spontaneous bacterial peritonitis • Hepatic encephalopathy

KEY POINTS

- In addition to disease-specific information, patients with chronic liver disease should receive counseling about nutrition, alcohol, medication safety, and monitoring needs.
- Patients with chronic liver disease should be monitored for progression to cirrhosis, because this diagnosis requires specific management, such as endoscopic screening for varices and screening for hepatocellular carcinoma.
- Cirrhosis is a clinical and often subtle diagnosis that integrates history, examination, laboratory and radiographic data, and occasionally liver biopsy or alternative noninvasive testing.
- In cirrhotic patients, protein-calorie malnutrition is common and is associated with complications and poorer prognosis. Patients should be encouraged to eat frequent meals and target protein intake of 1.2 to 1.5 g/kg per day.
- Development of ascites, jaundice, variceal bleeding, or hepatic encephalopathy marks a transition to decompensated cirrhosis and is associated with a significant decline in transplant-free survival.
- New-onset ascites requires diagnostic paracentesis to assess cause and exclude infection.
- New-onset or acute hepatic encephalopathy requires careful assessment to exclude infection and other alternative diagnoses and address contributing factors.
- Patients with cirrhosis, and many patients with chronic hepatitis B, should undergo ultrasonography imaging every 6 months for hepatocellular carcinoma screening.

Disclosures: The authors have no commercial or financial disclosures.
[a] Division of General Internal Medicine, Department of Medicine, Harborview Medical Center, University of Washington, Box 359892, 325 9th Avenue, Seattle, WA 98104, USA; [b] Division of Gastroenterology, Department of Medicine, University of Washington, Box 356175, 1959 Northeast Pacific Street, Seattle, WA 98195, USA
* Corresponding author.
E-mail address: jorose@uw.edu

Med Clin N Am 99 (2015) 913–933
http://dx.doi.org/10.1016/j.mcna.2015.05.001
0025-7125/15/$ – see front matter © 2015 Elsevier Inc. All rights reserved.

medical.theclinics.com

INTRODUCTION

Liver disease is the 12th leading cause of mortality in the United States, as reported by the National Center for Health Statistics.[1] A broad variety of disease processes can affect the liver and produce a range of health consequences, from subclinical abnormalities on liver tests to cirrhosis and death. The liver has important roles in many vital processes, including metabolism, coagulation, immune function, and nutrition.

The end stage of any chronic insult to the liver (**Box 1**) is cirrhosis; a progressive, diffuse fibrotic process characterized by nodule formation and disruption of the normal liver architecture (**Fig. 1**). Globally, cirrhosis caused more than 1 million deaths in 2010, roughly 2% of the global total.[2] Complications of cirrhosis relate to 2 primary syndromes: hepatic insufficiency and portal hypertension. Reduced liver function contributes to altered drug metabolism and hepatic encephalopathy (HE). Portal hypertension leads to collateralization and varix formation and is associated with dilation of the splanchnic and peripheral vasculature, decreased peripheral arterial resistance, and a hyperdynamic circulatory state. Portal hypertension and its hemodynamic consequences predispose patients to gastrointestinal bleeding, ascites, renal injury, and circulatory failure.

Comprehensive primary care of patients with chronic liver disease incorporates both harm reduction measures common to all patients and vigilant management of the specific complications of cirrhosis.

CHRONIC LIVER DISEASE AT ANY STAGE: MANAGEMENT GOALS
Harm Reduction

Transmission
Patients with chronic viral hepatitis should be educated about risk of transmission. Patients with hepatitis B and/or C can share food, glasses, and utensils; hug, kiss, and hold hands with others; and participate in sports and school activities. However, they should cover open cuts and avoid sharing toothbrushes or razors. Patients with hepatitis B should also clean blood spills with detergent or bleach and use barrier

---

Box 1
Diseases that affect the liver

Hemochromatosis

Viral hepatitis

Inherited metabolic disorders: Wilson disease, alpha-1-antitrypsin deficiency, and others

Autoimmune hepatitis

Bacterial, parasitic, and fungal infections

Cysts

Vascular diseases, including Budd-Chiari syndrome

Cholestatic liver diseases: primary sclerosing cholangitis, primary biliary cirrhosis, and cystic fibrosis

Alcoholic liver disease

Nonalcoholic steatohepatitis

Liver disease caused by medications and drugs

Primary and secondary malignancies

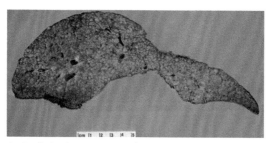

Fig. 1. Liver cirrhosis. Pathologic specimen of a cirrhotic liver. (*Courtesy of* Matthew Yeh, MD, Pathology, University of Washington.)

protection during sexual intercourse if the partner is not immune. Patients with hepatitis C who are injection drug users should be counseled about safe needle practices and provided resources on addiction treatment and needle exchange programs.

Weight, exercise, and nutrition

- Maintaining a healthy weight and lifestyle is recommended for patients with chronic liver disease, including patients with cirrhosis. Protein-calorie malnutrition (PCM) has been found to affect 50% to 100% of patients with cirrhosis and is most prevalent in those with decompensated disease.[3] It is associated with all the serious complications of cirrhosis and with reduced overall survival.[4]
- Clinicians should emphasize the importance of adequate protein intake. Frequent meals, including breakfast and a nighttime snack, targeting a daily total of 1.2 to 1.5 g/kg protein, may be beneficial.[5] The danger of protein malnutrition far outweighs the risk of worsening HE caused by increased protein intake. Referral to a dietician should be considered.
- Patients with alcoholic liver disease (ALD) are likely to also have deficiencies in many vitamins and minerals, including thiamine, folate, zinc, pyridoxine, and the fat-soluble vitamins A, D, E, and K. They should be monitored for signs or symptoms of these conditions and may require supplementation. Some experts recommend routine use of an oral multivitamin containing thiamine, folate, and pyridoxine in all patients with sustained heavy alcohol use.[6]
- Patients with Wilson disease should avoid intake of foods and water with high concentrations of copper (shellfish, nuts, chocolate, mushrooms, organ meats), at least during the first year of treatment.[7]
- In patients with nonalcoholic fatty liver disease (NAFLD), exercise and weight loss may improve laboratory parameters and hepatic steatosis.[8] NAFLD is a risk factor for progression of fibrosis in patients with hepatitis C.[9] Patients with hepatitis C who are overweight or obese or have insulin resistance should be counseled accordingly.
- In patients with nonalcoholic steatohepatitis (NASH) who do not have diabetes, treatment with vitamin E is associated with improvement in aminotransferase levels and histology; however, no effect has been shown on hepatic fibrosis, and some meta-analyses suggest that treatment with greater than 400 international units (IU) per day is associated with increased all-cause mortality.[10,11] There are also recent data suggesting that there is an increased risk of prostate cancer in healthy men using 400 IU per day.[12] The American Association for the Study of Liver Diseases (AASLD) acknowledges the limitations in data but

recommends treating biopsy-proven NASH in nondiabetic adults without cirrhosis with vitamin E 800 IU daily.[13]

Alcohol and tobacco

- Patients with liver disorders should limit intake of alcohol, which is itself a risk factor for liver disease. In patients with cirrhosis, alcoholism, or both, drinking greater than 4 alcoholic drinks per day is associated with a greatly increased risk of death.[14]
- Patients with hepatitis C or ALD should abstain from alcohol. In hepatitis C infection, alcohol seems to have synergistic effects on the liver at an intake of 50 g/d, but smaller amounts may also increase risk of progression to cirrhosis.[15] In ALD, abstinence decreases progression to cirrhosis, reduces portal pressure, and improves survival.[16]
- To best support abstinence, patients should be evaluated for an alcohol use disorder and referred for treatment, which differs according to the severity of the disorder. Patients with moderate to severe alcohol use disorders may be candidates for pharmacologic therapy with naltrexone; acamprosate; or, rarely, disulfiram,[17] although this assessment must incorporate the pattern of drinking, hepatic and renal function, and comorbidities. Disulfiram should be avoided in patients with cirrhosis because of risk of hepatotoxicity. Referral to an addiction specialist should be considered.
- Cigarette smoking and regular marijuana use may also increase progression of fibrosis in patients with chronic hepatitis C.[18,19] Patients should be counseled to quit and offered appropriate resources.
- In patients with ALD, abstaining from alcohol for a minimum of 6 months is required by most liver transplantation programs. Ongoing illicit substance use is another contraindication for liver transplantation. Assessment by an addiction specialist is frequently also required and is recommended by the AASLD.

Screening and immunizations

- Patients with hepatitis C should be screened for hepatitis B and human immunodeficiency virus. Those who are not immune to hepatitis A or B should be vaccinated accordingly. The immunologic response to the hepatitis B vaccine is reduced in the setting of cirrhosis; confirmation of immunity is particularly important in patients awaiting transplant.[20]
- Household members and steady sexual partners of patients with hepatitis B should be screened for hepatitis B and, if negative, vaccinated. HBsAg (surface antigen of the hepatitis B virus)-positive pregnant women should inform their providers so that hepatitis B immune globulin and hepatitis B vaccine can be given to the newborn.
- First-degree relatives of patients with *HFE*-related hereditary hemochromatosis should be screened with iron studies and *HFE* mutation analysis. Similarly, first-degree relatives of any patient with Wilson disease must be screened.
- Patients with advanced chronic liver disease should receive pneumococcal and annual influenza vaccinations.

Bone disease

Osteopenia and osteoporosis are common in patients with chronic liver disease caused by a combination of hypogonadism, malnutrition, inactivity, alcohol excess, and disease-specific factors, as in cholestasis and hemochromatosis, and may affect more than 50% of patients with cirrhosis in the United States. Screening for osteoporosis should be considered in these patients.[21] As in other patients with osteoporosis, contributing factors should be addressed; adequate calcium intake and vitamin D supplementation are recommended. Patients with cholestasis are at risk for fat-soluble vitamin deficiency, such as vitamin D, and should be screened accordingly. Bisphosphonate therapy may be less effective in the setting of cirrhosis, improving bone density but not risk of fractures, and suppressing bone formation that is already low from liver disease.[22] Referral to a specialist should be considered for patients with advanced liver disease and osteoporosis.

Surgical risk

Patients with cirrhosis have increased risk of perioperative complications and mortality. Emergent, cardiac, and intra-abdominal surgeries confer particularly high risk.[23]

- Portal hypertension and its associated conditions (decreased peripheral vascular resistance and hyperdynamic circulatory state) increase risk of hemodynamic instability and renal injury.
- Ascites predisposes to renal injury, volume shifts, and respiratory compromise.
- Poor nutrition and reticuloendothelial cell dysfunction increase risk of infection, impaired wound healing, and other complications.
- Hepatic insufficiency leads to altered and sometimes unpredictable metabolism of anesthetic agents and other medications.
- Coagulopathy, thrombocytopenia, and varices increase risk of bleeding.

Therefore, in patients with liver disease of any cause, clinical assessment to evaluate for cirrhosis and its complications and to weigh the risks and benefits of surgery should be performed before elective procedures.

- In patients with cirrhosis, the Child-Turcotte-Pugh (CTP) (**Table 1**) and Model for End-Stage Liver Disease (MELD) scores (calculated from serum bilirubin level, International Normalized Ratio [INR], and serum creatinine level) correlate well with operative morbidity and mortality.[24] **Table 2** shows mortality risk in relation to

Table 1 CTP classification of cirrhosis			
Points Assigned	1	2	3
Encephalopathy	None	Grade 1–2	Grade 3–4
Ascites	Absent-slight (detectable on imaging only)	Moderate (or diuretic responsive)	Severe (or diuretic refractory)
Albumin (g/dL)	>3.5	2.8–3.5	<2.8
Bilirubin (mg/dL)	1–2	2–3	>3
Prothrombin time	—	—	—
Seconds more than control	1–4	4–6	>6
Or INR	<1.7	1.8–2.3	>2.3

Class A, 5 to 6 points; class B, 7 to 9 points; and class C, 10 to 15 points.
Abbreviation: INR, International Normalized Ratio.
Data from Child CI, Turcotte J. Surgery and portal hypertension. In: Child CI, editor. The liver and portal hypertension. Philadelphia: WB Saunders; 1964. p. 50; and Pugh RN, Murray-Lyon IM, Dawson JL, et al. Transection of the esophagus for bleeding esophageal varices. Br J Surg 1973;60:646–9.

Table 2	
CTP classification and mortality in patients with cirrhosis undergoing abdominal surgery	
Child Class	**Surgical Mortality (%)**
A: 5–6 points	10
B: 7–9 points	30
C: 10–15 points	82

Data from Mansour A, Watson W, Shayani V, et al. Abdominal operations in patients with cirrhosis: still a major surgical challenge. Surgery 1997;122:730–5.

CTP classification. Most complications of cirrhosis (ascites, jaundice, encephalopathy, renal insufficiency, coagulopathy, gastrointestinal bleeding, anemia, infection) also increase surgical risk.[23]

- Primary care providers should assist in assessing and counseling patients with liver disease regarding surgical risk. Strategies to avoid or reduce surgical risk are listed in **Table 3**. Additional perioperative measures in patients with cirrhosis may be implemented during hospitalization.

Medication management

Patients with chronic liver disease are likely to have compromised synthetic function and hepatic metabolism, especially with advanced disease. Patients with portal hypertension may have hyperdynamic circulation, with low arterial pressure and decreased peripheral vascular resistance, which increase susceptibility to bleeding, renal failure, hemodynamic shifts, encephalopathy, and accumulation or delayed clearance of some medications (**Table 4**).

- Patients with cirrhosis and/or low platelet counts or coagulopathy should avoid nonsteroidal antiinflammatory drugs (NSAIDs), including aspirin, because of risk of bleeding and renal injury. NSAIDs can decrease glomerular filtration rate and impair renal function. Because NSAIDs are tightly bound to serum albumin, patients with cirrhosis are at risk for increased drug bioavailability and toxicity. In cirrhotic patients who are not actively drinking alcohol, acetaminophen at doses of up to 2 g/d is preferred.

Table 3	
Strategies to avoid or reduce perioperative risk in patients with chronic liver disease	
Strategy	**Patient Population**
Defer surgery	Patients with acute hepatitis, severe alcoholic hepatitis, CTP class C cirrhosis, and/or severe complications of liver disease
Delay elective procedures	Some patients with Child class B cirrhosis
Choose less invasive alternatives when available	All
Request preoperative gastroenterology/ hepatology consultation	Patients with class C cirrhosis or class B cirrhosis (with high risk of complications) who need to proceed with surgery
Evaluate and manage volume status before surgery	All

Data from Wong CJ, Hamlin NP. The perioperative medicine consult handbook. New York: Springer; 2013.

Table 4
Medications that should be avoided or used cautiously in advanced chronic liver disease or cirrhosis

Medication/Class	Concerns	Considerations	Alternatives
Antiplatelet agents	Bleeding	Weigh risk/benefit	NA
NSAIDs, including ASA	Bleeding, renal failure, toxicity	Avoid use	Acetaminophen ≤ 2 g daily
Opioids	Toxicity, increased HE, respiratory depression	Fentanyl or hydromorphone preferred Morphine requires dose and frequency reduction and should be avoided in renal failure Oxycodone, hydrocodone, and tramadol have unpredictable interindividual variability and should be avoided or used at lower and less frequent doses	Acetaminophen, gabapentin, topical lidocaine
Carbamazepine, phenytoin, and valproate	Hepatic decompensation, drug accumulation	Avoid use	Levetiracetam, topiramate
Lamotrigine	Drug accumulation	Requires dose reduction	Same as above
Bupropion	Drug accumulation caused by reduced clearance, increased half-life	Safe for use in early liver disease at reduced dose of $\leq$75 mg/d	SSRIs, dose reduced
Duloxetine	Drug accumulation caused by reduced clearance, increased half-life	Avoid use	Same as above
Macrolides (clarithromycin, erythromycin)	Drug accumulation, cholestasis, prolonged QTc	Avoid use	Fluoroquinolones (use with caution in patients with prolonged QT intervals) β-Lactams, carbapenems (monitor for leukopenia)
Tetracyclines	Drug accumulation	Avoid use	Same as above
Azoles	Hepatic dysfunction, drug interactions	Avoid ketoconazole; reduce doses of fluconazole and voriconazole	—

(continued on next page)

Table 4 *(continued)*			
Medication/Class	**Concerns**	**Considerations**	**Alternatives**
Metformin	Lactic acidosis	Avoid in decompensated cirrhosis, comorbid renal insufficiency, or excess alcohol use. Probably safe in compensated cirrhosis	Sulfonylureas (use with caution in older patients or those with renal insufficiency) Insulin
Amiodarone	Drug accumulation/ toxicity	Dose reduction likely necessary	—
β-Blockers and calcium channel blockers	Altered pharmacokinetics	Start at low doses and titrate gradually	—
ACE-inhibitors and angiotensin receptor blockers	Renal injury, hypotension, and increased mortality	Avoid use in decompensated cirrhosis with ascites	—

Abbreviations: ACE, angiotensin-converting enzyme; ASA, acetylsalicylic acid; NA, not available; NSAID, nonsteroidal antiinflammatory drug; SSRI, selective serotonin reuptake inhibitor.

Data from Hamilton JP, Goldberg E, Chopra S. Management of pain in patients with advanced chronic liver disease or cirrhosis. In: Runyon BA, Travis AC, editors. UpToDate. Waltham (MA): Wolters Kluwer; 2014; and Goldberg E, Chopra S. Cirrhosis in adults: Overview of complications, general management, and prognosis. In: Runyon BA, Travis AC, editors. UpToDate. Waltham (MA): Wolters Kluwer; 2014.

- All opioids can provoke or worsen HE and should be avoided or used judiciously in patients with this condition. In patients with cirrhosis who require opioids for pain control, dose reductions of 25% to 50% are recommended. Fentanyl and hydromorphone are generally safer than alternatives. Oxycodone, hydrocodone, and tramadol are hepatically metabolized to active metabolites, resulting in prolonged time to onset, variable efficacy, and risk of accumulation. They are best avoided in patients with advanced chronic liver disease. Morphine should be reduced in dose and frequency, because its oral bioavailability is increased up to 100% and its half-life is doubled. It should be avoided in patients with cirrhosis and renal failure.
- Risks and benefits of antiplatelet agents should be considered carefully, and decisions about therapy should involve shared decision making.
- Statin medications should not be withheld in patients with atherosclerotic disease or other indications.

MONITORING
Progression to Cirrhosis

Patients with chronic liver disease should be monitored clinically for progression to cirrhosis. Cirrhosis can be subtle in the absence of decompensation. Physical examination findings, laboratory parameters, and imaging findings that may assist in the diagnosis are listed in **Table 5**. Monitoring intervals should be guided by clinical judgment, in the absence of data regarding optimal frequency.

Table 5
Findings suggestive of clinically significant fibrosis or cirrhosis in patients with chronic liver disease

	Notes	Predictive Value
Physical Examination Findings		
Spider angiomata	Central arteriole surrounded by smaller vessels Found on trunk, face, arms	Independently predictive of esophageal varices
Palmar erythema	—	—
Gynecomastia and/or testicular atrophy	—	—
Digital clubbing	—	—
Splenomegaly	—	Discussed later
Caput medusa or other abdominal wall collateral circulation	—	—
Asterixis and/or HE	—	—
Ascites	Abdominal distention Flank dullness to percussion Fluid wave	—
Palpable, hard left lobe of liver	—	—
Jaundice	—	—
Laboratory Parameters		
Thrombocytopenia	<175,000	Platelet count may correlate with portal hypertension and esophageal varices
Hypoalbuminemia	Albumin level <3.8 g/dL	—
Increased INR	>1.3	—
Increased aminotransferase levels	Reversal of AST/ALT ratio	—
Calculated Laboratory Indices		
Age-platelet index	Fibrosis and cirrhosis	—
APRI	Fibrosis and cirrhosis	—
Imaging Findings		
Nodular liver or coarse echogenicity	—	Sensitivity, 55%–91%; specificity, 82%–95%
Portosystemic collateralization of vessels	—	Specific, not sensitive
L > R lobe ratio >1.3	—	Specific, not sensitive
Caudate lobe/R lobe ratio >0.65	—	Specific, not sensitive
Splenomegaly	—	Spleen length >12 cm: 93% sensitive, 36% specific for cirrhosis Likely predictive of esophageal varices

Abbreviations: APRI, aspartate aminotransferase-platelet ratio index; L, left; R, right.
Data from Chou R, Wasson N. Blood tests to diagnose fibrosis or cirrhosis in patients with chronic hepatitis C virus infection: a systematic review. Ann Intern Med 2013;158:807–20; and Berzigotti A, Ashkenazi E, Reverter E, et al. Non-invasive diagnostic and prognostic evaluation of liver cirrhosis and portal hypertension. Dis Markers 2011;31:129–38.

- Most patients with any stage of chronic liver disease merit at least yearly monitoring of serum aminotransferase levels. If advanced fibrosis or cirrhosis is suspected, prothrombin time, albumin level, and platelet count are also important, to assess synthetic function and evaluate for portal hypertension. Signs or symptoms of cirrhosis or decompensation of liver disease should also prompt comprehensive laboratory assessment.
- Numerous calculated indexes have been developed and tested in the diagnosis of fibrosis and cirrhosis. In hepatitis C infection, blood tests are more helpful in evaluating for clinically significant fibrosis or cirrhosis than in excluding it.[25]
- Liver ultrasonography is not required but may be helpful in some cases. Ultrasonography findings are more helpful in confirming rather than excluding cirrhosis.[26]
- Liver biopsy remains a cornerstone for staging liver disease, although it is frequently deferred when other clinical data are deemed sufficient, because of risk of complications and sampling variability. Noninvasive alternatives include vibration-controlled elastography, which measures liver stiffness; however, its clinical utility has not been firmly established.

Hepatocellular Carcinoma

Worldwide, hepatocellular carcinoma (HCC) is the second most frequent cause of cancer-related death among men and the sixth most frequent cause among women.[27] The highest risk of HCC is in patients with hereditary hemochromatosis, chronic hepatitis B, and chronic hepatitis C with cirrhosis. In the United States, the annual incidence of HCC is roughly 6 per 100,000 people; the most common cause is hepatitis C.[28]

The AASLD recommends that the following groups be screened for HCC[29]:

- Hepatitis B carriers
  - Asian men more than 40 years of age
  - Asian women more than 50 years of age
  - African and African American men and women of any age
  - Relative of patient with HCC
- Stage 4 primary biliary cirrhosis
- Most patients with severe fibrosis or cirrhosis

In patients who merit screening, liver ultrasonography every 6 months is recommended.[30] There is good evidence that alpha-fetoprotein should not be used alone for HCC monitoring, based on poor sensitivity and specificity.[31]

When screening ultrasonography shows a lesion concerning for HCC, the next step is usually dynamic contrast-enhanced computed tomography or MRI. Referral to a gastroenterologist/hepatologist or oncologist is appropriate for indeterminate or abnormal findings.

Treatment of Associated Conditions

To prevent progression in all patients with chronic liver disease, treatment of primary or associated conditions that affect the liver should be optimized. In many cases, referral to subspecialist providers is appropriate.

SPECIFIC MANAGEMENT OF CIRRHOSIS AND ITS COMPLICATIONS
Ascites

Evaluation of new ascites

Ascites is the most common complication of cirrhosis. Clinically apparent ascites in a patient with cirrhosis can occur because of progression of liver disease, but it can also indicate infection, malignancy, or another primary medical condition. Therefore, evaluation of new-onset ascites requires abdominal paracentesis and ascitic fluid analysis. Routine studies are shown in **Table 6**. Other ascitic fluid studies can be considered if there is suspicion for alternative causes of ascites.

Prophylactic blood products are not required before paracentesis in patients with cirrhosis with thrombocytopenia and coagulopathy.[32]

Basic management of ascites

- Cessation of alcohol use is vital in ascites caused by ALD. Treating autoimmune hepatitis and chronic hepatitis B may also improve or resolve ascites.
- Sodium restriction and diuretics are the mainstays of treatment of ascites caused by cirrhosis with portal hypertension (**Box 2**).
- New-onset large-volume ascites should be treated with single large-volume paracentesis (LVP) followed by dietary sodium restriction and initiation of diuretics.[33]

Management of tense or refractory ascites

Refractory ascites is unresponsive to dietary sodium restriction and maximal diuretic dosing or recurs rapidly after therapeutic paracentesis. It occurs in a minority of patients with cirrhosis and ascites but is associated with increased mortality.[34]

- If a patient becomes diuretic resistant, diuretics should be discontinued, and management relies on serial LVP alone.[33]
- LVP of up to 10 L removed every 2 weeks typically controls ascites in a patient who is compliant with dietary sodium restriction. Need for more frequent paracenteses suggests nonadherence.
- Only cell count and differential studies are recommended with serial therapeutic paracenteses.
- Postparacentesis circulatory dysfunction (PCD) is the largest predictor of mortality after LVP. Patients with ascites have decreased effective arterial volume; increased renin-angiotensin-aldosterone level, antidiuretic hormone level, and sympathetic nervous system activity; and renal vasoconstriction. LVP can

Table 6
Evaluation of new-onset ascites in patients with chronic liver disease and cirrhosis

Ascitic Fluid Study	Clinical Utility
Albumin	Calculate SAAG by subtracting the ascitic fluid albumin value from the serum albumin • A SAAG value $\geq$1.1 g/dL indicates portal hypertension but does not exclude additional causes of ascites • A SAAG value <1.1 suggests that portal hypertension is not the cause of ascites
Total protein	$\leq$ 2.5 g/dL is consistent with ascites from cirrhosis $\geq$2.5 indicates another cause of ascites
Cell count and differential Bacterial cultures	A PMN count of <250 cells/mm^3 and a negative culture generally exclude infection Asymptomatic patients with positive culture and normal PMN count (bacterascites) may have transient colonization. Paracentesis should be repeated to ensure that SBP has not developed

Abbreviations: PMN, polymorphonuclear leukocyte; SAAG, serum-ascites albumin gradient; SBP, spontaneous bacterial peritonitis.

Box 2
Basic management of ascites caused by cirrhosis

1. Limit dietary sodium to less than 2000 mg per day. Further restriction risks malnutrition caused by poor palatability of foods.

2. Initiate and titrate diuretics:

   a. Start with furosemide 40 mg daily and spironolactone 100 mg daily.

   b. Titrate at this ratio to maximum of furosemide 160 mg and spironolactone 400 mg.

   c. Limit weight loss to 0.5 kg per day in patients without peripheral edema. In those with significant peripheral edema, there is no daily weight loss limit.

   d. Monitor renal function and electrolytes with medication initiation and dose changes.

   e. If painful gynecomastia develops, consider amiloride 10 to 60 mg daily in place of spironolactone.

3. In case of new-onset large-volume ascites, a single large-volume paracentesis should precede the measures listed earlier.

Data from Runyon BA; AASLD. Introduction to the revised American Association for the Study of Liver Diseases Practice Guideline management of adult patients with ascites due to cirrhosis 2012. Hepatology 2013;57:1651–3.

---

exaggerate these processes and is associated with ascites recurrence, hepatorenal syndrome (HRS), dilutional hyponatremia, and decreased survival. If more than 5 L are removed during paracentesis, 6 to 8 g of at least 20% intravenous albumin per liter of ascitic fluid should be administered during or immediately after the procedure, because this practice has been shown to reduce PCD, hyponatremia, and mortality.[35]

- Transjugular intrahepatic portosystemic shunt (TIPS), a side-to-side portocaval shunt, controls ascites more effectively than LVP but has several contraindications and uncertain impact on transplant-free survival. It can also induce or worsen HE.[36] The decision to recommend this procedure is usually made by a liver specialist.

Important complications of ascites include spontaneous bacterial peritonitis (SBP; discussed later), dilutional hyponatremia, and HRS, each of which negatively influences survival. **Box 3** provides more information on the complications of ascites.

SBP occurs in up to 30% of patients with cirrhosis and ascites and has an estimated prevalence of 1.5% to 3.5% in cirrhotic outpatients.[37]

- In a patient with ascites, development of renal failure, HE, worsening liver function, or local and/or systemic signs or symptoms of infection (**Box 4**) should prompt diagnostic paracentesis to exclude SBP. Hospital admission should be considered for empiric treatment.
- Some patients (**Box 5**) are at increased risk of developing SBP and merit primary prophylaxis; an episode of SBP is an indication for secondary prophylaxis. Prophylaxis reduces risk of recurrence at 1 year from 70% to 20%.[38]
- Antibiotic options for SBP prophylaxis are shown in **Box 6**.

VARICES

In patients with cirrhosis, architectural distortion, intrahepatic vasoconstriction, and splanchnic arteriolar vasodilatation combine to enhance and increase resistance to

---

Box 3
Additional complications of ascites

1. Dilutional hyponatremia

   a. Activation of the renin-angiotensin and sympathetic nervous systems triggers sodium and water retention and release of antidiuretic hormone.

   b. Specific treatment not necessary unless hyponatremia leads to neurologic symptoms or the serum sodium level decreases to less than 120 mmol/L.

   c. Treatment involves relative fluid restriction (1000–1500 mL free water per day) and discontinuation of diuretics.

2. HRS

   a. Type-1 HRS: rapidly progressive renal failure frequently triggered by infection or intravascular volume contraction; leads to acute deterioration and a median survival of 2 weeks.[40] Manage in the inpatient setting.

   b. Type 2 HRS: slower, progressive decline in renal function associated with refractory ascites. Serum creatinine ranges from 1.5 to 2.5 mg/dL. Median survival is 4 to 6 months. Treatment centers on management of refractory ascites. Should prompt evaluation by a liver specialist.

3. Umbilical hernia. Patients should wear an abdominal binder to minimize strain and enlargement of the hernia and should be educated on the warning symptoms of an incarcerated hernia.

4. Hepatic hydrothorax. Treatment should start with dietary sodium restriction and diuretics. Therapeutic thoracentesis can be done for dyspnea.

Data from Gines P, Guevara M, Arroyo V, et al. Hepatorenal syndrome. Lancet 2003;362:1819–27.

---

portal blood flow. Collaterals develop at sites of communication between the portal and systemic circulations. Gastroesophageal varices are important because of risk of rupture.

Primary Variceal Prophylaxis

Screening esophagogastroduodenoscopy (EGD) should be performed on diagnosis of cirrhosis.

Box 4
Indications for diagnostic paracentesis

Emergency room visit or hospital admission

Local signs or symptoms of peritonitis: abdominal pain or tenderness, vomiting, diarrhea, ileus

Systemic signs or symptoms of infection: fever, hypothermia, hypotension, leukocytosis, acidosis

HE

Renal failure

Worsening of liver function

Data from Runyon BA; AASLD. Introduction to the revised American Association for the Study of Liver Diseases Practice Guideline management of adult patients with ascites due to cirrhosis 2012. Hepatology 2013;57:1651–3.

Box 5
Indications for SBP prophylaxis in outpatients

1. Prior episodes of SBP
2. Ascitic fluid total protein level less than 1.5 g/dL and at least 2 of the following:
   a. Serum creatinine level greater than 1.2 mg/dL
   b. Blood urea nitrogen level greater than 25 mg/dL
   c. Serum sodium level greater than 130 mEq/L
   d. Child-Pugh score greater than or equal to 9 points with bilirubin level greater than or equal to 3 mg/dL

Data from Runyon BA; AASLD. Introduction to the revised American Association for the Study of Liver Diseases Practice Guideline management of adult patients with ascites due to cirrhosis 2012. Hepatology 2013;57:1651–3.

- Individuals already taking a nonselective β-blocker (NSBB) need not undergo screening EGD. Those taking a selective β-blocker for other reasons should consider switching to an NSBB or carvedilol (for which there are promising data).
- Monitoring, surveillance, and treatment recommendations regarding varices are based on the result of screening EGD (**Table 7**).
- NSBBs decrease cardiac output (beta-1 effect) and induce splanchnic vasoconstriction (beta-2 effect) to decrease venous portal blood inflow; they reduce the incidence of first variceal hemorrhage and are recommended in higher-risk populations.[39]
- Medications and dosing for primary prophylaxis of variceal bleeding are shown in **Table 8**. Patients receiving variceal prophylaxis need to continue the NSBB indefinitely, but they do not need follow-up EGD.

Secondary Prophylaxis of Variceal Bleeding

Untreated cirrhotic patients with a history of variceal bleeding have a 60% risk of rebleeding within 2 years and a 20% risk of death with each episode.[40] Many patients receive endoscopic variceal ligation (EVL) and/or NSBB therapy. Both measures reduce variceal rebleeding rate, particularly in combination.[41] NSBB and endoscopic surveillance should be continued indefinitely.

Box 6
Outpatient management of primary and secondary SBP prophylaxis

Treatment with one of the following should be continued as long as ascites is present:

1. Norfloxacin 400 mg by mouth daily (preferred)
2. Double-strength trimethoprim/sulfamethoxazole, 1 tablet daily
3. Ciprofloxacin 500 mg by mouth daily
4. Levofloxacin 250 mg by mouth daily

Data from Runyon BA; AASLD. Introduction to the revised American Association for the Study of Liver Diseases Practice Guideline management of adult patients with ascites due to cirrhosis 2012. Hepatology 2013;57:1651–3.

Table 7
Variceal monitoring, surveillance, and treatment according to results of screening EGD

Result of Screening EGD	Treatment	Monitoring/Surveillance
No varices	NA	Repeat EGD annually for patients with decompensated cirrhosis Repeat EGD every 2–3 y for patients with compensated cirrhosis
Small varices	Treat with NSBB only in those with red wale marks or with Child class B or C cirrhosis	Repeat EGD only for patients not receiving NSBB therapy • Repeat in 2 y for compensated patients • Repeat annually for decompensated patients • Repeat if decompensating event occurs
Large varices	NSBB indefinitely and/or endoscopic variceal ligation until varices are eradicated	Repeat EGD every 6–12 mo only in those who are unable to take NSBBs

Data from Garcia-Tsao G, Sanyal AJ, Grace ND, et al. Practice and management of gastroesophageal varices and variceal hemorrhage in cirrhosis. Hepatology 2007;46:922–38.

HEPATIC ENCEPHALOPATHY

HE is the result of hepatic insufficiency or portosystemic shunting. Ammonia can lead to accumulation of glutamine in brain astrocytes, producing swelling. HE can present with a range of neuropsychiatric abnormalities of varying severity; clinically apparent HE occurs in at least 30% to 45% of cirrhotic patients.[42]

Diagnosis of HE requires excluding other causes of altered mental status (**Box 7**) and is based on the combination of impaired mental status and impaired neuromotor function, such as hyperreflexia, hypertonicity, and asterixis. Precipitating factors for HE should be explored and treated (**Box 8**). Patients with HE may show personality changes, decreased energy levels, impaired sleep-wake cycles, and diminished consciousness.

Patients with HE have increased serum ammonia levels, but these levels do not correlate with the severity of HE beyond a certain point and there are many nonhepatic causes of hyperammonemia.[43] Serial ammonia levels are not routinely used to follow patients; the clinical presentation and response to treatment are more meaningful.

Table 8
Primary medical prophylaxis against first variceal hemorrhage

Regimen	Starting Dose/Frequency	Goal	Monitoring
Propranolol	20 mg bid	Maximal tolerance or HR 55 bpm	Assess HR at every visit
Nadolol	20–40 mg once daily (adjust for renal insufficiency)	Maximal tolerance or HR 55 bpm	Assess HR at every visit
Carvedilol	6.25 mg once daily	Maximal tolerance or HR 55 bpm, up to a dose of 12.5 mg daily	Assess HR at every visit

Abbreviations: bid, twice a day; bpm, beats per minute; HR, heart rate.
Data from Garcia-Tsao G, Bosch J. Management of varices and variceal hemorrhage in cirrhosis. N Engl J Med 2010;362:823–32.

Box 7
Differential diagnosis of HE

Alternative causes of altered mental status to consider in patients with suspected HE:

Hypoxia

Hypercapnia

Acidosis

Uremia

Medications or intoxication

Electrolyte disturbances

Central nervous system abnormalities (eg, seizure, stroke, intracerebral hemorrhage, meningitis)

Hypoglycemia

Delirium tremens

Wernicke-Korsakoff syndrome

Delirium

Data from Prakash R, Mullen KD. Mechanisms, diagnosis and management of hepatic encephalopathy. Nat Rev Gastroenterol Hepatol 2010;7:515–25.

Treatment of acute HE requires supportive care, identifying and treating any precipitating causes, reducing nitrogenous load in the gut, and assessing the need for long-term therapy. Severe HE should prompt consideration of hospitalization. More chronic or mild HE can be treated on an outpatient basis.

Lactulose, a nonabsorbable disaccharide, remains the first-line treatment of HE based on extensive clinical experience. Lactulose acts in the gut to decrease ammonia absorption and increase fecal nitrogen waste. In mild HE treated in the outpatient setting, lactulose 10 to 30 g (15–45 mL) 2 to 4 times a day can be titrated to induce 2 to 3 soft bowel movements daily.[44] Therapy may be continued indefinitely for patients with recurrent or persistent HE. Lactulose can be difficult to tolerate; nonadherence to treatment is common and is associated with recurrence of HE.[45] Strategies to improve adherence and prevent recurrence include educating the patient, family members, and caregivers, and arranging close follow-up care. Education should include effects of the medication, potential side effects, importance of adherence, signs of recurrent HE, and how to manage recurrent HE.[44]

Box 8
Precipitating causes of HE

1. Increased nitrogen load: gastrointestinal bleed, infection, excess dietary protein
2. Decreased toxin clearance: hypovolemia, renal failure, constipation, portosystemic shunt, medication noncompliance, acute-on-chronic liver failure
3. Altered neurotransmission: sedating medication, alcohol, hypoxia, hypoglycemia

Data from Mullen KD. Review of the final report of the 1998 Working Party on definition, nomenclature and diagnosis of hepatic encephalopathy. Aliment Pharmacol Ther 2007;25 Suppl 1:11–6.

Rifaximin is a minimally absorbed (less than 0.4%) antibiotic with broad-spectrum in vitro activity. In patients with recurrent bouts of HE, rifaximin 550 mg twice daily can be added to lactulose therapy to maintain remission and reduce hospitalizations.[46]

Dietary protein restriction is not advised for the management of HE. Patients with cirrhosis are recommended to consume a high-protein diet of at least 1.0 g/kg to 1.5 g/kg daily.[47] Eating 4 to 6 small meals daily with a nighttime snack may help avoid protein loading.

HEPATOCELLULAR CARCINOMA

Patients with cirrhosis are at risk for developing HCC. Screening and diagnosis of HCC are discussed earlier. Treatment is usually managed by a gastroenterologist/hepatologist, surgical oncologist, or oncologist. Prognosis and liver transplantation are discussed later.

PROGNOSIS, LIVER TRANSPLANTATION, AND PALLIATIVE CARE
Prognosis in Patients with Chronic Liver Disease

Prognosis in patients with chronic liver disease ranges widely according to the underlying condition, availability and access to treatment, and disease severity. As in other conditions, providing prognostic assessment for individual patients is challenging; however, it is important in guiding liver transplantation assessment and other goals-of-care discussions. Studies suggest that the following considerations may be helpful:

- CTP class and MELD score. CTP classification (**Table 9**) and MELD scores are the best validated tools to predict short-term and overall survival in patients with cirrhosis.[48,49] Abnormalities of the individual CTP components (albumin, bilirubin, ascites, encephalopathy, and prothrombin time) have also been associated with increased mortality, even in compensated patients.[48]
- Compensated versus decompensated state. Patients with cirrhosis can remain asymptomatic for many years. However, prognosis worsens significantly when a decompensating event (eg, jaundice, ascites, SBP, variceal hemorrhage, HE) occurs. This transition occurs at a rate of 5% to 7% per year[48] and is associated with decline in 5-year survival from 90% to 50% and with 20% mortality at 1 year.[50]
- Renal failure. In cirrhotic patients, renal failure has been associated with significantly increased mortality.[48,51]
- Infection. Infection has also been associated with poor prognosis in cirrhotic patients, increasing mortality up to 4-fold.[52]
- HCC confers poor prognosis, decreasing 5-year survival to around 10% to 15%. Survival is even worse when HCC is detected after onset of symptoms.

Table 9
Modified CTP classification of severity of cirrhosis and corresponding estimated short-term survival

CTP Class	CTP Score	1-y % Survival	2-y % Survival
A	5–6	95	90
B	7–9	80	70
C	10–15	45	38

Data from D'Amico G, Garcia-Tsao G, Pagliaro L. Natural history and prognostic indicators of survival in cirrhosis: a systematic review of 118 studies. J Hepatol 2006;44:217–31.

Box 9
Reasons to refer for liver transplantation evaluation
1. Occurrence of decompensating event, such as ascites, variceal bleeding, HE, SBP, or hepatorenal syndrome
2. Hepatopulmonary syndrome attributed to cirrhosis
3. Newly diagnosed HCC meeting Milan criteria
4. MELD score of 10 or greater or CTP score of 7 or greater. (In the United States in 2002, the modified MELD score replaced the CTP score in prioritizing patients for liver transplantation.)

LIVER TRANSPLANTATION

Liver transplantation is a lifesaving surgery for patients with chronic liver disease with advanced cirrhosis. In the United States, chronic hepatitis C virus infection is the most common indication.

When considering referral for liver transplantation, the natural history of the disease should be compared with the expected survival after transplantation. Because the transplant evaluation may take weeks to months to complete, it is ideal to refer early in the clinical course rather than late.

Reasons to refer for evaluation of liver transplantation candidacy are listed in **Box 9**.

PALLIATIVE AND END-OF-LIFE CARE IN PATIENTS WITH CHRONIC LIVER DISEASE

Patients with advanced cirrhosis who are not candidates for liver transplantation require care that incorporates principles of palliative medicine, such as symptom management, discussion of end-of-life preferences, and planning for surrogate decision making. Discussions might incorporate prognosis, care options and goals (including comfort care), and care setting (home, nursing home, inpatient, or intensive care unit). Nausea, vomiting, HE, and massive ascites require aggressive symptom management. Hospice referral may be appropriate. Cirrhotic patients may develop complications or symptoms that are difficult to manage in the outpatient setting and can be traumatic for patients and families, such as massive gastrointestinal or other bleeding. In this case, admission to a hospital or inpatient hospice program should be considered.

SUMMARY

Comprehensive care of patients with all forms of chronic liver disease requires education, counseling, and harm reduction practices, as well as monitoring for progression to cirrhosis. For patients with advanced liver disease, specific management is required.

REFERENCES

1. Deaths: final data for 2010. National Vital Statistics Reports. Available at: http://cdc.gov/nchs/data/nvsr/nvsr61/nvsr61_04.pdf.
2. Lozano R, Naghavi M, Foreman K, et al. Global and regional mortality from 235 causes of death for 20 age groups in 1990 and 2010: a systematic analysis for the Global Burden of Disease Study 2010. Lancet 2012;380(9859):2095–128.

3. Mendenhall C, Roselle GA, Gartside P, et al. Relationship of protein calorie malnutrition to alcoholic liver disease: a reexamination of data from two Veterans Administration Cooperative Studies. Alcohol Clin Exp Res 1995;19(3): 635–41.

4. Caregaro L, Alberino F, Amodio P, et al. Malnutrition in alcoholic and virus-related cirrhosis. Am J Clin Nutr 1996;63(4):602–9.

5. Swart GR, Zillikens MC, van Vuure JK, et al. Effect of a late evening meal on nitrogen balance in patients with cirrhosis of the liver. BMJ 1989;299(6709):1202–3.

6. Gramlich L, Tandon P, Rahman A. Nutritional status in patients with sustained heavy alcohol use. Waltham (MA): Up To Date; 2014. Available at: http://www.uptodate.com/contents/nutritional-status-in-patients-with-sustained-heavy-alcohol-use. Accessed September, 2014.

7. Roberts EA, Schilsky ML, American Association for Study of Liver Diseases (AASLD). Diagnosis and treatment of Wilson disease: an update. Hepatology 2008;47(6):2089–111.

8. Ueno T, Sugawara H, Sujaku K, et al. Therapeutic effects of restricted diet and exercise in obese patients with fatty liver. J Hepatol 1997;27(1):103–7.

9. Everhart JE, Lok AS, Kim HY, et al. Weight-related effects on disease progression in the hepatitis C antiviral long-term treatment against cirrhosis trial. Gastroenterology 2009;137(2):549–57.

10. Miller ER 3rd, Pastor-Barriuso R, Dalal D, et al. Meta-analysis: high-dosage vitamin E supplementation may increase all-cause mortality. Ann Intern Med 2005;142(1):37–46.

11. Bjelakovic G, Nikolova D, Gluud LL, et al. Mortality in randomized trials of antioxidant supplements for primary and secondary prevention: systematic review and meta-analysis. JAMA 2007;297(8):842–57.

12. Klein EA, Thompson IM Jr, Tangen CM, et al. Vitamin E and the risk of prostate cancer: the Selenium and Vitamin E Cancer Prevention Trial (SELECT). JAMA 2011;306(14):1549–56.

13. Chalasani N, Younossi Z, Lavine JE, et al. The diagnosis and management of non-alcoholic fatty liver disease: practice guideline by the American Gastroenterological Association, American Association for the Study of Liver Diseases, and American College of Gastroenterology. Gastroenterology 2012;142(7):1592–609.

14. Thun MJ, Peto R, Lopez AD, et al. Alcohol consumption and mortality among middle-aged and elderly U.S. adults. N Engl J Med 1997;337(24):1705–14.

15. Corrao G, Arico S. Independent and combined action of hepatitis C virus infection and alcohol consumption on the risk of symptomatic liver cirrhosis. Hepatology 1998;27(4):914–9.

16. Pessione F, Ramond MJ, Peters L, et al. Five-year survival predictive factors in patients with excessive alcohol intake and cirrhosis. Effect of alcoholic hepatitis, smoking and abstinence. Liver Int 2003;23(1):45–53.

17. Jonas DE, Amick HR, Feltner C, et al. Pharmacotherapy for adults with alcohol use disorders in outpatient settings: a systematic review and meta-analysis. JAMA 2014;311(18):1889–900.

18. Hezode C, Lonjon I, Roudot-Thoraval F, et al. Impact of smoking on histological liver lesions in chronic hepatitis C. Gut 2003;52(1):126–9.

19. Hezode C, Zafrani ES, Roudot-Thoraval F, et al. Daily cannabis use: a novel risk factor of steatosis severity in patients with chronic hepatitis C. Gastroenterology 2008;134(2):432–9.

20. Dominguez M, Barcena R, Garcia M, et al. Vaccination against hepatitis B virus in cirrhotic patients on liver transplant waiting list. Liver Transpl 2000;6(4):440–2.

21. Carey EJ, Balan V, Kremers WK, et al. Osteopenia and osteoporosis in patients with end-stage liver disease caused by hepatitis C and alcoholic liver disease: not just a cholestatic problem. Liver Transpl 2003;9(11):1166–73.
22. Susan Ott. In: James J, editor. Patient documentation. 2014.
23. Mansour A, Watson W, Shayani V, et al. Abdominal operations in patients with cirrhosis: still a major surgical challenge. Surgery 1997;122(4):730–5 [discussion: 735–6].
24. Farnsworth N, Fagan SP, Berger DH, et al. Child-Turcotte-Pugh versus MELD score as a predictor of outcome after elective and emergent surgery in cirrhotic patients. Am J Surg 2004;188(5):580–3.
25. Chou R, Wasson N. Blood tests to diagnose fibrosis or cirrhosis in patients with chronic hepatitis C virus infection: a systematic review. Ann Intern Med 2013; 158(11):807–20.
26. Berzigotti A, Ashkenazi E, Reverter E, et al. Non-invasive diagnostic and prognostic evaluation of liver cirrhosis and portal hypertension. Dis Markers 2011; 31(3):129–38.
27. Jemal A, Bray F, Center MM, et al. Global cancer statistics. CA Cancer J Clin 2011;61(2):69–90.
28. El-Serag HB, Kanwal F. Epidemiology of hepatocellular carcinoma in the United States: Where are we? Where do we go? Hepatology 2014;60(5):1767–75.
29. Bruix J, Sherman M, Practice Guidelines Committee, American Association for the Study of Liver Diseases. Management of hepatocellular carcinoma. Hepatology 2005;42(5):1208–36.
30. Bruix J, Sherman M, American Association for the Study of Liver Diseases. Management of hepatocellular carcinoma: an update. Hepatology 2011;53(3):1020–2.
31. Lok AS, Sterling RK, Everhart JE, et al. Des-gamma-carboxy prothrombin and alpha-fetoprotein as biomarkers for the early detection of hepatocellular carcinoma. Gastroenterology 2010;138(2):493–502.
32. Runyon BA. Paracentesis of ascitic fluid. A safe procedure. Arch Intern Med 1986;146(11):2259–61.
33. Gines P, Arroyo V, Quintero E, et al. Comparison of paracentesis and diuretics in the treatment of cirrhotics with tense ascites. Results of a randomized study. Gastroenterology 1987;93(2):234–41.
34. Heuman DM, Abou-Assi SG, Habib A, et al. Persistent ascites and low serum sodium identify patients with cirrhosis and low MELD scores who are at high risk for early death. Hepatology 2004;40(4):802–10.
35. Bernardi M, Caraceni P, Navickis RJ, et al. Albumin infusion in patients undergoing large-volume paracentesis: a meta-analysis of randomized trials. Hepatology 2012;55(4):1172–81.
36. Gines P, Uriz J, Calahorra B, et al. Transjugular intrahepatic portosystemic shunting versus paracentesis plus albumin for refractory ascites in cirrhosis. Gastroenterology 2002;123(6):1839–47.
37. Evans LT, Kim WR, Poterucha JJ, et al. Spontaneous bacterial peritonitis in asymptomatic outpatients with cirrhotic ascites. Hepatology 2003;37(4): 897–901.
38. Gines P, Rimola A, Planas R, et al. Norfloxacin prevents spontaneous bacterial peritonitis recurrence in cirrhosis: results of a double-blind, placebo-controlled trial. Hepatology 1990;12(4 Pt 1):716–24.
39. Garcia-Tsao G, Sanyal AJ, Grace ND, et al, Practice Guidelines Committee of the American Association for the Study of Liver Diseases, Practice Parameters Committee of the American College of Gastroenterology. Prevention and management

of gastroesophageal varices and variceal hemorrhage in cirrhosis. Hepatology 2007;46(3):922–38.

40. Bosch J, Garcia-Pagan JC. Prevention of variceal rebleeding. Lancet 2003; 361(9361):952–4.

41. Gonzalez R, Zamora J, Gomez-Camarero J, et al. Meta-analysis: Combination endoscopic and drug therapy to prevent variceal rebleeding in cirrhosis. Ann Intern Med 2008;149(2):109–22.

42. Poordad FF. Review article: the burden of hepatic encephalopathy. Aliment Pharmacol Ther 2007;25(Suppl 1):3–9.

43. Ong JP, Aggarwal A, Krieger D, et al. Correlation between ammonia levels and the severity of hepatic encephalopathy. Am J Med 2003;114(3):188–93.

44. Vilstrup H, Amodio P, Bajaj J, et al. Hepatic encephalopathy in chronic liver disease: 2014 Practice Guideline by the American Association for the Study of Liver Diseases and the European Association for the Study of the Liver. Hepatology 2014;60(2):715–35.

45. Bajaj JS, Sanyal AJ, Bell D, et al. Predictors of the recurrence of hepatic encephalopathy in lactulose-treated patients. Aliment Pharmacol Ther 2010;31(9): 1012–7.

46. Bass NM, Mullen KD, Sanyal A, et al. Rifaximin treatment in hepatic encephalopathy. N Engl J Med 2010;362(12):1071–81.

47. Plauth M, Cabre E, Riggio O, et al. ESPEN guidelines on enteral nutrition: liver disease. Clin Nutr 2006;25(2):285–94.

48. D'Amico G, Garcia-Tsao G, Pagliaro L. Natural history and prognostic indicators of survival in cirrhosis: a systematic review of 118 studies. J Hepatol 2006;44(1): 217–31.

49. Kamath PS, Wiesner RH, Malinchoc M, et al. A model to predict survival in patients with end-stage liver disease. Hepatology 2001;33(2):464–70.

50. Gines P, Quintero E, Arroyo V, et al. Compensated cirrhosis: natural history and prognostic factors. Hepatology 1987;7(1):122–8.

51. Fede G, D'Amico G, Arvaniti V, et al. Renal failure and cirrhosis: a systematic review of mortality and prognosis. J Hepatol 2012;56(4):810–8.

52. Arvaniti V, D'Amico G, Fede G, et al. Infections in patients with cirrhosis increase mortality four-fold and should be used in determining prognosis. Gastroenterology 2010;139(4):1246–56, 1256.e1–5.

Primary Care of the Patient with Chronic Kidney Disease

 CrossMark

Meghan M. Kiefer, MD, MPH[a],*, Michael J. Ryan, MD[b]

KEYWORDS

- Chronic kidney disease • Chronic disease management • Primary care • Proteinuria
- Albuminuria

KEY POINTS

- Patients with chronic kidney disease (CKD) are more likely to die of cardiovascular (CV) disease than progressing to end-stage renal disease (ESRD).
- Prevention, early detection, and proper treatment of CKD helps reduce the risk of CKD complications and progression to ESRD.
- Persistent albuminuria or proteinuria should always be evaluated and is an independent marker for disease progression and mortality.
- Angiotensin blockade is a cornerstone of therapy for CKD.
- Kidney specialist referral should be initiated for all patients with rapidly progressing CKD, with stage 4 CKD, or with uncertain etiology.

Case

Jack Francis, a 52-year-old gentleman of European descent, is scheduled to see you for follow-up of an emergency department visit. You skim his chart before walking in the room and see his emergency visit was for left toe pain, ultimately leading to a diagnosis of gout. Further chart review reveals no past medical history other than mild knee osteoarthritis, overweight (body mass index of 27 kg/m²), and borderline high blood pressure (BP). He takes no prescribed medications. Laboratory results drawn at the emergency visit reveal a serum creatinine level of 1.8 mg/dL. Looking through his chart, the only other creatinine value in the records is 1.5 mg/dL 2 years ago.

How do you approach this creatinine value in this patient?

Conflicts of interest: nothing to disclose.
[a] Division of General Internal Medicine, Department of Medicine, University of Washington School of Medicine, Seattle, WA, USA; [b] Division of Nephrology, Department of Medicine, University of Washington School of Medicine, Seattle, WA, USA
* Corresponding author. Harborview Medical Center, 325 9th Avenue, Box 359780, Seattle, WA 98104.
E-mail address: meghanm@uw.edu

Med Clin N Am 99 (2015) 935–952
http://dx.doi.org/10.1016/j.mcna.2015.05.003
0025-7125/15/$ – see front matter © 2015 Elsevier Inc. All rights reserved.

medical.theclinics.com

BACKGROUND

While it is tempting for the busy clinician to overlook the modestly elevated creatinine level in this individual, particularly given his more acute and symptomatic complaint, further evaluation is critical. In the primary care setting, it can be challenging to recognize CKD as a distinct entity from its co-occuring conditions; in most studies, less than half of patients with CKD have it documented in their medical record.[1] International guidelines define CKD as at least 3 months of either reduced glomerular filtration rate (GFR<60 mL/min/1.73 m^2) or evidence of kidney damage.[2] Current recommendations classify kidney disease based on the underlying cause,[1] GFR category,[2] and albuminuria category.[3] Each of these is important for predicting the risk of complications from CKD.

Kidney disease severity is divided into 5 stages, based on the estimated GFR; CKD is defined as kidney damage or GFR less than 60 mL/min/1.73 m^2 for 3 months or more, irrespective of the cause (**Box 1, Fig. 1**). The 2012 guidelines have been updated to emphasize the importance of albuminuria, dividing it into 3 stages, with stages 2 to 3 definitive for CKD. ESRD, or kidney failure, is generally defined by dependence on renal replacement therapy (RRT) or transplant.

Mr Francis' GFR can be quickly calculated using Modification of Diet in Renal Disease (MDRD) and Chronic Kidney Disease Epidemiology Collaboration (CKD-EPI) tools available online (such as at nephromatic.com); it is 42 mL/min/1.73 m^2, placing him in CKD category G3b.

EPIDEMIOLOGY

CKD affects approximately 13.6% of all US adults, making it more common than diabetes.[3] The prevalence increases with age; among adults aged 60 to 69 years, nearly 25% have either albuminuria or reduction in GFR, and among adults older than 70 years, nearly 50% do.[4] Some decline in GFR is expected with age and may reflect normal aging processes, potentially leading to some overdiagnosis of CKD in the elderly; however, advanced CKD and ESRD rates are also higher in this group.[5] Among persons with hypertension, the prevalence of CKD is approximately 20%, and one-third of adults with diabetes have CKD.[6] Among adults who develop ESRD, the vast majority of cases (>70%) are thought to be due to either hypertension or diabetes.[6]

CKD is also more common among African-American and Latino individuals.[3] Women have higher rates of overall CKD, but ESRD is more common among men.[6] Other risk factors for CKD include obesity, CV disease, a family history of renal disease, or a history of acute kidney injury (AKI).[3]

Despite overall improvement in the management of CKD risk factors such as hypertension, smoking, and diabetes, the proportion of Americans with CKD has been

---

Box 1
CKD definitions

- CKD is defined by 3 months or more of reduced GFR (<60 mL/min/1.73 m^2) or evidence of kidney damage (such as albuminuria, abnormal pathology, imaging, or urine sediment)

- Albuminuria is defined by a urine albumin-to-creatinine ratio of 30 mg/g or more (or ≥30 mg/mmol)

- Each of these (reduced GFR and albuminuria) can be broken down into further categories, with more dysfunction corresponding to higher risks of CKD progression and complications

		Albuminuria category (UACR, in mg/g)		
		A1 (<30) Normal/mildly increased	A2 (30–299) Moderately increased	A3 (>300) Severely increased
GFR Category (mL/min/1.73 m²)	G1 (≥90)	n/a	1	1
	G2 (60–89)	n/a	2	2
	G3a (45–59)	3a	3a	3a
	G3b (30–44)	3b	3b	3b
	G4 (15–29)	4	4	4
	G5 (<15)	5	5	5

Fig. 1. Classification of CKD, by GFR and albuminuria, along with "heat map" of risk of adverse CKD outcomes. Green, low risk (no CKD if no other markers of kidney disease); yellow, moderate risk; orange, high risk; red, very high risk. UACR, urine albumin-to-creatinine ratio. (*Adapted from* Kidney Disease: Improving Global, Outcomes (KDIGO) CKD Work Group. KDIGO 2012 clinical practice guideline for the evaluation and management of chronic kidney disease. Kidney Int Suppl 2013;3:6; with permission.)

rising, primarily attributed to the aging of the US population. In adults older than 40 years, glomerular filtration decreases at a rate of approximately 1% annually, and older adults have higher rates of diabetes, hypertension, and other risk factors for CKD.[7]

Determining the precise cost burden of CKD on the US health care system is limited because of several factors, including its underdiagnosis as well as its synergistic role in the morbidity and mortality of those with CV disease, diabetes, and infection. Medicare data suggest that although those who carry a formal diagnosis of CKD account for 10% of Medicare beneficiaries, this group incurs nearly 20% of the costs. Patients with CKD without diabetes or heart failure still have per-person per-year costs almost 50% greater than the average Medicare recipient.[3]

Despite the significance of CKD and the modifiable nature of progression, few are aware of their diagnosis. Among patients with stage 3 CKD or albuminuria, less than 10% are aware of their diagnosis.[3] Among patients with stage 4 CKD, almost half are unaware of having this condition.

NATURAL HISTORY

When you tell Mr Francis that he may have kidney disease, he stares at you blankly. "What? Nobody ever told me that. What does that mean? Are they going to stop working? Do I have to go on dialysis?"

Mortality

Although renal disease is the ninth leading cause of death in the United States,[8] most patients with CKD die of CV disease.[3] Even when adjusted for age, sex, race, and other comorbidities, CV mortality is 10 to 30 times higher in individuals with end-stage kidney disease than in the general population.[9,10] The mortality rate is higher with more advanced CKD stages.[3] Although older people are more likely to have CKD, when younger people have CKD, the diagnosis carries a higher proportional risk of death or ESRD when compared with their non-CKD counterparts of the same age. Mr Francis' GFR of 42 mL/min at the relatively young age of 52 years gives him an approximately 8-fold increase in mortality risk, compared with his counterpart with normal renal function (**Box 2**).[11]

Progression to End-Stage Renal Disease

The more advanced the kidney disease at the time of diagnosis (the greater the degree of albuminuria or reduction in GFR), the higher the risk of progression to ESRD; both lower GFR and higher degree of albuminuria independently predict development of ESRD.[2,11] The underlying cause of CKD also influences the rate of progression.[12] Other predictors of progression to ESRD significantly overlap with risk factors for CKD development, and include elevated BP, smoking, obesity, hyperglycemia, and exposure to nephrotoxins. When adjusted for age and sex, African Americans have 3 times the incidence of ESRD as whites, and the rates of incidence in Native Americans are 1.5 times greater than those in whites. Rates of developing ESRD in Hispanics are also 50% higher than those in non-Hispanics.[3] Some of these disparities may be due to recently identified genetic variations.[13,14] Furthermore, derangements in certain laboratory values, again suggestive of the degree of renal dysfunction (hemoglobin [Hb], calcium, phosphate, bicarbonate, and albumin), can also identify those at higher risk for CKD progression.[2] Calculators such as the kidney risk equation[15] incorporate these values to provide an estimate of the risk of progression to ESRD.

What can be told to Mr Francis about his risk of death and ESRD? Regarding ESRD, on an average 1% to 2% of people with stage 3 or higher are on dialysis at 5 years; the proportion is much higher (>17%) for those with stage 4 CKD, and the risk is also higher at any stage for those with albuminuria.[16,17] For persons with stage 4 CKD (who are often older, with CV disease), the risk of death remains higher than the risk of progressing to ESRD,[16] although this may not be the case in younger, healthier people without CVD, such as Mr Francis.[17]

EVALUATION

Kidney disease, particularly in its earlier stages, is often asymptomatic. This fact poses a particular challenge, because these are the stages in which clinicians and patients have the greatest chance of halting its progression. Signs and symptoms associated with renal disease include edema, hypertension, anemia, and uremic symptoms (nausea, pericarditis, anorexia, neuropathy, altered mental status). However, less-severe renal disease has also been associated with greater infection risk, increased risk of adverse surgical outcomes, higher rates of drug-related adverse events, as well as physical and cognitive decline.[2,18] Patients with CKD are also at increased risk of AKI, which is itself a source of morbidity and mortality as well as a precipitant of CKD progression.[19]

Box 2
Risk of progression to ESRD and mortality risk

- The lower the GFR and/or the greater the albuminuria, the higher the risk of all-cause and CV mortality and risk of progression to ESRD

- Most patients with CKD are over 10 times more likely to die of CV disease than progressing to ESRD

Screening

Given the asymptomatic nature and modifiable course of the disease, one might think that screening for renal disease would be recommended in major guidelines. However, there is disagreement about the role of screening in the general population, because the benefits of screening are not entirely clear.[20] The 2012 report of the United States Preventive Services Task Force considers the evidence as insufficient to warrant screening in the general population (although this recommendation does not extend to those with hypertension or diabetes). The American College of Physicians found the evidence insufficient to screen even those with risk factors.[21] However, the American Society of Nephrology strongly disagrees with these recent recommendations.[22] The American Diabetes Association recommends screening all adults with diabetes for CKD with annual albumin-creatinine ratios and serum creatinine levels.[23] The American College of Cardiology and American Heart Association (AHA) jointly recommend annual measurement of serum creatinine levels for patients with ischemic heart disease.[24]

New Diagnosis

The history and examination of a person with newly diagnosed kidney disease should focus on 3 areas: the determination of the underlying cause of CKD, the presence of risk factors for CKD progression and CV disease, and the presence of complications of CKD. History should include past medical history (CV disease, diabetes, hypertension, autoimmune disease, human immunodeficiency virus [HIV], hepatitis C, myeloma, episodes of AKI, recurrent urinary tract infections, lower urinary tract/obstructive symptoms), family history (CKD, polycystic kidney disease), social history (smoking), and medications, including herbal and over-the-counter remedies (**Box 3**). The complete medication list is critical for proper diagnosis and risk reduction: this list should be reviewed for common nephrotoxins (such as nonsteroidal antiinflammatory drugs [NSAIDs]), agents that predispose to hypovolemia (diuretics), as well as medications that may require renal dosing (such as atenolol or allopurinol) and medications that, below a certain GFR, are contraindicated (bisphosphonates, factor Xa anticoagulants, metformin) or ineffective (hydrochlorothiazide) (**Table 1**). A few

Box 3
Common medications that require renal adjustment

Atenolol	Gabapentin
Acyclovir	Glyburide
Allopurinol	Levofloxacin
Amoxicillin	Metformin
Bisphosphonates	Metoclopramide
Cefpodoxime	Morphine
Cephalexin	Ranitidine
Clarithromycin	Rosuvastatin
Ciprofloxacin	Simvastatin
Codeine	Thiazides
Colchicine	Tramadol
Fluconazole	Trimethoprim/sulfamethoxazole

Table 1 Measurement of proteinuria	
Test	**Comments**
Urine dipstick	Measures albumin; typically only detects moderately or severely increased proteinuria; prone to false-positive results
UACR	Spot test; estimates daily albumin excretion; standardized across laboratories
UPCR	Also detects nonalbumin proteins; not standardized
24-h urine protein testing	Not routinely indicated in primary care of patents with CKD

Abbreviations: UACR, urine albumin-to-creatinine ratio; UPCR, urine protein-to-creatinine ratio.

medications, such as trimethoprim, cimetidine, and cefoxitin, are also known to interfere with the serum creatinine assay. Patients should also be assessed for signs/symptoms associated with renal disease complications, including anemia and edema. A careful physical examination should include auscultation for bruits and assessment of volume status, including edema. More targeted components of examination, such as looking for vasculitis or rheumatic processes or cardiac or hepatic dysfunction, may be indicated by history.

ASSESSING RENAL DYSFUNCTION
Glomerular Filtration Rate

Initial evaluation of patients with CKD should include a limited set of laboratory studies in an attempt to determine the cause and degree of dysfunction. Accurate estimation of the GFR is key to assessing renal function and establishing a diagnosis of kidney disease (**Box 4**). Serum creatinine concentration is a function of (1) production (creatinine is a breakdown product of muscle, and its level may also be affected by dietary meat consumption)[25] and (2) GFR (creatinine is freely filtered by the kidneys). Measurement of creatinine clearance using a timed urine sample is both cumbersome and impractical for the primary care provider. Instead, GFR is estimated using equations based on creatinine and other factors. The equations most commonly recommended by national groups are the MDRD and the CKD-EPI. Both include a patient's serum creatinine, age, sex, and race (black vs nonblack). Comparison studies suggest that the CKD-EPI may be more accurate in those with higher GFR and there is some suggestion that MDRD is more accurate for persons with stage 3 or more severe CKD.[26,27]

However, it is of primary importance for clinicians to actually estimate the GFR with one of these calculators, rather than rely on the serum creatinine level alone. This fact is particularly true for serum creatinine level in the 1 to 2 mg/dL range. If, for example, Mr Francis was a 25-year-old African American, his serum creatinine level of 1.8 mg/dL would reflect a GFR of 60 mL/min/1.73 m^2. A 75-year-old nonblack woman with the

Box 4 Interpreting serum creatinine
• GFR (or estimated GFR) is the best single marker of kidney function.
• Age, sex, and race have such a significant effect on GFR estimates that GFR must be calculated, rather than "eyeballed" from serum creatinine
• A single numerical value of creatinine may represent normal GFR for one person and severely decreased GFR for another

same creatinine level would have a GFR less than half that, of approximately 28 mL/min/1.73 m^2. Mr Francis likely had his prior serum creatinine level of 1.5 mg/dL overlooked as normal, even though this also reflected CKD.

Proteinuria

There are 3 main types of persistent proteinuria: glomerular (in which proteins leak through the glomerulus in glomerular disease), tubular (small proteins that normally are filtered through the glomerulus are not resorbed as they should be), and overflow (the volume of small proteins, such as myeloma light chains, overwhelm the resorption mechanisms).

Albuminuria, defined as greater than 30 mg albumin/24 hours, is due to glomerular disease and is the type of proteinuria in most cases of CKD.[2] There are several options for estimating the quantity of proteinuria or albuminuria (**Box 5**; see **Table 1**). A 24-hour urine sample is rarely the test of choice, because 24-h excretion can be well estimated by a spot or random untimed sample. From the measured levels of albumin and creatinine in this single sample, a urine albumin-to-creatinine ratio (UACR) is calculated. A UACR greater than or equal to 30 mg/mmol (or 300 mg/g) is considered evidence of albuminuria and may be characterized as moderately increased (30–299 mg/mmol) or severely increased (>300 mg/mmol, see **Fig. 1**).

For calculating total protein excretion, a similar urine protein-to-creatinine ratio (UPCR) is used. For this, a UPCR greater than or equal to 50 mg/mmol (or 500 mg/g) is the threshold for proteinuria. However, a limitation of this modality is that UPCR testing is not standardized across laboratories.

Any initial evidence of proteinuria, whether by urine dipstick or UACR, merits confirmation via repeat UACR testing, because certain common scenarios (fever, exercise) can lead to a transient increase in urinary protein excretion, and other scenarios (gross hematuria, highly alkaline or concentrated urine) may also lead to a false-positive result on urine dipstick.[2,28,29]

Other Laboratory Studies

In patients with a new CKD diagnosis, further testing should include a basic metabolic panel, calcium, phosphate, serum albumin, Hb/hematocrit, and lipids, used to evaluate prognosis and assess for complications (**Table 2**).

Further laboratory testing is usually done in order to help determine the cause of CKD and look for treatable causes. For patients with longstanding hypertension or diabetes, additional testing is often unnecessary. However, further testing (hepatitis B/C serologies, HIV antibody testing, serum protein electrophoresis (SPEP), and rapid plasma reagin) should be carried out in patients who are young, have rapid progression, severe disease, or uncertain diagnosis. This testing should also be considered in patients who have diabetes known to be of recent onset and without evidence of

---

Box 5
Assessing proteinuria

- UACR is the preferred monitoring test for albuminuria in patients with CKD

- Detection of protein, either on urine dipstick or by UACR, should be repeated to determine if the proteinuria is transient or persistent

- Persistent proteinuria is an independent predictor of CKD progression and mortality; the greater the degree of proteinuria, the worse the prognosis

Table 2
Laboratory evaluation of CKD

Test	Indication	Frequency
Basic metabolic panel	Prognosis, hyperkalemia	At diagnosis and periodically
Calcium, phosphate	Prognosis, metabolic bone disease	At diagnosis and again when GFR<45 mL/min/1.73 m^2
Serum albumin	Prognosis	At diagnosis
PTH, alkaline phosphatase, vitamin D	Metabolic bone disease	When GFR<45 mL/min/1.73 m^2
Hemoglobin/hematocrit	Prognosis, anemia	At diagnosis and then annually if eGFR≥30 mL/min/1.73 m^2; q 6 mo if eGFR<30 mL/min/1.73 m^2
Lipids	CV risk stratification	At diagnosis and periodically
UACR, serum creatinine	Prognosis, progression	At least yearly, more frequently in more advanced CKD or when it will affect management
HIV, HBV, HCV, RPR, SPEP	If unclear cause	At diagnosis
Complement, ANA, ANCA, anti-GBM	Only if specific syndrome suspected	At diagnosis

Abbreviations: ANA, anti-neutrophilic antibody; ANCA, anti-neutrophil cytoplasm antibody; anti-GBM, anti-glomerular basement membrane; eGFR, estimated GFR; HBV, hepatitis B virus; HCV, hepatitis C virus; PTH, parathyroid hormone; RPR, rapid plasma reagin; SPEP, serum protein electrophoresis.

other microvascular disease. Kidney biopsy is considered if the patient has rapid-onset proteinuria, hematuria, active urinary sediment, rapidly progressive disease, or suspicion of nephropathy secondary to systemic disease.[30] If the features suggest a nephritic syndrome, kidney specialists should be involved and may perform further testing, such as for complement, anti-neutrophilic antibody (ANA), anti-neutrophil cytoplasm antibody (ANCA) and anti-glomerular basement membrane (anti-GBM).

The frequency of laboratory monitoring for CKD progression and complications is generally based on the degree of CKD; more advanced disease requires more frequent monitoring. Recommendations suggest at least annual UACR and creatinine testing for all patients with CKD, with increased frequency for those with lower GFR or higher albuminuria.[2] A patient with stage 3b CKD such as Mr Francis would likely benefit from serum creatinine testing every 3 to 4 months.

TREATMENT

Just as CKD affects multiple physiologic domains, care of the patient with CKD must also take a multifaceted approach. Although certain aspects of patient care are often best handled by a renal specialist (titrating immunosuppressants in nephritic syndrome, offering erythropoietin-stimulating agents [ESAs] for CKD-associated anemia), most of the monitoring and management (particularly of the most common causes of CKD, hypertension, and diabetes) is coordinated by the primary care provider (PCP) (**Box 6**).

The management of CKD has multiple aims: to slow CKD progression, to reduce the CV and infectious morbidity/mortality, and to screen for and manage the associated metabolic and endocrine complications. Additional responsibilities include avoiding medication-related harms, including AKI, and, for patients with advanced CKD, to discuss and prepare for RRT. Given this panoply of responsibilities, it is perhaps

---

Box 6
Specific interventions that slow progression of CKD

BP control in patients with hypertension

Glycemic control in diabetic patients

Angiotensin blockade in those with proteinuric CKD

Avoiding nephrotoxins and AKI

Bicarbonate therapy if serum HCO_3 level is less than 22 mmol/L

---

reassuring that, for most patients, the mechanisms for achieving the first 2 aims are well within the scope of everyday primary care: managing hypertension, heart disease, and diabetes. However, seeing these problems within the context of CKD allows for a more complete and improved care of the patient.

The destruction of substantial (>50%) renal mass in and of itself places the patient at risk for increased renal destruction, through structural damage mediated by hypertension, hyperlipidemia, hyperfiltration, proteinuria, and hyperactivation of the renin-angiotensin-aldosterone system (RAAS).[17] Thus management of these mediators can help slow CKD progression, regardless of the original cause (**Box 7**).

Renin-Angiotension-Aldosterone System Inhibition

For persons with hypertension and CKD, angiotensin-converting enzyme inhibitors (ACEIs) or angiotensin receptor blockers (ARBs) are the treatment of choice and have demonstrated reduction in CKD progression.[31] For persons with proteinuria, Kidney Disease: Improving Global, Outcomes (KDIGO) target BPs are less than 130/less than 80 mm Hg; for persons without proteinuria, these targets are slightly higher, at less than 140/less than 90 mm Hg. It should be noted that each target must be adjusted for the individual patient, accounting for age and comorbidities, and that older patients in particular should be assessed for orthostasis and other adverse reactions associated with lowering BP.[2] Joint National Commission 8 guidelines, by contrast, have a target BP of less than 140/90 for patients with CKD, regardless of proteinuria. For those older than 65 years, this represents a more conservative goal than that of 150/90 for the general population.[32]

In normotensive patients with diabetes, there is no strong evidence that prophylactic RAAS inhibition helps prevent the development of proteinuria. However, in hypertensive patients with diabetes, there is good evidence that RAAS inhibition can reduce

---

Box 7
RAAS inhibitor use

- ACEIs/ARBs are first-line antihypertensive agents for persons with CKD, particularly those with diabetes or severely increased albuminuria (UACR>300 mg/g, UPCR>500 mg/g)

- Use of ACEI and ARB in combination is contraindicated; it does not improve outcomes and increases incidence of hyperkalemia and AKI

- GFR should be assessed and serum potassium levels should be measured at baseline and again within 1 week of starting or following any dose escalation

- Serum creatinine level rise after initiation is to be expected; rise of up to 30% of baseline is tolerated

the risk of albuminuria onset[33] or progression of microalbuminuria to overt proteinuria.[34,35]

ACEI or ARB therapy (combination therapy is not recommended because it carries an elevated risk of AKI and hyperkalemia)[36,37] is a mainstay of secondary prevention for both diabetic and nondiabetic kidney disease. Although generally well tolerated, these agents have several potential side effects, which range from the irritating to the life threatening. The primary adverse effects to note are cough (ACEI), AKI, hyperkalemia, and angioedema. A dry cough is one of the most common side effects, affecting nearly 20% of ACEI users. Onset is typically within 1 to 2 weeks of initiation but may not occur until after 6 months of therapy; after ACEI discontinuation, cough typically resolves within a week but may persist as long as 3 months.[38] If cough is due to ACEI and angiotensin blockade is indicated, patients should be switched to an ARB, because cough with ARB is rare and cough is common with reinitiation of any agent within the ACEI class. Bradykinin-mediated angioedema, characterized by dermal/mucosal swelling of gradual onset, without rash, involving the extremities, face, gastrointestinal tract (leading to abdominal pain), and/or larynx (leading to the feared airway obstruction), is very rare, occurring in approximately 0.3% to 0.7% of cases.[39] The incidence of ARB-mediated angioedema is less than half of that of bradykinin-mediated angioedema can be considered with close monitoring and discussion with the patient.[37,39] Hyperkalemia (K^+ >5 mmol/L) occurs in an estimated 3% of patients using angiotensin blockers; however, this occurs primarily in those predisposed to this complication, such as persons using NSAIDs or potassium-sparing diuretics, persons with advanced CKD, persons with baseline K^+ greater than 4.5 mmol/L, or persons with other causes of hypoaldosteronism.[40,41]

Reduction in GFR is commonly seen after initiation of angiotensin blockade. It is not surprising that this occurs—angiotensin blockade dilates the efferent arteriole, thus reducing intraglomerular pressure and hence glomerular filtration. However, in those with renal artery stenosis, advanced heart failure, or other reasons for relying on angiotensin II to maintain GFR, the resulting rise in creatinine levels/decline in GFR can be marked. An increase in serum creatinine of up to 30% within the first 2 months of treatment should be tolerated by the primary care physician, because this is associated with a long-term preservation of renal function.[42] Again, serum creatinine levels should be measured within 1 week of dose initiation or escalation. In the case of Mr Francis, then, if a serum creatinine level of 1.8 mg/dL is determined to be his baseline, a rise to a creatinine level of 2.3 mg/dL should be tolerated with ACEI initiation.

Risk Factor Modification

Glycemic control can also reduce the risk of progression from normoalbuminuria to microalbuminuria in both type 1 and type II diabetic patients,[43,44] although the target glycated hemoglobin A_{1c} (HbA$_{1c}$) of 7.0% may need to be adjusted given the patient's age, comorbidities, and risks of hypoglycemia.[23,29] There has been some question as to the reliability of HbA$_{1c}$ in CKD and ESRD, particularly given the alterations in red blood cell (RBC) turnover, hemolysis, and transfusions. Although there is some suggestion that HbA$_{1c}$ underestimates average glucose levels in patients with advanced CKD, the primary finding has been that of significant individual variability in the correlation between HbA$_{1c}$ and average glucose,[2] and thus correlating HbA$_{1c}$ findings with blood glucose monitoring is recommended.

Regarding the use of metformin in diabetic patients with CKD, there is a growing consensus that the serum creatinine level cutoffs of 1.4 mg/dL and 1.5 mg/dL for women and men, respectively, are too restrictive[45] and that the risk for lactic acidosis remains very low for most patients with these creatinine values. Many providers suggest continuing metformin at reduced dose in patients with mild to moderate renal impairment, withdrawing the drug at a creatinine clearance of less than 30 mL/min/1.73 m². [46]

Other interventions to reduce progression include reducing salt intake (<2 g sodium/day). The beneficial effect of protein restriction, if any, is probably modest, and there are clinically important risks. However, patients with CKD are advised to avoid excessive protein intake (>1.3 g/kg/d). Meeting with a nutritionist or other educator is recommended to discuss sodium, protein, and (if indicated) phosphate or potassium intake. Smoking cessation is critical in patients with CKD, both because of the increased CV mortality risk and because smoking may accelerate CKD as well as contribute to the arterial calcification of ESRD. [47] Management of metabolic acidosis, when present, can also slow progression of CKD, and alkali therapy, in the form of sodium bicarbonate, is generally safe and well tolerated, although it should notably be initiated in those with hypocalcemia or hypokalemia. Sodium bicarbonate is often dosed by weight at 0.5 to 1 mg/kg daily, and one reasonable starting dose is 600 mg thrice daily. [48] Hyperuricemia has also been associated with CKD in epidemiologic studies, but further studies are needed before xanthine oxidase inhibitors are routinely recommended. [49]

A final method of slowing CKD progression is avoiding AKI where possible. Although much of AKI prevention is beyond the scope of this article, it is worth noting that patients with CKD are at progressively increased risk of AKI (and in turn, worsening of their CKD). [19] Much of this susceptibility can be attributed to intrinsic dysfunction leading to decreased renal blood flow, but it can also be caused or exacerbated by prescription medications. Decreases in the flow or volume of renal circulation can be caused by antihypertensive agents, NSAIDs, RAAS inhibitors, or diuretics. Withholding such agents before procedures associated with volume shifts or administration of other nephrotoxins (eg, radiocontrast) can help avoid AKI. [50] Caution with NSAIDs should be exercised in all persons with CKD, particularly those on angiotensin inhibitors, because of the resulting impaired autoregulation of blood flow and increased risk of AKI, particularly in the setting of dehydration.

Recalling that patients with CKD are at increased risk of CV disease, it is important to ensure appropriate CV risk reduction. Recommendations for patients with CKD are not necessarily different from those for the general population. All patients with CKD should be given appropriate counseling on lifestyle, including exercise and a heart-healthy diet, as well as smoking cessation. The KDIGO 2012 guidelines recommend statins for all patients with CKD older than 50 years. Although the AHA/American College of Cardiology guidelines from 2013 do not specifically recommend that patients with CKD receive statins, the vast majority (>90%) of patients with CKD older than 50 years do meet AHA criteria for statin administration through other criteria. Statins reduce the risk of major CV events in patients with CKD, [51,52] and risk stratification should occur in all patients with CKD, with statin therapy considered in all patients with other CV risk factors or with stage 3 to 4 CKD. There are some data that suggest that statins did not improve mortality when initiated in patients with ESRD, partly due to a higher incidence of hemorrhagic stroke, [53,54] so for those with ESRD, the discussion regarding statin therapy should be made in conjunction with a kidney specialist. If aspirin is indicated for primary prevention of CV disease, providers should be reassured that the morbidity/mortality benefits are also seen in patients with CKD and, in aggregate, outweigh the risk of bleeding, although this should be assessed for each individual patient. [2,55]

Persons with CKD, because of multiple mechanisms, have an acquired immunosuppression and are at increased risk of infection. [56,57] Ensuring that these patients are protected against common and preventable diseases is a key role for providers. All patients with CKD should receive an annual flu vaccine; this should be one of the inactivated forms, and the live attenuated vaccine is considered contraindicated.[58]

Patients with stage 4 or more severe CKD should receive 2 pneumococcal vaccines: PPSV23 and the newer PCV13. The timing of these 2 vaccines can be complex, but in patients without prior pneumococcal immunization, the ideal initial timing is PCV13 followed by PPSV23 after 8 weeks. In patients who have recently been administered PPSV23 vaccine, it is recommended that PCV13 be deferred for 1 year. This coordination is to ensure maximal immune response generated to each vaccine. Patients with stage 4 or more severe CKD should also receive the hepatitis B immunization series, in anticipation of the greatly reduced (but still present) risk of hepatitis B virus (HBV) acquisition via hemodialysis. Of note, owing to their immunosuppressed state, patients with advanced CKD who acquire HBV are at increased risk of chronic infection.[58] These patients are also at increased risk of failing to mount an appropriate immune response to vaccination, and a surface antibody (hepatitis B surface antibody) should be checked after completion of the series to ensure immunity.

COMPLICATIONS

The principal metabolic and endocrine complications of CKD are unlikely to manifest before stage 3. However, their presence/absence should be assessed routinely as part of the comprehensive care of the patient with CKD (**Box 8**).

Anemia

Anemia affects approximately 12% of those with stage 3a CKD, and greater than 50% of those with advanced (stage 4 or 5) CKD.[2] It is slightly more common among persons with diabetes.[59] Anemia of CKD is normocytic and is primarily because of reduced erythropoietin synthesis by the kidney as well as decreased RBC half-life. However, anemia of CKD is primarily a diagnosis of exclusion, and consideration of other relatively common causes of anemia, particularly iron deficiency anemia, should occur before diagnosis. Cutpoints for anemia are the same as those given by the World Health Organization: Hb levels less than 13 g/dL for men and less than 12 g/dL for women. Although some of the symptoms attributed to CKD (fatigue, lethargy) may be exacerbated by or be caused by anemia, treatment of anemia with ESAs has become more judicious, initiated at lower Hb levels and with lower Hb targets, because of the increased risk of CV events[60] and failure to meaningfully improve quality of life[61] when aiming to fully correct anemia. For anemia screening, KDIGO guidelines recommend testing every 12 months for persons with stage 3 CKD and every 6 months for patients with stage 4 to 5 CKD.

Box 8
Complications of CKD

- Complications of CKD are increasingly common with advanced stages
- Anemia of CKD is a diagnosis of exclusion: iron deficiency must first be considered
- Persistent metabolic acidosis increases risk of kidney disease progression
- Mineral bone disease is complex and should be managed with a nephrologist
- DXA scans are not reliable in patients with stage 3b or more severe CKD; bisphosphonates are contraindicated in patients with stage 4 or more severe disease

Abbreviation: DXA, dual-energy X-ray absorptiometry.

Metabolic Acidosis

The metabolic acidosis of CKD is primarily due to impaired renal ammonia synthesis and acid excretion. This condition affects nearly 20% of patients at stage 4 to 5, although it can occur earlier in patients with other tubular disorders or hypoaldosteronism.[62] Metabolic acidosis can lead to malaise, fatigue, acceleration of bone disease (due to bone acting as an acid buffer), impaired renal synthesis of 1,25-dihydroxyvitamin D, muscle catabolism, and inflammation, which in turn are implicated in CV disease and renal dysfunction itself.[62,63] As noted above, there is some evidence to suggest that alkali treatment can help slow CKD progression.

Chronic Kidney Disease-Mineral and Bone Disorder

Chronic kidney disease-mineral and bone disorder (CKD-MBD) is a complex and multifactorial process. The onset is typically seen with stage 3b or more severe CKD (GFR<45 mL/min/1.73 m^2). Secondary hyperparathyroidism is the major abnormality seen in CKD-MBD and is due to a complex interplay of multiple factors: hyperphosphatemia (due to impaired phosphate excretion), reduced 1,25-dihydroxyvitamin D levels, hypocalcemia, increased fibroblast growth factor (FGF)-23 concentration, reduced expression of vitamin D receptors, calcium-sensing receptors, FGF receptors, and klotho in the parathyroid glands.

Complications of CKD-MBD include various forms of renal osteodystrophy, tertiary (autonomous) hyperparathyroidism, vascular calcification, and calciphylaxis. As primary care providers, emphasis should not be on managing the complexities of CKD-MBD, but rather on prevention, through assessment of serum parathyroid hormone (PTH), calcium, phosphate, and alkaline phosphatase levels. If an elevated level of PTH is detected, attention should first be on ensuring that normal values of calcium, phosphate, and vitamin D are achieved. It is worth noting that patients with GFR less than 45 mL/min/1.73 m^2 may have bone disease, which prevents accurate bone mineral density testing, and as such dual-energy X-ray absorptiometry scanning is best avoided in these groups.[2] Furthermore, bisphosphonates should not be prescribed for patients with stage 4 to 5 CKD without the guidance of a specialist in bone health or CKD-MBD. KDIGO guidelines recommend PTH, calcium, phosphate, and alkaline phosphatase be checked at least once for all patients with stage 3b or more severe disease to establish a baseline.[2] Calcitriol, or 1,25-dihydroxyvitamin D, has typically been limited to use in those with secondary hyperparathyroidism. However, there is some suggestion that it may slow CKD progression and may be used by renal specialists for this purpose.[64]

Volume overload and hyperkalemia are complications of advanced CKD; these rarely occur before stage 5. However, hyperkalemia can occur earlier, particularly in the setting of a high-potassium diet; angiotensin blockade, underlying type 4 renal tubular acidosis (RTA), potassium-sparing diuretics, and NSAIDs can also exacerbate hyperkalemia in this setting.[2]

WHEN TO REFER

Timely referral to nephrology improves clinical outcomes and reduces costs. For patients with CKD, the optimal timing of referral is often stage 3 to 4 CKD. The earlier end of the spectrum is appropriate for anyone who has developed the abnormalities described above (anemia of CKD, hyperparathyroidism, metabolic acidosis, or other persistent electrolyte abnormalities). Nephrology specialist care is indicated for anyone with stage 4 CKD, regardless of the cause. In addition, patients with CKD of any stage and severely increased proteinuria (UACR>300 mg/g or >30 mg/mmol),

---

Box 9
Advanced CKD management/planning

- All patients with stage 4 CKD or complicated CKD should be referred to a nephrologist
- In patients who develop ESRD, delayed nephrology referral is associated with increased mortality
- Venipuncture and, particularly, PICCs should be avoided in patients with advanced CKD in order to preserve hemodialysis access options

Abbreviation: PICC, peripherally inserted central catheter.

---

evidence of nephritic syndrome, rapid progression of CKD (defined as GFR decline of >5 mL/min/1.73 m^2 in 1 year), hereditary kidney disease, or refractory hypertension should also be referred to a nephrologist.[2]

Earlier nephrology referral has shown a survival benefit for patients with stage 3 to 4 CKD[65]; referral greater than 4 months before initiating dialysis has a survival benefit for patients who develop ESRD.[66] Despite this, only a minority (~37%) of patients at stage 4 CKD have been referred to a nephrologist,[7] and only 27% of patients with ESRD were under a nephrologist's care in the year before initiating RRT.[67] Predictors of nonreferral include nonwhite race/ethnicity, lower socioeconomic status, female sex (among elderly), and multiple comorbidities.[2,52] Given that 20% of patients with stage 4 CKD will go on to develop ESRD, early referral helps patients prepare for consideration of methods of RRT, including transplant. Anticipating and preparing for ESRD requires planning and decision making on the part of patient and providers. All forms of RRT require further referral and evaluation (surgeons, transplant centers); time is therefore critical for care coordination and decision making. Nephrologists can offer counseling, patient education, dialysis access planning, and help determine if and when to initiate dialysis. Patient education in persons with CKD is ideally comprehensive and longitudinal and ranges from avoiding peripherally inserted central catheter lines and blood draws in the nondominant arm (to preserve future vascular access sites) to dietary counseling and medication review.

The decision to initiate dialysis is a complex one and merits careful consideration, particularly in the elderly. The mortality and quality of life benefits of elderly patients with baseline poor functioning are uncertain at best.[68,69] Primary care providers are in an excellent position to elicit patient goals and expectations and communicate these with the nephrologist to ensure shared decision making and advanced planning (**Box 9**).

SUMMARY

CKD is a common condition and is frequently underrecognized by providers. Early and accurate diagnosis can slow the progression of CKD and reduce the incidence of ESRD. Recognition of the increased CV risks for persons with CKD may allow for improved treatment and CV outcomes. By diagnosing CKD, primary care providers can help reduce the risk of AKI and adverse effects of renally cleared or nephrotoxic agents. Timely referral to nephrologists allow for diagnostic assistance, comprehensive education regarding progression, management of complications, and appropriate referrals for dialysis and/or transplant.

REFERENCES

1. Plantinga LC, Tuot DS, Powe NR. Awareness of chronic kidney disease among patients and providers. Adv Chronic Kidney Dis 2010;17(3):225–36.

2. Kidney Disease: Improving Global, Outcomes (KDIGO) CKD Work Group. KDIGO 2012 clinical practice guideline for the evaluation and management of chronic kidney disease. Kidney Int Suppl 2013;3:1–150.

3. CKD in the United States: an overview of USRDS annual data report volume 1. Ann Arbor (MI): United States Renal Data System. Available at: http://www.usrds.org/2014/view/v1_00.aspx. Accessed December 30, 2014.

4. Chronic kidney disease (CKD) surveillance project: tracking kidney disease in the United States. Atlanta (GA): Centers for Disease Control and Prevention. Available at: http://nccd.cdc.gov/CKD/detail.aspx?QNum=Q9. Accessed December 30, 2014.

5. Nitta K, Okada K, Yanai M, et al. Aging and chronic kidney disease. Kidney Blood Press Res 2013;38(1):109–20.

6. National chronic kidney disease fact sheet. Atlanta (GA): Centers for Disease; 2014. Available at: http://www.cdc.gov/diabetes/pubs/pdf/kidney_factsheet.pdf. Accessed December 30, 2014.

7. Chronic kidney disease (CKD) surveillance project: tracking kidney disease in the United States. risk factor and theme: age. Atlanta (GA): Centers for Disease Control and Prevention. Available at: http://nccd.cdc.gov/CKD/FactorsOfInterest.aspx?type=Age. Accessed December 30, 2014.

8. Hoyert D, Xu J. Deaths: Preliminary data for 2011. National Vital Statistics Reports, vol. 61. Hyattsville (MD): National Center for Health Statistics; 2012. no 6. Available at: http://www.cdc.gov/nchs/data/nvsr/nvsr61/nvsr61_06.pdf. Accessed December 30, 2014.

9. Gansevoort RT, Correa-Rotter R, Hemmelgarn BR, et al. Chronic kidney disease and cardiovascular risk: epidemiology, mechanisms, and prevention. Lancet 2013;382(9889):339–52.

10. Go AS, Chertow GM, Fan D, et al. Chronic kidney disease and the risks of death, cardiovascular events, and hospitalization. N Engl J Med 2004;351(13):1296–305.

11. Hallan SI, Matsushita K, Sang Y, et al. Age and the association of kidney measures with mortality and end-stage renal disease. JAMA 2012;308(22):2349–60.

12. Ekart R, Ferjuc A, Furman B, et al. Chronic kidney disease progression to end stage renal disease: a single center experience of the role of the underlying kidney disease. Ther Apher Dial 2013;17(4):363–7.

13. Genovese G, Friedman DJ, Pollak MR. APOL1 variants and kidney disease in people of recent African ancestry. Nat Rev Nephrol 2013;9(4):240–4.

14. Kao WHL, Klag MJ, Meoni LA, et al. MYH9 is associated with nondiabetic end-stage renal disease in African Americans. Nat Genet 2008;40(10):1185–92.

15. Tangri N, Stevens LA, Griffith J, et al. A predictive model for progression of chronic kidney disease to kidney failure. JAMA 2011;305(15):1553–9.

16. Keith DS, Nichols GA, Gullion CM, et al. Longitudinal follow-up and outcomes among a population with chronic kidney disease in a large managed care organization. Arch Intern Med 2004;164(6):659–63.

17. Abboud H, Henrich WL. Stage IV chronic kidney disease. N Engl J Med 2010;362(1):56–65.

18. Roshanravan B, Robinson-Cohen C, Patel KV, et al. Association between physical performance and all-cause mortality in CKD. J Am Soc Nephrol 2013;24(5):822–30.

19. Chawla LS, Eggers PW, Star RA, et al. Acute kidney injury and chronic kidney disease as interconnected syndromes. N Engl J Med 2014;371(1):58–66.

20. Fink HA, Ishani A, Taylor BC, et al. Screening for, monitoring, and treatment of chronic kidney disease stages 1 to 3: a systematic review for the U.S. preventive

services task force and for an American college of physicians clinical practice guideline. Ann Intern Med 2012;156(8):570–81.

21. Qaseem A, Hopkins J, Robert H, et al. Screening, monitoring, and treatment of stage 1 to 3 chronic kidney disease: a clinical practice guideline from the American college of physicians. Ann Intern Med 2013;159(12):835–47.

22. ASN emphasizes need for early detection of kidney disease, a silent killer. Washington, DC: American Society of Nephrology; 2013. Available at: http://www.asn-online.org/news/2013/ASN_COMM_ACP_Screening_Response_102213_R12.pdf. Accessed December 30, 2014.

23. American Diabetes Association. Standards of medical care in diabetes–2014. Diabetes Care 2014;37(Suppl 1):S14–80.

24. Fihn SD, Gardin JM, Abrams J, et al. 2012 ACCF/AHA/ACP/AATS/PCNA/SCAI/STS guideline for the diagnosis and management of patients with stable ischemic heart disease a report of the American College of Cardiology Foundation/American Heart Association Task Force on Practice Guidelines, and the American College of Physicians, American Association for Thoracic Surgery, Preventive Cardiovascular Nurses Association, Society for Cardiovascular Angiography and Interventions, and Society of Thoracic Surgeons. J Am Coll Cardiol 2012;60(24):e44–164.

25. Butani L, Polinsky MS, Kaiser BA, et al. Dietary protein intake significantly affects the serum creatinine concentration. Kidney Int 2002;61(5):1907.

26. Stevens LA, Schmid CH, Greene T, et al. Comparative Performance of the CKD Epidemiology Collaboration (CKD-EPI) and the Modification of Diet in Renal Disease (MDRD) study equations for estimating GFR levels above 60 mL/min/1.73 m^2. Am J Kidney Dis 2010;56(3):486–95.

27. Michels WM, Grootendorst DC, Verduijn M, et al. Performance of the Cockcroft-Gault, MDRD, and new CKD-EPI Formulas in Relation to GFR, age, and body size. Clin J Am Soc Nephrol 2010;5(6):1003–9.

28. Carroll MF, Temte JL. Proteinuria in adults: a diagnostic approach. Am Fam Physician 2000;62(6):1333–40.

29. Levey AS, de Jong PE, Coresh J, et al. The definition, classification, and prognosis of chronic kidney disease: a KDIGO controversies conference report. Kidney Int 2011;80(1):17–28.

30. Gonzalez Suarez ML, Thomas DB, Barisoni L, et al. Diabetic nephropathy: is it time yet for routine kidney biopsy? World J Diabetes 2013;4(6):245–55.

31. Sarafidis PA, Khosla N, Bakris GL. Antihypertensive therapy in the presence of proteinuria. Am J Kidney Dis 2007;49(1):12–26.

32. James PA, Oparil S, Carter BL, et al. 2014 evidence-based guideline for the management of high blood pressure in adults: report from the panel members appointed to the eighth joint national committee (JNC 8). JAMA 2014;311(5):507–20.

33. Patel A, ADVANCE Collaborative Group, MacMahon S, et al. Effects of a fixed combination of perindopril and indapamide on macrovascular and microvascular outcomes in patients with type 2 diabetes mellitus (the ADVANCE trial): a randomised controlled trial. Lancet 2007;370(9590):829–40.

34. Parving HH, Lehnert H, Bröchner-Mortensen J, et al. The effect of irbesartan on the development of diabetic nephropathy in patients with type 2 diabetes. N Engl J Med 2001;345(12):870–8.

35. Kitada M, Kanasaki K, Koya D. Clinical therapeutic strategies for early stage of diabetic kidney disease. World J Diabetes 2014;5(3):342–56.

36. Fried LF, Emanuele N, Zhang JH, et al. Combined angiotensin inhibition for the treatment of diabetic nephropathy. N Engl J Med 2013;369(20):1892–903.

37. Mann JFE, Schmieder RE, McQueen M, et al. Renal outcomes with telmisartan, ramipril, or both, in people at high vascular risk (the ONTARGET study): a multi-centre, randomised, double-blind, controlled trial. Lancet 2008;372(9638):547–53.

38. Dicpinigaitis PV. Angiotensin-converting enzyme inhibitor-induced cough: ACCP evidence-based clinical practice guidelines. Chest 2006;129(1 Suppl): 169S–73S.

39. Bezalel S, Mahlab-Guri K, Asher I, et al. Angiotensin converting enzyme inhibitor induced angioedema. Am J Med 2015;128:120–5. Available at: http://www.amjmed.com/article/S0002934314005919/abstract. Accessed December 31, 2014.

40. Reardon LC, Macpherson DS. Hyperkalemia in outpatients using angiotensin-converting enzyme inhibitors: How much should we worry? Arch Intern Med 1998;158(1):26–32.

41. Khosla N, Kalaitzidis R, Bakris GL. Predictors of hyperkalemia risk following hypertension control with aldosterone blockade. Am J Nephrol 2009;30(5):418–24.

42. Bakris GL, Weir MR. Angiotensin-converting enzyme inhibitor-associated elevations in serum creatinine: is this a cause for concern? Arch Intern Med 2000; 160(5):685–93.

43. Holman RR, Paul SK, Bethel MA, et al. 10-year follow-up of intensive glucose control in type 2 diabetes. N Engl J Med 2008;359(15):1577–89.

44. ADVANCE Collaborative Group, Patel A, MacMahon S, et al. Intensive blood glucose control and vascular outcomes in patients with type 2 diabetes. N Engl J Med 2008;358(24):2560–72.

45. Inzucchi SE, Bergenstal RM, Buse JB, et al. Management of hyperglycemia in type 2 diabetes, 2015: a patient-centered approach: update to a position statement of the American diabetes association and the European association for the study of diabetes. Diabetes Care 2015;38(1):140–9.

46. Lipska KJ, Bailey CJ, Inzucchi SE. Use of metformin in the setting of mild-to-moderate renal insufficiency. Diabetes Care 2011;34(6):1431–7.

47. Orth SR, Hallan SI. Smoking: a risk factor for progression of chronic kidney disease and for cardiovascular morbidity and mortality in renal patients—absence of evidence or evidence of absence? Clin J Am Soc Nephrol 2008; 3(1):226–36.

48. Łoniewski I, Wesson DE. Bicarbonate therapy for prevention of chronic kidney disease progression. Kidney Int 2014;85(3):529–35.

49. Johnson RJ, Nakagawa T, Jalal D, et al. Uric acid and chronic kidney disease: which is chasing which? Nephrol Dial Transplant 2013;28(9):2221–8.

50. Jo S-H, Lee JM, Park J, et al. The impact of Renin-Angiotensin-aldosterone system blockade on contrast-induced nephropathy: a meta-analysis of 12 studies with 4,493 patients. Cardiology 2015;130(1):4–14.

51. Baigent C, Landray MJ, Reith C, et al. The effects of lowering LDL cholesterol with simvastatin plus ezetimibe in patients with chronic kidney disease (study of heart and renal protection): a randomised placebo-controlled trial. Lancet 2011; 377(9784):2181–92.

52. Navaneethan SD, Pansini F, Perkovic V, et al. HMG CoA reductase inhibitors (statins) for people with chronic kidney disease not requiring dialysis. Cochrane Database Syst Rev 2009;(2):CD007784.

53. Wanner C, Krane V, März W, et al. Atorvastatin in patients with type 2 diabetes mellitus undergoing hemodialysis. N Engl J Med 2005;353(3):238–48.

54. Fellström BC, Jardine AG, Schmieder RE, et al. Rosuvastatin and cardiovascular events in patients undergoing hemodialysis. N Engl J Med 2009;360(14): 1395–407.

55. Jardine MJ, Ninomiya T, Perkovic V, et al. Aspirin is beneficial in hypertensive patients with chronic kidney disease: a post-hoc subgroup analysis of a randomized controlled trial. J Am Coll Cardiol 2010;56(12):956–65.

56. Kurts C, Panzer U, Anders H-J, et al. The immune system and kidney disease: basic concepts and clinical implications. Nat Rev Immunol 2013;13(10):738–53.

57. Dalrymple LS, Katz R, Kestenbaum B, et al. The risk of infection-related hospitalization with decreased kidney function. Am J Kidney Dis 2012;59(3):356–63.

58. Guidelines for vaccinating kidney dialysis patients and patients with chronic kidney disease. Atlanta (GA): Centers for Disease Control and Prevention; 2006. Available at: http://www.cdc.gov/diabetes/pubs/pdf/CKD_vaccination.pdf. Accessed December 30, 2014.

59. El-Achkar TM, Ohmit SE, McCullough PA, et al. Higher prevalence of anemia with diabetes mellitus in moderate kidney insufficiency: the kidney early evaluation program. Kidney Int 2005;67(4):1483–8.

60. Palmer SC, Navaneethan SD, Craig JC, et al. HMG CoA reductase inhibitors (statins) for people with chronic kidney disease not requiring dialysis. Cochrane Database Syst Rev 2014;(5):CD007784.

61. Clement FM, Klarenbach S, Tonelli M, et al. The impact of selecting a high hemoglobin target level on health-related quality of life for patients with chronic kidney disease: a systematic review and meta-analysis. Arch Intern Med 2009;169(12):1104–12.

62. Dobre M, Rahman M, Hostetter TH. Current status of bicarbonate in CKD. J Am Soc Nephrol 2015;26:515–23.

63. Drawz P, Rahman M. Chronic kidney disease. Ann Intern Med 2009;150(3):ITC2-1–15.

64. Mirković K, van den Born J, Navis G, et al. Vitamin D in chronic kidney disease: new potential for intervention. Curr Drug Targets 2011;12(1):42–53.

65. Tseng C-L, Kern EFO, Miller DR, et al. Survival benefit of nephrologic care in patients with diabetes mellitus and chronic kidney disease. Arch Intern Med 2008;168(1):55–62.

66. Kazmi WH, Obrador GT, Khan SS, et al. Late nephrology referral and mortality among patients with end-stage renal disease: a propensity score analysis. Nephrol Dial Transplant 2004;19(7):1808–14.

67. Healthy people 2020. Chronic kidney disease: objectives. Washington, DC: Office of Disease Prevention and Health Promotion, Dept of Health and Human Services. Available at: https://www.healthypeople.gov/2020/topics-objectives/topic/chronic-kidney-disease/objectives. Accessed December 30, 2014.

68. Singh P, Germain MJ, Cohen L, et al. The elderly patient on dialysis: geriatric considerations. Nephrol Dial Transplant 2014;29(5):990–6.

69. Treit K, Lam D, O'Hare AM. Timing of dialysis initiation in the geriatric population: toward a patient-centered approach. Semin Dial 2013;26(6):682–9.

Primary Care of the Patient with Asthma

Michael J. Lenaeus, MD, PhD[a],*, Jan Hirschmann, MD[b]

KEYWORDS

- Asthma • Adult-onset asthma • Asthma exacerbation • COPD

KEY POINTS

- Adult-onset asthma is common and different from classical, early-onset disease associated with atopy.
- Diagnosis of adult-onset asthma is challenging, particularly in older adults or those with coexistent chronic obstructive pulmonary disease.
- Adult-onset asthma is often difficult to treat and has a poorer prognosis than childhood disease.

BACKGROUND

Asthma is a common chronic disease in the United States, affecting 8% of the population in 2012.[1] It usually begins in childhood, especially before the age of 6.[2] Atopy, defined as a measurable immunoglobulin E (IgE) titer to 1 or more antigens, is present in most of these patients and contributes to the development of asthma, as well as allergic rhinitis and atopic dermatitis.[3] Other features suggesting an immunologic basis for childhood asthma are the high rates of immediate skin test responses to molds and other inhaled allergens[4] and an association between serum IgE levels, skin test reactivity, and asthma.[5,6] Furthermore, control of allergens brings substantial relief for many patients. For unknown reasons, disease remission is common in this group (a longitudinal study found a rate of 66%).[7]

Asthma in adults may occur as persistent or relapsed childhood disease, but often begins in adulthood. Compared with childhood asthmatics, fewer of these patients have an allergic component,[8] and more have decreased lung function and persistent, refractory disease.[9] Indeed, most asthma-related deaths occur in older adults.

[a] Department of General Internal Medicine, University of Washington Medical Center, 1959 Northeast Pacific Street, Box 356429, Seattle, WA 98195-6429, USA; [b] Department of General Internal Medicine, Puget Sound VA Medical Center, University of Washington School of Medicine, 1660 South Columbian Way, Seattle, WA 98108, USA
* Corresponding author.
E-mail address: mlenaeus@uw.edu

Med Clin N Am 99 (2015) 953–967
http://dx.doi.org/10.1016/j.mcna.2015.05.007
0025-7125/15/$ – see front matter © 2015 Elsevier Inc. All rights reserved.

medical.theclinics.com

Patients with adult-onset asthma are more heterogeneous than those with early onset disease, and several classification schemes have been proposed to help guide clinical care and investigation of adults. Rackemann in the 1940s proposed the first classification,[10] which remains instructive today. He described "extrinsic" (or allergic) asthma as typical in those younger than 30 and used the term "intrinsic" (or nonallergic) asthma for those who developed the disease after age 30. Subsequent study has revealed the presence of new-onset "extrinsic" asthma in adults as well as a number of subgroups of nonallergic or "intrinsic" asthma, including those with nonatopic asthma and persistent eosinophilia, often with aspirin sensitivity,[11] nonatopic obese female asthmatics,[12] a chronic obstructive pulmonary disease (COPD)–overlap syndrome that includes nonatopic patients with a history of cigarette smoking[13] and many others. Some adult-onset disease may also be considered "extrinsic" in nature, particularly among patients with occupational asthma.[14] Indeed, the heterogeneity in adults with asthma is so great that some authors have argued that the term "asthma" merely represents the final, common pathway for diverse disease processes.[15]

The precise prevalence of adult-onset asthma is unknown (being clouded by estimates that include those with long-standing disease from childhood), although the disease prevalence is 8% in American adults as a whole and probably increases with age, suggesting that a substantial portion of older patients with asthma have developed the disease later in life.[1] The estimated incidence of new-onset asthma in the elderly is 95 cases per 100,000 people[16] and there was an estimated case burden of approximately 2 million in the elderly in 2011.[17]

RISK FACTORS
Occupational Exposure

Patients with established asthma may have symptoms worsen at work because of nonspecific bronchial hyperactivity to such factors as smoke, dust, fumes, or exposure to cold. In about 10% to 25% of patients with adult-onset asthma, however, occupational conditions seem to initiate the disease.[14] One form of this adult-onset "extrinsic" asthma is induced by an immunologic reaction to specific sensitizers, such as wheat flour, chemicals, or metals, usually after chronic, low-level exposure.[18] In these patients, symptoms occur during or after work and improve on nonworking days, such as weekends and holidays. Irritant asthma (or reactive airway dysfunction syndrome) is another form of occupational asthma and is a response to compounds without an identified immunologic mechanism.[14] It typically occurs after a large exposure and can cause rapid-onset disease, sometimes within 24 hours. In some instances of either type, symptoms persist for many years after exposure ceases.[19]

Smoking and Second-Hand Smoke

Inhalation of tobacco smoke is a significant risk factor for developing adult-onset asthma.[3] Cigarette smoking approximately doubles the risk of a subsequent asthma diagnosis in adults.[20] Smoking probably also interacts with other predisposing factors, as demonstrated by increased diagnosis of asthma in patients with a family history of asthma and exposure to second-hand smoke,[21] as well as in adult smokers with allergic rhinitis.[22]

Female Sex

Female sex hormones are predisposing factors for developing adult-onset asthma.[12] It is more common and more severe in women than men, decreases with menopause and oral contraceptive use, and increases with the number of pregnancies and post-menopausal female hormone replacement therapy.[23]

Obesity

Support for a role of obesity in asthma pathogenesis comes from large epidemiologic studies[24] as well as improvement in asthma control after weight loss or bariatric surgery.[25] Several studies suggest a dose–response relationship between obesity and asthma: a 1995 analysis of survey data from the Nurses Health Study II, for example, showed that incident asthma diagnosis was 2 to 3 times more likely in patients with a body mass index (BMI) of greater than 30 kg/m² when compared with those with a BMI of 20 to 22 kg/m² and that there was an increasing incidence of asthma as BMI increased in adult women.[26] Similar findings were noted in a cohort of 88,000 California Teachers: overweight women had an adult-onset asthma odds ratio of 1.45 when compared with women of normal weight, and extremely obese women had an odds ratio of 3.66.[27]

Other Risk Factors, Including Infection

Genetics may be important, although a family history is often absent. Other risk factors include infections,[28] upper respiratory disease (particularly allergic rhinitis),[29] and life stress.[30] Infectious disease may be the most common of these: a longitudinal study suggested that up to 70% of incident adult-onset asthma was related to infection,[31] usually from presumed viral causes, although *Chlamydophila* (formerly *Chlamydia*) *pneumoniae* and *Mycoplasma pneumoniae* have been implicated in some investigations.[32,33] Often, the first attack of asthma develops after typical symptoms of a viral respiratory infection, such as rhinitis, pharyngitis, and cough, but, rather than abating, the cough persists, accompanied by wheezing and dyspnea.

DIAGNOSIS OF ADULT-ONSET ASTHMA
Patient History and Physical Examination

Diagnosis of adult-onset asthma may be straightforward in early adulthood, although it may be challenging at older ages, given the frequent presence of comorbidities, such as congestive heart failure. Accurate distinction of asthma from other causes of dyspnea, wheeze, or cough is paramount, given differences in prognosis and expected responses to treatment. Assessment of these patients begins with a detailed history and physical examination. Intermittent symptoms of dyspnea, wheeze, chest tightness, or cough should be noted and particular attention paid to the activities of daily life and possible exposure at home, with recreation, and in the workplace. Many patients have a history of worsening symptoms with specific provoking factors, such as apparent viral respiratory infections, cold air, and exposure to dust, smoke, and fumes (eg, perfume). They may notice increased cough, wheezing, and dyspnea with exercise, either beginning after a few minutes of exertion or, often, only after completion of the activity. These exacerbations typically resolve within 30 minutes. For some patients, exercise-induced symptoms are the major or only manifestation of their asthma. For others, the preeminent symptom is cough alone, and asthma is a common cause for unexplained chronic cough in adults.

Wheeze is the characteristic examination finding in asthma, although it may be absent between exacerbations and even during severe bronchoconstriction, when airflow is too low to generate the sound. Patients should be examined both when upright and recumbent, because wheezing is often apparent only when the patient is supine, or it is much more intense in that position. Wheezing is typically heard during exhalation. It may also be present during inhalation, when substantial bronchoconstriction occurs, but in such cases it is wise to listen with the stethoscope over the neck because upper airway obstruction causing stridor is often transmitted to the lungs as inspiratory wheezing and can mimic asthma. The wheezing of asthma is a widespread, high-pitched musical noise; alternative patterns, such as a focal wheeze, may indicate other causes of bronchial obstruction, including lung cancer. Wheezing is a nonspecific finding that can be present in other respiratory disorders and congestive heart failure.

Additional features that may help in diagnosing asthma include the presence of allergic rhinitis, atopy, or nasal polyps, which are particularly common in those with aspirin-sensitive disease.[11] Extrapulmonary findings that indicate an alternative cause of symptoms include clubbing, jugular venous distention, edema, or liver failure.

Imaging and Additional Testing

Chest radiology should be performed in patients with suspected adult-onset asthma because of the relatively common presence of mimicking conditions, such as cardiac disease, interstitial lung disease, cancer, or bronchiectasis.[34] The radiograph is nearly always normal in patients with pure adult-onset asthma, and in the absence of atypical features, such as weight loss, hemoptysis, or clubbing, CT is unnecessary.

Spirometry findings in adult-onset asthma are similar to those with early-onset asthma—a reduced forced expiratory volume in 1 second (FEV_1)/forced vital capacity ratio (<0.7) with an FEV_1 that improves by >200 mL or 12% after the administration of a bronchodilator.[35] The distinction between asthma and COPD often rests primarily on the absence of such reversible airflow obstruction. Using that definition, the pulmonary disease of some patients with longstanding asthma evolves into COPD as the obstruction becomes fixed. Furthermore, as many as 20% of patients with the diagnosis of COPD, based on such characteristics as a substantial smoking history and chronic productive cough, have asthmalike features and postbronchodilator reversibility on spirometry.[36] These issues demonstrate that asthma and COPD, particularly in the elderly, often overlap. The distinction in most patients, however, is unimportant therapeutically, because treatment for the 2 diseases is similar.

False-negative spirometry results are common in asthmatics with nearly normal spirometry at baseline, and a bronchoprovocation test may be administered to aid in diagnosis in these subjects. Bronchial hyperresponsiveness may be diagnosed if a concentration of 8 mg/mL or less of methacholine induces a 20% decrease in FEV_1.[37] In elderly patients and those with atopy, however, both false-positive and false-negative results are common, and the test is unsafe in those with cardiac comorbidity or low FEV_1.[37]

A white cell count with differential is worthwhile to detect blood eosinophilia, which is often present in adult-onset asthma and generally does not require further evaluation in the absence of clinical features that suggest another cause, such as residence in a tropical country. Two important exceptions exist. Blood eosinophilia in an asthmatic that is associated with such features as recurrent febrile exacerbations, pulmonary consolidation on thoracic imaging, and the expectoration of brownish mucus plugs should suggest the diagnosis of allergic bronchopulmonary aspergillosis, for which further appropriate investigations are serum IgE levels, precipitating serum antibodies to *Aspergillus fumigatus*, and chest CT to look for parenchymal disease, mucoid impaction, and the characteristic bronchiectasis of central airways.[38] Second, in patients with longstanding asthma and upper respiratory disorders such as nasal polyposis, serous otitis media, allergic rhinitis, and recurrent sinusitis, blood eosinophilia may indicate the presence of Churg–Strauss syndrome (eosinophilic granulomatosis with polyangiitis). Other common features are migratory or transient pulmonary opacities, skin nodules or palpable purpura, abdominal pain, and painful peripheral neuropathy. Further investigations include anti-neutrophilic antibodies, which are positive in about 50% of cases, serum IgE levels, and biopsy of an affected organ.[39]

Because few adult-onset asthmatics have an identifiable allergen responsible for their disease, skin or serologic testing for allergens is not routinely recommended. Even when one is present, subcutaneous immunotherapy is not very effective.[40]

MANAGEMENT OF ADULT-ONSET ASTHMA
Management Goals

The goals of management include (1) avoiding or reducing precipitating and provoking factors, (2) providing symptomatic relief, and (3) controlling the chronic inflammation and disease progression that may ultimately cause fixed, obstructive disease. The National Heart, Lung and Blood Institute has published guidelines on the diagnosis, classification, and management of asthma in adults, which can be referenced for further review.[35]

Nonpharmacologic Strategies

Nonpharmacologic strategies of disease control are particularly effective in managing asthma. A written action plan, along with home peak flow monitoring and other aspects of self-management, reduces asthma exacerbations, hospitalizations, self-reported symptoms, unexpected physician visits, and mortality.[41] Teaching proper inhaler use and providing appropriate equipment can improve asthma severity scores and quality of life.[42] For obese patients, weight loss, whether achieved by dieting and increased exercise or by bariatric surgery, leads to substantial improvement in lung function. In those with concurrent sleep apnea, use of continuous positive airway pressure at night reduces asthmatic symptoms. Gastroesophageal reflux disease is common in asthmatics, particularly in the obese, but treatment with proton pump inhibitors does not affect lung function and should be reserved for those with symptomatic gastroesophageal reflux disease.

Asthmatics should try to shun provoking factors such as dust, fumes, and smoke, whether at work or leisure. With unavoidable exposure, a face mask or respirator may be useful. Those who smoke tobacco or marijuana should quit, and clinicians can help to provide assistance through smoking cessation programs and, as appropriate, by prescribing medications such as nicotine, bupropion, or varenicline. Asthmatics should also try to avoid people with viral respiratory infections and should get annual influenza vaccination, which decreases asthma exacerbations and hospitalization in older adults.[43] Vaccination against *Streptococcus pneumoniae* is also recommended for adults with asthma and COPD based on longitudinal studies in older adults,[44] although several COPD-specific trials and a metaanalysis have found no benefit in morbidity or mortality for such vaccination.[45]

For patients with exercise-induced symptoms, a period of warmup before intense activity helps to avert bronchoconstriction. Use of a facemask or scarf with exercise in cold environments may also be beneficial. Inhalation of a short-acting β-agonist such as albuterol 5 to 20 minutes before exertion commonly prevents symptoms. With frequent exercise, regular use of a combination of an inhaled corticosteroid (ICS) and long-acting β-agonist, such as budesonide/formoterol or fluticasone/salmeterol, is appropriate. For the occasional patient who fails to respond to these approaches, the oral leukotriene inhibitor, montelukast, is often helpful, as is preexercise inhalation of the mast cell stabilizer, cromolyn sodium.[46] Certain medications may precipitate asthma attacks. From 5% to 20% of adult asthmatics are intolerant of aspirin, especially those with concurrent allergic rhinitis and nasal polyps. Many also have worsening respiratory function when exposed to nonsteroidal antiinflammatory drugs (NSAIDs),[11] and they should be counseled to avoid NSAIDs or referred for desensitization if NSAID therapy is necessary for cardiovascular disease or another indication. Some patients, particularly those with severe asthma, may not tolerate β-blockers, but most adult-onset asthmatics or patients with COPD can receive the cardioselective ones, such as atenolol and metoprolol, safely.[47] Although narcotics and benzodiazepines do not precipitate asthma attacks or worsen lung function, they must also be prescribed carefully to patients with severe COPD or asthma. One prospective study found that increasing dosages of benzodiazepines and narcotics were each associated with increasing mortality in a dose–response fashion, but that low dosages of narcotics (<30 mg or oral morphine equivalents per day) were generally safe.[48]

Pharmacologic Strategies

Initial pharmacologic therapy for chronic, adult-onset asthma is determined by the severity of symptoms—short-acting relief medications may be sufficient for intermittent disease, whereas multiple, long-acting medications may be necessary for severe, persistent disease. Standardized definitions of asthma severity have been published by National Heart, Lung and Blood Institute and include the categories of intermittent disease for those with symptoms fewer than 2 days per week and varying degrees of persistent disease for those with more frequent symptoms.[35]

Short-acting β₂-agonists

Symptomatic relief in adults with adult-onset asthma may occur with inhaled albuterol, a short-acting β₂-agonist that induces bronchodilation, and its use alone is sufficient for many patients with intermittent asthma. There is no advantage to a fixed schedule of inhaling short-acting β₂-agonists in stable asthma and patients should use them on an as-needed basis. With exacerbations, a regular schedule of every 3 to 4 hours may help to relieve symptoms, along with prescribing oral corticosteroids, as discussed elsewhere in this article.

Many patients use inhalers improperly. Patients should shake the inhaler for about 5 seconds and then exhale completely, followed by putting the mouthpiece between their lips. They should begin inhaling, simultaneously activate the inhaler, and then slowly fill their lungs to full capacity. They should hold their breath for 10 seconds or as long as is comfortable and then exhale through their nose, preferably, or through their mouth. They should wait for about 30 to 60 seconds before administering a second dose. They should rinse their mouth with water and then expectorate the material after using ICS to help prevent oral thrush. Some patients have difficulty coordinating inhaler activation with inhalation. In these patients, a spacer may be helpful. The instructions are the same, but the timing is not so critical. Although nebulizers generally offer no advantages over inhalers, some patients, particularly the elderly or those with certain disabilities, find them easier to manage, especially with acute exacerbations. They can be prescribed small portable units for use at home or during travel.

Inhaled corticosteroids

Control of inflammation can be accomplished by administering antiinflammatory therapy, of which ICS are the most commonly used. ICS, such as mometasone, budesonide, and fluticasone, are the first-line controller medication for adult patients with adult-onset asthma. They have proven effectiveness in adult and elderly populations, although high doses may be necessary in those with severe disease, and some asthmatics do not respond at all.[49] ICS may increase the incidence of pneumonia in patients with respiratory disease, based on a systematic review of studies of COPD,[50] and a case-control investigation in asthmatics.[51] Additional potential side effects include thrush, dysphonia/hoarseness, and osteoporosis, if used in high doses, particularly in elderly patients. There is no difference among the various ICS agents studied, although asthma control is improved when combination products that include a long-acting β-agonist are compared with ICS alone.[52]

Long-acting $β_2$-agonists

Additional symptomatic relief may occur with long-acting $β_2$-agonists (LABA), such as formoterol or salmeterol. They are not recommended as monotherapy in asthma, however, because of a slightly increased risk for serious adverse events, including death or severe asthma exacerbations.[53,54] Combination inhaler products that use a moderate-dose ICS in addition to a LABA, such as budesonide/formoterol 80/4.5 or fluticasone 250 µg/salmeterol 50 µg, are safer and more effective than monotherapy with a LABA[55] and should be prescribed for those with symptoms that persist despite at least moderate-dose ICS.[35]

Oral corticosteroids

Systemic corticosteroids are the mainstay for treating severe asthma exacerbations, but chronic oral corticosteroids are often needed in adult asthma, particularly in the elderly.[8] Because many adverse effects occur with prolonged systemic corticosteroids, they should be provided in the minimum necessary dosage and tapered as symptoms improve. Often, asthmatic control can be attained with a small daily maintenance dose, such as 5 to 10 mg of prednisone. Prednisone is usually administered as a single morning dose, but sometimes patients with that schedule notice relief of symptoms during the day, but worsening during the evening or early morning. For these patients, prescribing the medication as a twice-daily program may be useful, with the second dose taken in the late afternoon or early evening.

Those requiring chronic systemic corticosteroids should receive vitamin D/calcium supplements to help prevent bone loss. Most individuals require 1200 mg of elemental calcium daily, total diet plus supplement, and 800 IU of vitamin D daily. Screening for osteoporosis with dual energy x-ray absorptiometry scans is appropriate in these patients, and prescription of bisphosphonates, such as alendronate, may be necessary with significant bone disease.

Inhaled anticholinergic agents

Inhaled anticholinergic agents improve symptom control for many patients with asthma, particularly those with long-standing disease.[56] In general, tiotropium is preferable to ipratropium, given its longer duration of action and once-daily administration. Ipratropium, however, may provide prompt control of symptoms when combined with albuterol, either in inhalers or in solutions mixed for nebulizer use. Side effects with these agents are infrequent based on data from patients with COPD.[57]

Leukotriene receptor antagonists

Leukotriene receptor antagonists, including montelukast and zafirlukast, are less effective than ICS for control of adult asthma. These medications are also slightly less effective than LABAs in patients with persistent symptoms despite ICS therapy, although LABAs cause slightly more adverse events in this population, and some clinicians favor long-term control with leukotriene receptor antagonists in those with cardiovascular disease.[58] Leukotriene receptor antagonists may also have a specific role in the treatment of NSAID-exacerbated asthma: a randomized trial found that 4 weeks of montelukast therapy improved lung function tests and asthma symptoms in a group already receiving a mixture of ICS, oral glucocorticoids, and theophylline.[59]

Theophylline

Theophylline can be helpful in patients who prefer oral medications to inhalers or whose disease has not been controlled with them. It may be especially beneficial in relieving nighttime symptoms. It is usually given as a sustained released tablet or capsule once or twice daily, depending on the pharmaceutical formulation. A good starting dose for adults is 300 mg daily, with monitoring of peak serum levels (obtained 3–7 hours after a morning dose of a twice daily preparation or 8–12 hours after a once-daily medication) to attain a level of 5 to 15 μg/mL. Most patients tolerate the medication well, but clinicians need to realize that theophylline clearance is decreased with age greater than 60, liver disease, pregnancy, congestive heart failure, recent smoking cessation, and certain concurrent drugs (**Box 1**).[60]

EVALUATION, ADJUSTMENT, AND RECURRENCE

Patients with newly diagnosed asthma should be seen frequently until their symptoms are controlled,[35] as gauged by frequency of rescue inhaler, dyspnea, nighttime awakenings, and activity limitations.[61] Once symptoms abate, the follow-up interval can be

---

Box 1
Drugs with major interactions with theophylline

Contraindicated

Dypyridamole

Febuxostat

Riociguat

Serious drug interaction—use alternative drug

Allopurinol

Bupropion

Carbamazepine

Ceritinib

Cimetidine

Ciprofloxacin

Erythromycin

Fluvoxamine

Itraconazole

Ivacaftor

Ketoconazole

Nefazodone

Regadenoson

Rifabutin

Rifampin

St John's wort

Tacrine

decreased to 3 to 6 months and consideration given to gradual and carefully monitored withdrawal of asthma medications to minimize side effects.

Treating Asthma Exacerbations

Asthma exacerbations, consisting of increased dyspnea, cough, and, sometimes, sputum production, typically have a less abrupt onset in adults than in children. Patients also commonly have a longer duration of symptoms before seeking care, often giving a history of gradual deterioration over days to weeks, and they typically have a less dramatic and slower response to therapy. Usually, the provoking factors for an exacerbation are obvious, such as a viral respiratory illness or exposure to smoke or dust, but sometimes the cause is unclear.

The major therapies for asthma exacerbations are inhaled bronchodilators and systemic corticosteroids. Albuterol with or without ipratropium may be given every 3 to 4 hours via inhaler or nebulizer. For systemic corticosteroids, prednisone 40 to 60 mg daily seems as effective as greater doses. The optimal duration of treatment is uncertain, and it may vary among patients and even among exacerbations in the same patient. A study in COPD indicated no difference between treatment for 5 or 10 days,[62] but its applicability to asthmatics is unclear, and some patients seem to require more protracted therapy. Tapering of the dose is unnecessary for short-course treatment and is often confusing to patients and practitioners alike. Even in patients with purulent sputum, antibiotics are unhelpful, unless pneumonia, a rare complication of asthma, is present. Routine chest radiographs and sputum cultures are unnecessary. In reliable patients, having a supply of prednisone on hand allows them to initiate therapy early in an exacerbation, which may avert visits to the emergency department and hospitalizations.

"Difficult-to-Control" Disease and Indications for Referral

Referral to a pulmonary specialist should be initiated with persistent symptoms, "difficult-to-control" disease or suspicion of alternative or coexistent disease.[35] It should also be considered for patients with frequent exacerbations or those requiring hospitalization. Before referral, primary care physicians should ensure accurate diagnosis, appropriate inhaler technique, medication adherence, and the absence of correctable factors that exacerbate disease. Clinicians should include pulmonary function tests and chest radiographs or order them if they have not been performed recently.

COMPLICATIONS OF OBSTRUCTIVE LUNG DISEASE

Patients with advanced COPD or asthma may experience complications of their lung disease, including "pulmonary cachexia," chronic hypoxemia, osteoporosis, pulmonary hypertension, and neurocognitive deficits. Hypoxemia, cachexia, and osteoporosis are a few of the most common of these complications and their management in primary care are discussed herein.

Weight Loss and Cachexia

Malnutrition, or "pulmonary cachexia," frequently accompanies COPD or asthma, with prevalence estimates of 20% to 40% in patients with advanced disease.[63] The cause of pulmonary cachexia is unknown, although its presence is an indicator of disease severity and an independent predictor of mortality in COPD.[64] Patients should be screened for weight loss at regular intervals and weighed at each follow-up visit. Diagnosis can be made based on the presence of an ideal body weight of less than 90% predicted or a BMI of less than 20 kg/m^2.[63] Treatment should include nutritional counseling and oral nutrition supplementation.[65] Pharmacotherapy with progesterone analogs may be considered in some cases as well, although modest benefit (weight gain of approximately 10 lbs, in 1 randomized, controlled trial[66]) must be weighed against increased risk of edema and a small increased risk of venous thromboemboli.

Osteoporosis

Osteoporosis frequently complicates COPD and asthma, with disease estimates ranging from approximately 30% to 60% depending on the population studied.[67,68] Risk factors for bone loss in those with COPD or asthma include traditional risk factors (including age, smoking, alcohol use, low BMI, female sex, and calcium and/or vitamin D deficiency) as well the severity of the underlying lung disease and the dose of oral glucocorticoid required.[69] ICS may also increase a patient's risk of osteoporosis, although this issue remains unsettled.

Patients with COPD should be tested for osteoporosis, as should those with asthma and certain high-risk features, including older age, frequent corticosteroid usage, high-dose ICS, vitamin D deficiency, or traditional risk factors. Dual energy x-ray absorptiometry allows direct measurements of bone mineral density, which helps to predict future fractures and treatment response. Those with suspected osteoporosis should also undergo evaluation for other secondary causes of osteoporosis with bloodwork to measure calcium, phosphate, liver function tests, serum creatinine, vitamin D, sex hormones and other testing (thyroid-stimulating hormone, parathyroid hormone, serum protein electrophoresis/urine protein electrophoresis) as guided by the history and physical examination.[70]

If osteoporosis is confirmed (T-score of <-2.5 by dual energy x-ray absorptiometry), treatment should be initiated with both nonpharmacologic and pharmacologic measures. All patients should receive counseling on smoking and alcohol cessation and physical activity, in addition to an assessment of fall risk and counseling on fall avoidance. Calcium and vitamin D intake should be supplemented to dosages of 1200 to 1500 mg/d and 800 to 1000 IU/d, respectively, and bisphosphonate therapy should be initiated with alendronate or risendronate.[71] Some patients with osteopenia or certain "high-risk" features (eg, history of fragility fracture, high-dose oral glucocorticoids, or other causes of secondary osteoporosis) may warrant treatment as well and should be treated as discussed. The World Health Organization's Frax calculator (http://www.shef.ac.uk/FRAX/tool.jsp) has been used to guide treatment in postmenopausal women and may provide additional information regarding fracture risk in patients with low bone mineral density, although it has not been validated in men, premenopausal women, or those with secondary or glucocorticoid-induced osteoporosis. Serial measurements of bone mineral density may be informative in patients at risk for accelerated bone loss, perhaps at 1- to 2-year intervals, although this issue is still being studied.

Hypoxemia

Chronic hypoxemia is frequently present in individuals with advanced COPD, is a marker of disease severity, and is associated with both increased mortality and decreased quality of life. Its presence is also associated with other complications of chronic obstructive lung disease: pulmonary hypertension, cor pulmonale, polycythemia, skeletal muscle dysfunction, and probably neurocognitive dysfunction.[72] Long-term oxygen therapy improves survival in patients with severe COPD whose resting PaO_2 is less than 55 mm Hg.[73] No survival benefit has been shown for oxygen therapy in patients with milder hypoxemia or hypoxemia with exertion, although oxygen therapy can be offered to many patients in the latter category in the United

States based on analogy with those with more severe resting hypoxemia. Resting oxygen saturation (Spo_2) should be measured at every follow-up visit with oxygen prescribed for those with an Spo_2 of less than 88% (or Pao_2 <55 mm Hg) or for those with an Spo_2 of less than 89% (or Pao_2 56–59 mm Hg) and evidence of cor pulmonale, pulmonary hypertension, or erythrocytosis. Oxygen therapy may also be considered during exercise or sleep if Pao_2 falls by more than 10 mm Hg or the Spo_2 is less than 88% during these periods.[74] Oxygen should be provided during air travel for those with a resting Spo_2 of less than 92% or those with an Spo_2 of less than 95% and certain risk factors, including severely diminished lung function (FEV_1 <50%) and those with hypoxemia on exertion during a 6-minute walk test. The latter groups should undergo specialty consultation and, perhaps, a hypoxic challenge test before air travel.[75] Patients with a resting oxygen requirement of greater than 4 L/min should not travel by air.[76]

SUMMARY

Asthma occurs in adults, even at an advanced age, particularly with certain occupations, tobacco smoke exposure, female sex, obesity, or recent upper respiratory disease. In adults, the disease can represent long-standing disease acquired in childhood or be a different, late-onset disorder associated with decreased lung function and fixed airway obstruction. Therapy of these 2 groups includes patient education, nonpharmacologic strategies, and avoidance of exacerbating or alleviating factors. Pharmacologic treatments should be aimed at rapid relief of symptoms, usually with bronchodilators, and control of chronic inflammation, typically with inhaled or oral corticosteroids. Frequent reevaluation is necessary as symptoms and complications are brought under control, and referral to a pulmonary specialist should be considered for those with severe symptoms or frequent exacerbations.

REFERENCES

1. Center for Disease Control and Prevention (CDC). Data, statistics and surveillance. Available at: http://www.cdc.gov/asthma/asthmadata.htm. Accessed January 6, 2015.
2. Yunginger JW, Reed CE, Connell EJO, et al. A community-based study of the epidemiology of asthma. Incidence rates, 1964–1983. Am Rev Respir Dis 1992;146:888–94.
3. Strachan DP, Butland BK, Anderson HR. Incidence and prognosis of asthma and wheezing illness from early childhood to age 33 in a national British cohort. BMJ 1996;312:1195–9.
4. Halonen M, Stern DA, Wright AL, et al. Alternaria as a major allergen for asthma in children raised in a desert environment. Am J Respir Crit Care Med 1997;155: 1356–61.
5. Burrows B, Martinez FD, Halonen M, et al. Association of asthma with serum IgE levels and skin-test reactivity to allergens. N Engl J Med 1989;320(5):271–7.
6. Sears M, Burrows B, Flannery E, et al. Relation between airway responsiveness and serum IgE in children with asthma and in apparently normal children. N Engl J Med 1991;325:1067–71.
7. Burgess JA, Matheson MC, Gurrin LC, et al. Factors influencing asthma remission: a longitudinal study from childhood to middle age. Thorax 2011;66:508–13.
8. Miranda C, Busacker A, Balzar S, et al. Distinguishing severe asthma phenotypes: role of age at onset and eosinophilic inflammation. J Allergy Clin Immunol 2004;113:101–8.

9. Rönmark E, Lindberg A, Watson L, et al. Outcome and severity of adult onset asthma–report from the obstructive lung disease in northern Sweden studies (OLIN). Respir Med 2007;101:2370–7.

10. Rackemann F. A working classification of asthma. Am J Med 1947;3:601–6.

11. Szczeklik A, Nizankowska E. Clinical features and diagnosis of aspirin induced asthma. Thorax 2000;55(Suppl 2):42–4.

12. Moore WC, Meyers DA, Wenzel SE, et al. Identification of asthma phenotypes using cluster analysis in the Severe Asthma Research Program. Am J Respir Crit Care Med 2010;181:315–23.

13. Kim TB, Jang AS, Kwon HS, et al. Identification of asthma clusters in two independent Korean adult asthma cohorts. Eur Respir J 2013;41:1308–14.

14. Tarlo SM, Lemiere C. Occupational asthma. N Engl J Med 2014;370:640–9.

15. Wenzel SE. Asthma phenotypes: the evolution from clinical to molecular approaches. Nat Med 2012;18:716–25.

16. Bauer BA, Reed CE, John W, et al. Incidence and outcomes of asthma in the elderly. A population-based study in Rochester, Minnesota. Chest 1997;111: 303–10.

17. Center for Disease Control and Prevention (CDC). Vital signs: asthma prevalence, disease characteristics, and self-management: United States, 2001–2009. MMWR Morb Mortal Wkly Rep 2011;60:547–52.

18. Malo J-L, Chan-Yeung M. Agents causing occupational asthma. J Allergy Clin Immunol 2009;123:545–50.

19. Aldrich T, Gustave J, Hall C, et al. Lung function in rescue workers at the World Trade Center after 7 years. N Engl J Med 2010;362:1263–72.

20. Aanerud M, Carsin AE, Sunyer J, et al. Interaction between asthma and smoking increases the risk of adult airway obstruction. Eur Respir J 2015;45:635–43.

21. Lajunen TK, Jaakkola JJ, Jaakkola MS. The synergistic effect of heredity and exposure to second-hand smoke on adult-onset asthma. Am J Respir Crit Care Med 2013;188:776–82.

22. Polosa R, Knoke JD, Russo C, et al. Cigarette smoking is associated with a greater risk of incident asthma in allergic rhinitis. J Allergy Clin Immunol 2008; 121:1428–34.

23. De Nijs SB, Venekamp LN, Bel EH. Adult-onset asthma: is it really different? Eur Respir Rev 2013;22:44–52.

24. Beuther DA, Sutherland ER. Overweight, obesity, and incident asthma: a meta-analysis of prospective epidemiologic studies. Am J Respir Crit Care Med 2007;175:661–6.

25. Al-Alwan A, Bates JH, Chapman DG, et al. The nonallergic asthma of obesity. A matter of distal lung compliance. Am J Respir Crit Care Med 2014;189:1494–502.

26. Camargo C, Weiss S, Zhang S, et al. Prospective study of body mass index, weight change, and risk of adult-onset asthma in women. Arch Intern Med 1999;159:2582–8.

27. Von Behren J, Lipsett M, Horn-Ross PL, et al. Obesity, waist size and prevalence of current asthma in the California Teachers Study cohort. Thorax 2009;64: 889–93.

28. Guilbert T, Denlinger L. Role of infection in the development and exacerbation of asthma. Expert Rev Respir Med 2010;4:71–83.

29. Shaaban R, Zureik M, Soussan D, et al. Rhinitis and onset of asthma: a longitudinal population-based study. Lancet 2008;372:1049–57.

30. Rod N, Kristensen T, Lange P. Perceived stress and risk of adult-onset asthma and other atopic disorders: a longitudinal cohort study. Allergy 2012;67:1408–14.

31. Sama SR, Hunt PR, Cirillo CI, et al. A longitudinal study of adult-onset asthma incidence among HMO members. Environ Health 2003;2:10.
32. Hahn D, Dodge R, Golubjatnikov R. Association of *Chlamydia pneumoniae* (strain TWAR) infection with wheezing, asthmatic bronchitis, and adult-onset asthma. JAMA 1991;266:225–30.
33. Yano T, Ichikawa Y, Komatu S, et al. Association of *Mycoplasma pneumoniae* antigen with initial onset of bronchial asthma. Am J Respir Crit Care Med 1994;149: 1348–53.
34. Patel MR, Janevic MR, Heeringa SG, et al. An examination of adverse asthma outcomes in U.S. Adults with multiple morbidities. Ann Am Thorac Soc 2013; 10:426–31.
35. National Asthma Education and Prevention Program Third Expert Panel on the Diagnosis and Management of Asthma. Expert Panel Report 3: guidelines for the diagnosis and management of asthma. Bethesda (MD): National Heart, Lung, and Blood Institute (US); 2007.
36. Barrecheguren M, Esquinas C, Miravitlles M. The asthma-chronic obstructive pulmonary disease overlap syndrome (ACOS): opportunities and challenges. Curr Opin Pulm Med 2015;21:74–9.
37. Crapo R, Casaburi R, Coates A, et al. American thoracic society guidelines for methacholine and exercise challenge testing — 1999. Am J Respir Crit Care Med 2000;161:309–29.
38. Agarwal R, Chakrabarti A, Shah A, et al. Allergic bronchopulmonary aspergillosis: review of literature and proposal of new diagnostic and classification criteria. Clin Exp Allergy 2013;43:850–73.
39. Vaglio A, Buzio C, Zwerina J. Eosinophilic granulomatosis with polyangiitis (Churg-Strauss): state of the art. Allergy 2013;68:261–73.
40. Creticos P, Reed C, Norman P, et al. Ragweed immunotherapy in adult asthma. N Engl J Med 1996;334:501–6.
41. Gibson P, Powell H, Coughlan J, et al. Self-management education and regular practitioner review for adults with asthma. Cochrane Database Syst Rev 2003;(1):CD001117.
42. Al-Alawi M, Hassan T, Chotirmall SH. Advances in the diagnosis and management of asthma in older adults. Am J Med 2014;127:370–8.
43. Voordouw B, van der Linden P, Simonian S, et al. Influenza vaccination in community-dwelling elderly: impact on mortality and influenza-associated morbidity. Arch Intern Med 2003;163:1089–94.
44. Moberley S, Holden J, Tatham D, et al. Vaccines for preventing pneumococcal infection in adults. Cochrane Database Syst Rev 2013;(1):CD000422.
45. Walters J, Smith S, Poole P, et al. Injectable vaccines for preventing pneumococcal infection in patients with chronic obstructive pulmonary disease. Cochrane Database Syst Rev 2010;(11):CD001390.
46. Parsons JP, Hallstrand TS, Mastronarde JG, et al. An official American Thoracic Society clinical practice guideline: exercise-induced bronchoconstriction. Am J Respir Crit Care Med 2013;187:1016–27.
47. Zeki A, Kenyon N, Yomeda K, et al. The adult asthmatic. Clin Rev Allergy Immunol 2012;43:138–55.
48. Ekström MP, Bornefalk-Hermansson A, Abernethy AP, et al. Safety of benzodiazepines and opioids in very severe respiratory disease: National prospective study. BMJ 2014;348:g445.
49. Adams N, Bestall J, Lasserson T, et al. Fluticasone versus placebo for chronic asthma in adults and children. Cochrane Database Syst Rev 2008;(4):CD003135.

50. Kew K, Seniukovich A. Inhaled steroids and risk of pneumonia for chronic obstructive pulmonary disease. Cochrane Database Syst Rev 2014;(3):CD010115.

51. McKeever T, Harrison TW, Hubbard R, et al. Inhaled corticosteroids and the risk of pneumonia in people with asthma: a case-control study. Chest 2013;144:1788–94.

52. Cates C, Kamer C. Combination formoterol and budesonide as maintenance and reliever therapy versus current best practice (including inhaled steroid maintenance), for chronic asthma in adults and children. Cochrane Database Syst Rev 2013;(4):CD007313.

53. Nelson HS, Weiss ST, Bleecker ER, et al. A comparison of usual pharmacotherapy for asthma or usual pharmacotherapy plus salmeterol. Chest 2006;129:15–6.

54. Cates C, Jaeschke R, Schmidt S, et al. Regular treatment with formoterol for chronic asthma: serious adverse events. Cochrane Database Syst Rev 2013;(6):CD006924.

55. Ducharme F, Ni Chroinin M, Greenstone I, et al. Addition of long-acting beta2-agonists to inhaled steroids versus higher dose inhaled steroids in adults and children with persistent asthma. Cochrane Database Syst Rev 2010;(4):CD005533.

56. Befekadu E, Onofrei C, Colice G. Tiotropium in asthma: a systematic review. J Asthma Allergy 2014;7:11–21.

57. Tashkin D, Celli B, Senn S, et al. A 4-year trial of tiotropium in chronic obstructive pulmonary disease. N Engl J Med 2008;359:1543–54.

58. Chauhan BF, Ducharme FM. Anti-leukotriene agents compared to inhaled corticosteroids in the management of recurrent and/or chronicasthma in adults and children. Cochrane Database Syst Rev 2012;(5):CD002314.

59. Dahlén S, Malmström K, Nizankowska EW, et al. Improvement of aspirin-intolerant asthma by montelukast, a leukotriene antagonist: a randomized, double-blind, placebo-controlled trial. Am J Respir Crit Care Med 2002;165:9–14.

60. Weinberger M, Hendeles L. Theophylline in asthma. N Engl J Med 1996;334:1380–8.

61. Nathan RA, Sorkness CA, Kosinski M, et al. Development of the asthma control test: a survey for assessing asthma control. J Allergy Clin Immunol 2004;113:59–65.

62. Leuppi JD, Schuetz P, Bingisser R, et al. Short-term vs conventional glucocorticoid therapy in acute exacerbations of chronic obstructive pulmonary disease: the REDUCE randomized clinical trial. JAMA 2013;309:2223–31.

63. Wagner P. Possible mechanisms underlying the development of cachexia in COPD. Eur Respir J 2008;31:492–501.

64. Cote CG. Surrogates of mortality in chronic obstructive pulmonary disease. Am J Med 2006;119:54–62.

65. Ferreira I, Brooks D, White J, et al. Nutritional supplementation for stable chronic obstructive pulmonary disease. Cochrane Database Syst Rev 2012;(12):CD000998.

66. Weisberg J, Wanger J, Olson J, et al. Megestrol acetate stimulates weight gain and ventilation in underweight COPD patients. Chest 2002;121:1070–8.

67. Graat-Verboom L, Wouters EF, Smeenk FW, et al. Current status of research on osteoporosis in COPD: a systematic review. Eur Respir J 2009;34:209–18.

68. Ferguson GT, Calverley PM, Anderson J, et al. Prevalence and progression of osteoporosis in patients with COPD: results from the TOwards a Revolution in COPD Health study. Chest 2009;136:1456–65.

69. De Vries F, van Staa TP, Bracke MS, et al. Severity of obstructive airway disease and risk of osteoporotic fracture. Eur Respir J 2005;25:879–84.

70. Watts NB, Adler RA, Bilezikian JP, et al. Osteoporosis in men: an Endocrine Society clinical practice guideline. J Clin Endocrinol Metab 2012;97:1802–22.

71. Grossman JM, Gordon R, Ranganath VK, et al. American College of Rheumatology 2010 recommendations for the prevention and treatment of glucocorticoid-induced osteoporosis. Arthritis Care Res (Hoboken) 2010;62:1515–26.
72. Kent BD, Mitchell PD, McNicholas WT. Hypoxemia in patients with COPD: cause, effects, and disease progression. Int J Chron Obstruct Pulmon Dis 2011;6: 199–208.
73. Nocturnal Oxygen Therapy Trial Group. Continuous or nocturnal oxygen therapy in hypoxemic chronic obstructive lung disease: a clinical trial. Ann Intern Med 1980;93:391–8.
74. Kim V, Benditt JO, Wise R, et al. Oxygen therapy in chronic obstructive pulmonary disease. Proc Am Thorac Soc 2008;5:513–8.
75. Edvardsen A, Akerø A, Christensen CC, et al. Air travel and chronic obstructive pulmonary disease: a new algorithm for pre-flight evaluation. Thorax 2012;67: 964–9.
76. Ahmedzai S, Balfour-Lynn IM, Bewick T, et al. Managing passengers with stable respiratory disease planning air travel: British Thoracic Society recommendations. Thorax 2011;66(Suppl 1):i1–30.

Primary Care of the Patient with Inflammatory Bowel Disease

 CrossMark

Jean R. Park, MD[a], Sheryl A. Pfeil, MD[b],*

KEYWORDS

- Inflammatory bowel disease • Ulcerative colitis • Crohn disease
- Extraintestinal manifestations • Routine health maintenance

KEY POINTS

- Inflammatory bowel disease (IBD) refers to the disorders ulcerative colitis and Crohn's disease.
- Patients with IBD can present with disease-related complications, extraintestinal manifestations, or treatment-related complications.
- Routine health maintenance in patients with IBD is of key importance. Preventive care should also be individualized, especially with regard to vaccinations, bone health, and cancer screening.

INTRODUCTION

Inflammatory bowel disease (IBD) includes 2 major disorders, ulcerative colitis and Crohn disease, both of which are due to inflammatory dysregulation in the gastrointestinal tract. The interaction of environment and human physiology necessitates a constant but controlled immunologic response in the gastrointestinal tract. When an imbalance occurs because of genetic and environmental factors, IBD may be precipitated.[1]

Ulcerative colitis and Crohn disease have many overlapping as well as distinguishing features in pathophysiology and management. This article highlights aspects of IBD that are most applicable to a primary care physician's practice. Also detailed

[a] Division of Hospital Medicine, Department of Internal Medicine, The Ohio State University College of Medicine and Wexner Medical Center, M112 Starling Loving Hall, 320 West 10th Avenue, Columbus, OH 43210, USA; [b] Division of Gastroenterology, Hepatology, and Nutrition, Department of Internal Medicine, Wexner Medical Center, The Ohio State University College of Medicine and Wexner Medical Center, 395 West 12th Avenue, Columbus, OH 43210, USA
* Corresponding author.
E-mail address: Sheryl.Pfeil@osumc.edu

Med Clin N Am 99 (2015) 969–987
http://dx.doi.org/10.1016/j.mcna.2015.05.009
0025-7125/15/$ – see front matter Published by Elsevier Inc.

are disease-related and treatment-related complications, and routine health maintenance practices for the patient with IBD.

DEMOGRAPHICS

North America, northern Europe, and the United Kingdom have the highest incidence rates and prevalence of IBD. Although IBD has historically presented in what was traditionally deemed as developed and Western countries, there has been an increase in IBD in southern and central Europe, Asia, Latin America, and Africa.[2]

Ulcerative Colitis

Ulcerative colitis has an incidence rate of 2.2 to 14.3 cases per 100,000 person-years. The prevalence rate is 37 to 246 cases per 100,000 persons.[2,3] Ulcerative colitis is slightly more prevalent in males. Although it can present at any age, the incidence of ulcerative colitis has traditionally been bimodal with a peak onset between 20 and 40 years of age and a lesser peak after 60 years of age.[4] Men are more likely than women to be diagnosed with ulcerative colitis in the later decades of life.[2] There is a higher incidence in urban areas.[4]

Crohn Disease

Crohn disease has an incidence rate of 3.1 to 14.6 cases per 100,000 person-years. The prevalence rate is 26 to 201 cases per 100,000 persons.[2,3] Crohn disease tends to be slightly more prevalent in females. Although it can present at any age, Crohn disease also has a traditionally bimodal disease onset that tends to be 5 to 10 years earlier than for ulcerative colitis.[2]

RISK FACTORS

Family history is a known risk factor that may be stronger in Crohn disease than ulcerative colitis.[5,6] Smoking has different effects on ulcerative colitis and Crohn disease, as detailed further in the Routine Health Maintenance section.[2]

CLINICAL PRESENTATION AND PATHOLOGY

Ulcerative Colitis

Ulcerative colitis is characterized by continuous mucosal inflammation beginning at the rectum and extending for a variable distance proximally. Endoscopically, the inflamed mucosa is friable, granular, ulcerated, and bleeds easily. Recurrent exacerbations can lead to inflammatory polyps and shortening of the colon caused by contractions of the muscle layer. Histologic findings on biopsies include lamina propria infiltration by inflammatory cells, vascular congestion, edema, mucin depletion of goblet cells, and crypt abscesses.[4]

Because of the inflamed and friable colonic mucosa, patients typically present with diarrhea, urgency, tenesmus, and hematochezia. In fact, hematochezia is so common that the lack of hematochezia on presentation should broaden the clinician's differential. Nocturnal episodes of diarrhea may also occur. In patients with primarily left-sided colitis, proximal constipation may be present even as the patient complains of passing bloody stool and mucus. Contrary to Crohn disease, abdominal pain is usually mild or absent, and weight loss is typically not severe. The physical examination can be unrevealing except for hematochezia on rectal examination.[4] Severe exacerbations of ulcerative colitis can lead to toxic megacolon, a condition that is characterized by dilatation of the colon and signs of severe systemic illness. Toxic megacolon requires intensive medical management, close observation, and early surgical consultation.

The overall rate of surgical intervention in ulcerative colitis has remained variable and ranges from 15% to 44% at 20 years.[7,8] In the era of medical therapy that includes biologic agents, the overall frequency of surgical intervention has declined.[9]

Crohn Disease

Crohn disease is characterized by transmural, patchy inflammation that can involve the entire gastrointestinal tract from the mouth to the anus. Typically, however, Crohn disease will involve the terminal ileum and right colon with variable involvement of other areas of the colon and small intestine. Endoscopically, the lesions have often been described as "skip lesions," because areas of inflammation are interspersed between normal mucosa. If deeper inflammation is present, "cobblestoning" can occur, which refers to a pattern of inflammation marked by linear or serpiginous ulcers separated by more elevated areas of normal or inflamed mucosa. Histologically, Crohn disease has been characterized by noncaseating granulomas, which can be found in approximately 25% of patients.[10] Fistulization and stricturing are also hallmarks that are rarely seen in ulcerative colitis.

Because of potential involvement throughout the entire gastrointestinal tract, the clinical presentation of Crohn disease can be varied. With small bowel involvement, patients can present with diarrhea, malabsorption, small bowel bacterial overgrowth, and protein-losing enteropathy. An important complication that can be seen is kidney stones, which occur because of malabsorption of fatty acids and bile salts, leading to increased oxalate absorption. With ileocecal involvement, patients can develop a palpable mass in the right lower quadrant caused by inflammation in and around the small bowel in this region. With perianal involvement patients can present with fistulas, fissures, or abscesses.[11]

Unlike ulcerative colitis, patients with Crohn disease often present with abdominal pain and weight loss resulting from malabsorption. Furthermore, because of the propensity for fistulization and strictures, the clinician should remain vigilant for possible obstructive symptoms. Fistulization can present as perianal disease (anorectal fistula), feculent skin discharge (enterocutaneous fistula), pneumaturia (enterovesical fistula), feculent vaginal discharge (enterovaginal fistula), and passage of undigested food or unexplained weight loss (enteroenteral fistula). Because of the transmural nature of the inflammation, abscesses can also occur in Crohn disease.

Approximately two-thirds of patients with Crohn disease will ultimately require surgical intervention during the course of their disease.[12,13] Similar to ulcerative colitis, the incidence of surgery in Crohn disease is likely changing with the use of biologic agents.[14]

Extraintestinal Manifestations

Both ulcerative colitis and Crohn disease are systemic diseases that can lead to extraintestinal manifestations in up to 25% of patients.[15] The most common organ systems involved are musculoskeletal, ocular, dermatologic, and hepatobiliary. Extraintestinal manifestations can occur before, during, or completely separate from IBD flares. Type 1 peripheral arthritis, episcleritis, erythema nodosum, and oral aphthous ulcers have been observed to occur during disease exacerbations. Type 2 peripheral arthritis, uveitis, pyoderma gangrenosum, and primary sclerosing cholangitis (PSC) seem to occur separately from IBD flares. Several extraintestinal manifestations have been associated with specific human leukocyte antigen alleles.[16]

The most common musculoskeletal manifestations of IBD include osteoporosis, sacroiliitis, ankylosing spondylitis, and peripheral arthritides. The arthritis associated with IBD is of particular interest and can be categorized into 2 types. Type 1 peripheral arthritis is pauciarticular and usually parallels the activity of the IBD; it typically involves less than 5 weight-bearing joints. Type 2 peripheral arthritis is polyarticular and affects the small joints; it typically manifests independent of IBD activity.[16]

The most common ocular manifestations of IBD include episcleritis, scleritis, and uveitis. Episcleritis presents with redness of one or both eyes and often parallels the activity of IBD. Uveitis is less common but more serious. It may occur independent of IBD flares and present with eye pain, redness, photophobia, and blurred vision. Ocular manifestations of IBD require prompt recognition and referral of the patient for an ophthalmologic evaluation.[16]

The most common cutaneous manifestations of IBD are erythema nodosum and pyoderma gangrenosum. Erythema nodosum is clinically evident as tender, red, or violet raised nodules, often along the anterior tibial region. The appearance of erythema nodosum typically parallels intestinal disease activity. Pyoderma gangrenosum (**Fig. 1**), on the other hand, is less common, more serious, and not always linked to intestinal disease activity. It appears as a single or multiple erythematous papules that progress to deep ulcerations with undermined, violaceous edges. Pyoderma gangrenosum is most commonly located on the legs but can occur anywhere on the body, including on the abdominal wall adjacent to a surgical stoma.

One of the more common hepatobiliary complications of IBD is PSC, a condition that leads to inflammation and scarring of the bile ducts, cholestasis, and sometimes further complications such as acute cholangitis or cholangiocarcinoma. Of patients who have PSC, up to 90% will have a diagnosis of IBD, most typically ulcerative colitis. Patients who have IBD and PSC are at increased risk for colonic dysplasia and cancer. Thus, annual surveillance colonoscopy is advised. Besides PSC, other hepatobiliary diseases that are associated with IBD include cholelithiasis, autoimmune hepatitis, and drug-induced liver injury. To detect hepatobiliary complications, patients who have IBD should undergo periodic monitoring of liver enzymes.

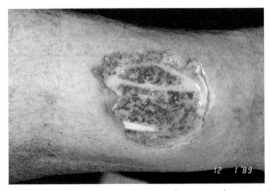

Fig. 1. Example of pyoderma gangrenosum. (*From* Callen JP, Jackson JM. Pyoderma gangrenosum: an update. Rheum Dis Clin North Am 2007;33(4):798, vi; with permission.)

In addition to the extraintestinal manifestations described here, it must be noted that patients with IBD have an increased risk of venous thromboembolism, particularly when hospitalized for an IBD flare.[17] There are also several less frequent extraintestinal manifestations, including pulmonary disease, digital clubbing, vasculitis, and pancreatitis, among others. The extraintestinal manifestations underscore the systemic nature of IBD. Patients may not associate these distant manifestations with their IBD; hence, the primary care physician may be the first to receive these complaints. Prompt recognition and appropriate management of extraintestinal manifestations is of key importance in preventing significant morbidity (**Table 1**).[16]

Table 1 Common extraintestinal manifestations in inflammatory bowel disease	
Cutaneous	Erythema nodosum Pyoderma gangrenosum
Hematologic	Venous thromboembolism
Hepatobiliary	Primary sclerosing cholangitis
Ocular	Episcleritis Scleritis Uveitis
Musculoskeletal	Sacroiliitis Ankylosing spondylitis Type 1 peripheral arthritis (pauciarticular) Type 2 peripheral arthritis (polyarticular) Osteoporosis

Data from Refs.[15–17]

DIFFERENTIAL DIAGNOSIS AND EVALUATION OF A PATIENT WITH A SUSPECTED FLARE OR COMPLICATION OF INFLAMMATORY BOWEL DISEASE

The diagnosis of a suspected flare or complication of ulcerative colitis or Crohn disease requires a comprehensive approach, including a thorough history and physical examination in addition to selected laboratory studies. Imaging and endoscopic evaluation may also be indicated. Initial diagnostic evaluation of suspected IBD flare or complications is outlined in **Table 2**. In addition, patients with IBD have a unique differential when presenting with abdominal pain or diarrhea, as outlined in **Boxes 1** and **2**.

It is important to exclude an infectious process such as *Clostridium difficile* infection, an intra-abdominal abscess complicating Crohn disease, or an infectious complication related to immunosuppressing therapy. *C difficile* has been increasing in frequency and severity in patients with IBD. Patients with ulcerative colitis or colonic Crohn disease are particularly vulnerable.[20] Clinically, *C difficile* infection may be difficult to distinguish from a flare of IBD. In addition, patients may not have the traditional risk criteria for *C difficile* infection such as antibiotic use or hospitalization.

When patients with Crohn disease present with symptoms suggestive of a disease flare, the differential diagnosis should also include bile salt diarrhea, bacterial overgrowth, fistulizing disease, symptomatic gallstones and renal stones, and other disease-related complications.[12,21]

Table 2
Initial diagnostic evaluation of suspected flare or complication of inflammatory bowel disease

Clinical Evaluation	
History	Fever, abdominal pain, diarrhea, number of stools per 24 h, nocturnal stools, bloody stool, tenesmus, fecal urgency, or obstructive symptoms
	Extraintestinal manifestations including eye, skin, or joint symptoms
	Precipitating factors, such as antibiotic exposure or travel
	Perianal complaints in Crohn patients
Vital Signs	Fever, tachycardia, or hypotension
Physical examination	Dehydration, malnutrition, or pallor
	Abdominal tenderness, rebound, signs of obstruction, or a palpable right lower quadrant mass
	Extraintestinal manifestations of eye, joint, or skin
	Perianal abscesses or fistulas in Crohn patients
Laboratory Evaluation	
Blood studies	Complete blood count, ferritin, iron, total iron-binding capacity
	Chemistry panel
	Acute phase reactants including ferritin, erythrocyte sedimentation rate (ESR), and C-reactive protein
	Liver function tests
	Albumin and prealbumin
	Cytomegalovirus (CMV) quantitative polymerase chain reaction
Stool studies	*Clostridium difficile* testing, parasite screening, stool cultures, Shiga toxin evaluation, *Escherichia coli* O157:H7 assays
	Fecal calprotectin and lactoferrin
Imaging Evaluation	
In ulcerative colitis	Consider plain film of abdomen (evaluate for toxic megacolon)
In Crohn disease	Consider plain film of abdomen, computed tomography (CT) of abdomen/pelvis, CT or MRI enterography (evaluate for obstruction, strictures, fistulas, abscesses)
Endoscopy Evaluation	
In ulcerative colitis	Consider colonoscopy or flexible sigmoidoscopy (evaluate for mucosal inflammation and rule out CMV colitis)
In Crohn disease	Consider colonoscopy (evaluate location and severity of mucosal inflammation in colon, terminal ileum)

Data from Refs.[4,11,12,18]

Box 1
Differential diagnosis of abdominal pain in patients with inflammatory bowel disease

- Abscess (Crohn disease)
- Cholangitis
- Cholelithiasis
- Inflammatory bowel disease flare
- Intestinal obstruction (due to adhesions or strictures)
- Nephrolithiasis
- Pancreatitis

Data from Williams H, Walker D, Orchard TR. Extraintestinal manifestations of inflammatory bowel disease. Curr Gastroenterol Rep 2008;10(6):597–605.

Box 2
Differential diagnosis of diarrhea in patients with inflammatory bowel disease

- Bile acid diarrhea
- Fistula
- Food intolerance (including lactose intolerance)
- Inflammatory bowel disease flare
- Infection (including *Clostridium difficile* or cytomegalovirus)
- Irritable bowel syndrome
- Malabsorption (including diarrhea due to terminal ileum resection)
- Medications (including aminosalicylates)
- Small intestinal bacterial overgrowth

Data from Refs.[12,18,19]

MANAGEMENT

Assessing Severity of Disease

In both ulcerative colitis and Crohn disease, the severity of IBD guides the approach to therapy. Among the several different clinical severity indices published, a clinically useful guide to assessing severity in ulcerative colitis can be found in the American College of Gastroenterology (ACG) ulcerative colitis practice guideline, outlined in **Table 3**.[18]

Table 3
Assessing clinical severity of ulcerative colitis

Disease Severity	Mild	Moderate	Severe	Fulminant
No. of bowel movements (BMs) per day	<4 BMs, with or without hematochezia	>4 BMs	>6 BMs, bloody	>10 BMs with continuous bleeding
Additional clinical characteristics	No systemic toxicity, normal ESR	Minimal evidence of systemic toxicity	Evidence of systemic toxicity including fever, tachycardia, anemia, or elevated ESR	Evidence of systemic toxicity, abdominal tenderness, abdominal distention, colonic dilatation on imaging, need for blood transfusions

Data from Kornbluth A, Sachar DB, The Practice Parameters Committee of the American College of Gastroenterology. Ulcerative colitis practice guidelines in adults: American College of Gastroenterology, Practice Parameters Committee. Am J Gastroenterol 2010;105(3):501–23; [quiz: 524].

Similar to ulcerative colitis, the clinical severity indices used for Crohn disease have primarily been used for research studies, and scoring systems are difficult to apply clinically. The most commonly used severity indices have been the Crohn Disease Activity Index[22] and the Harvey-Bradshaw Index.[23,24] A more clinically oriented severity index has been described in the 2009 ACG Crohn disease practice guideline, summarized in **Table 4**.[12]

Table 4
Assessing clinical severity of Crohn disease

	Mild to Moderate	Moderate to Severe	Severe to Fulminant
Crohn disease activity index (CDAI) correlation	CDAI 150–220	CDAI 220–450	CDAI >450
Clinical characteristics	Ambulatory, tolerating an oral diet, without significant morbidities	Failed therapy for mild-moderate disease; systemic toxicity including fever, weight loss, abdominal pain or tenderness, nausea or vomiting (without obstruction), or significant anemia	Persistent symptoms even with outpatient corticosteroid or biologic agent use; cachexia; severe systemic toxicity including high fevers; persistent vomiting; intestinal obstruction; peritoneal signs including guarding, rebound tenderness; evidence of abscess

Data from Lichtenstein GR, Hanauer SB, Sandborn WJ, et al. Management of Crohn's disease in adults. Am J Gastroenterol 2009;104(2):465–83; [quiz: 464, 484].

Medical Therapeutics

With the advent of advanced immunologic and biologic therapy, the current approach toward management of IBD has been one of either accelerated step-up approaches whereby advanced therapies are introduced rapidly, or aggressive top-down treatment approaches whereby advanced therapies are initiated and then tapered.[25] The goal of management is to first induce remission and then maintain remission.

The current medical therapies can be loosely divided into the following categories:

- Corticosteroids, including systemic (eg, methylprednisolone and prednisone), enteric (ie, budesonide), and topical (eg, hydrocortisone enemas) steroids
- 5-Aminosalicylates including mesalamine (oral, enemas, suppositories), sulfasalazine (which is a mesalamine prodrug), olsalazine, and balsalazide
- Immunomodulators, including thiopurines (6-mercaptopurine, azathioprine) and methotrexate
- Antibiotics, including ciprofloxacin and metronidazole
- Biologics, including the anti–tumor necrosis factor (TNF) agents infliximab, adalimumab, and certolizumab pegol

In both ulcerative colitis and Crohn disease, chronic steroids such as prednisone should not be used as maintenance therapy. 5-Aminosalicylate agents are generally less effective in Crohn disease than in ulcerative colitis. Surgery should also be considered for appropriate clinical cases before emergent situations arise.[25–27]

Although specific therapy guidelines are beyond the scope of this article, **Table 5** summarizes medications commonly used to treat IBD.[12,18,28]

Table 5
Review of medical therapies in inflammatory bowel disease

Medication	Adverse Effects	Monitoring Recommendations
Corticosteroids		
Systemic Corticosteroids		
Prednisone, hydrocortisone, methylprednisolone	Iatrogenic Cushing syndrome (moon facies, fat redistribution, etc), opportunistic infections, adrenal suppression, diabetes, weight gain, striae, impaired wound healing, osteopenia, osteoporosis, avascular necrosis, glaucoma, cataracts	Blood pressure Blood glucose Electrolytes Dual-energy x-ray absorptiometry if patients have indications as detailed in Routine Health Maintenance Annual ophthalmologic examination
Enteric Corticosteroids		
Budesonide	Although budesonide is less systemically available, it has a similar adverse effect profile if used for a prolonged period of time	See above
5-Aminosalicylates (5-ASA)		
5-ASA in its original form is highly absorbed in the small bowel. Several formulations have been developed to deliver 5-ASA to more distal areas of the gastrointestinal tract		
Azo compounds: sulfasalazine, balsalazide, olsalazine Mesalamine: Pentasa, Asacol, Apriso, Lialda, Rowasa enema, Canasa suppository	5-ASA agents are generally well tolerated but can rarely lead to nephrotoxicity, pancreatitis, hypersensitivity reactions. Sulfasalazine can cause gastrointestinal upset, folate deficiency, abnormal sperm counts	Complete blood count with differential periodically Chemistry panel, specifically renal function, periodically Liver function tests periodically Urinalysis periodically
Antimetabolites		
Thiopurines		
Azathioprine, 6-mercaptopurine	Opportunistic infections, gastrointestinal intolerance, macrocytic anemia, hepatic toxicity, bone marrow suppression with leukopenia, anemia, thrombocytopenia. Hypersensitivity reactions can cause fever, rash, pancreatitis. Increased risk of lymphoma, including non-Hodgkin lymphoma and hepatosplenic T-cell lymphoma	Thiopurine methyltransferase (TPMT) level before initiation of therapy. Absent TPMT contraindicates thiopurine use Complete blood count with differential, weekly on initiation and then regular monitoring Chemistry panel, including renal function, periodically Liver function tests periodically Monitor for signs of infection or malignancy

(continued on next page)

Table 5 (continued)		
Medication	**Adverse Effects**	**Monitoring Recommendations**
Folate Antagonists		
Methotrexate	Bone marrow suppression (including leukopenia), nausea, opportunistic infections, hepatic toxicity, hypersensitivity pneumonitis	Pregnancy category X medication. Contraception required Complete blood count with differential periodically Liver function tests periodically Chest radiograph at baseline
Anti–Tumor Necrosis Factor (TNF) Therapy		
Infliximab, adalimumab, certolizumab pegol	Opportunistic infections including tuberculosis, hepatitis B reactivation, others. Hepatotoxicity, demyelinating disorders, hematologic reactions, worsening congestive heart failure in patients with preexisting heart disease, development or exacerbation of multiple sclerosis. Development of antibodies to the antibody, serum sickness-like reaction, lupus-like syndrome, development of antinuclear antibodies, anti–double-stranded DNA. May increase risk of lymphoma. The combination of immunomodulators with anti-TNF monoclonal antibodies has been associated with hepatosplenic T-cell lymphomas in young males	Tuberculosis screening (tuberculin skin testing or interferon-γ release assay) before treatment and annually during treatment Complete blood counts with differential periodically Chemistry panel periodically Liver function tests Hepatitis B screening before treatment Chest radiograph before treatment Monitor for symptoms of infection, heart failure, lupus-like syndromes, and malignancy

Data from Refs.[12,18,28]

ROUTINE HEALTH MAINTENANCE

Preventive health maintenance is essential to the optimum care of patients with IBD. Patients with chronic illnesses, including IBD, are at higher risk of not obtaining health maintenance care and screening. As such, both the primary care physician and gastroenterologist should remain vigilant in preventive health service counseling.[29,30] This section reviews the specific screening and health maintenance caveats associated with IBD.

Vaccinations

In recent years, our approach to the treatment of IBD has changed with increasing and earlier use of immunosuppressing medications, particularly biologic agents. IBD patients who are treated with immunosuppressing medications are at increased risk for infectious complications, some of which are vaccine preventable. Nevertheless, IBD patients may be inadequately vaccinated for a variety of reasons, which may be related to fewer primary care visits or hesitance by either gastroenterologists or primary care physicians to take ownership of vaccinating these patients. Moreover, immunosuppressed patients, especially those on combination immunosuppression, may have a diminished response to vaccination or may be anergic.[31] Thus, it is opportune to vaccinate patients before initiating immunosuppressive therapy.

Adult patients with IBD should follow the vaccination schedules as recommended by the Centers for Disease Control and Prevention Advisory Committee on Immunization Practices (ACIP), with the important caveat that live vaccines should not be administered to an immunosuppressed patient.[32,33] Immunosuppressed patients include those who are on corticosteroids, immunomodulators, or biologic agents, and patients who have received such therapies in the last 3 months. Patients with significant protein-calorie malnutrition are also considered immunosuppressed.[34]

As per the ACIP 2011 general vaccination recommendation guidelines, live vaccines should not be administered for 3 months after immunosuppressive therapy has been stopped.[33] The administration of live vaccines presents a unique concern when a patient is expected to be immunosuppressed in the future. Although data are lacking, waiting at least 12 to 24 weeks after administering a live vaccine before beginning immunosuppressive therapy has been suggested **(Table 6)**.[31,35]

Table 6 Live vaccines	
Live bacterial vaccines	BCG (bacillus Calmette-Guérin) and oral Ty21a *Salmonella Typhi* vaccine
Live viral vaccines	MMR (measles, mumps, and rubella), MMRV (measles, mumps, rubella, and varicella), OPV (oral polio vaccine), LAIV (live, attenuated influenza vaccine), yellow fever, zoster, rotavirus, varicella, and vaccinia (smallpox)

Do not administer live vaccines to immunosuppressed patients.
Data from National Center for Immunization and Respiratory Diseases. Respiratory. General recommendations on immunization—recommendations of the Advisory Committee on Immunization Practices (ACIP). MMWR Recomm Rep 2011;60(2):1–64.

In general, patients with IBD should receive the influenza vaccine annually, the pneumococcal vaccine if chronically immunosuppressed, and the tetanus and diphtheria vaccine every 10 years (with tetanus, diphtheria, and acellular pertussis given once). As per ACIP guidelines, substantial steroid immunosuppression is defined as taking 20 mg of prednisone or more daily for ≥ 2 weeks. When age-appropriate, the human papillomavirus (HPV) vaccine should be administered. Furthermore, patients must be screened for hepatitis B before starting biologic therapy. If patients are not immune, they should receive the hepatitis B vaccine (3 doses) with postvaccine titers checked to assure adequate response. Other vaccinations may be appropriate based on special circumstances, such as the meningococcal vaccine for first-year college students.[31–33,36]

When patients are diagnosed with IBD, it is important to check and update their vaccination histories. Though not always feasible, the most opportune time to vaccinate patients is before any form of immunosuppression. When caring for a patient who has IBD, the primary care physician can play a crucial role in assuring that the patient receives appropriate vaccines.

Mycobacterium tuberculosis Screening

Patients with IBD in whom the use of TNF-α inhibitors is being considered require testing for latent tuberculosis (TB) before the initiation of therapy. The TNF-α inhibitors increase the risk of reactivation of latent TB, which may result in serious and disseminated infection.[37] Appropriate screening includes a tuberculin skin test or interferon-γ release assay (IGRA), and a chest radiograph in patients who have a history suggestive of tuberculosis, positive skin test, or positive IGRA.[36]

Osteoporosis

Patients with IBD are at increased risk for osteopenia and osteoporosis. The reported rates of osteoporosis in IBD patients vary but may be in the range of 15%.[38] Low bone density may occur in both ulcerative colitis and Crohn disease. The etiology seems to be multifactorial, including the effect of inflammation on bone, corticosteroid use, calcium and vitamin D malabsorption, and other factors such as low body mass index.[31] Because corticosteroids are the strongest risk factor for decreased bone density, every effort should be made to limit exposure to corticosteroids.

The American Gastroenterological Association (AGA) published a medical position statement on osteoporosis in 2003.[39,40] The guideline recommends bone mineral density screening with dual-energy x-ray absorptiometry (DXA) scanning in postmenopausal women or men older than 50 years, in patients with prolonged corticosteroid use (>3 consecutive months or recurrent courses), patients with a history of a low-trauma fracture, or patients with hypogonadism.[40] When a patient has osteoporosis or sustains a low-trauma fracture, screening for secondary causes of low bone density should also be performed.[40] According to the ACG practice guidelines on ulcerative colitis published in 2010, smoking, low body mass index, sedentary lifestyle, nutritional deficiencies, or family history of bone density abnormalities should also prompt consideration for DXA scanning.[18]

Although specific treatment of osteoporosis is beyond the scope of this review, some general preventive measures include lifestyle modifications such as smoking cessation, regular weight-bearing exercise, and minimizing alcohol use. Adequate calcium intake and vitamin D intake should be ensured.[36] Patients with IBD may avoid dairy products or have malabsorption. Measuring a 25-hydroxyvitamin D level may identify patients in whom vitamin D supplementation would be beneficial. Again, as corticosteroid use is the most common variable associated with decreased bone density in IBD patients, minimizing corticosteroid use can be one of the most effective interventions.

By recognizing risk factors and implementing screening and preventive measures, the primary care physician can play an important role in maintaining the bone health of IBD patients.

Cervical Cancer and Dysplasia Screening

There is an increased prevalence of abnormal Papanicolaou smears in women with IBD, particularly those on immunomodulators.[31,36] Rungoe and colleagues[41] compared a Danish cohort of 27,408 patients with IBD with controls, and found an increased risk of cervical dysplasia in both Crohn disease and ulcerative colitis patients. An increased risk of cervical cancer in patients with Crohn disease was also observed. Accordingly, women with IBD who are immunocompromised should undergo annual gynecologic examinations, annual cervical cancer screening,[42] and receive HPV vaccination when appropriate.

Skin Cancer Screening

Nonmelanoma skin cancers (NMSC), which include squamous cell and basal cell carcinoma, are one of the most common malignancies in the United States. Among IBD patients there is an increased risk of nonmelanoma skin cancer, particularly in those who have been treated with thiopurines.[43] In a large study, Long and colleagues[44] found an increased risk of both NMSC and melanoma in patients with IBD. The risk of melanoma was increased by the use of biologics, and the risk of NMSC was increased by the use of thiopurines. Because of this increased risk, patients with IBD, particularly those who are immunosuppressed, should be counseled and monitored for skin cancer. Patients should be advised to use broad-spectrum sun protection. Although to date there are no clear guidelines on skin cancer screening for IBD patients, some practitioners suggest that annual skin examinations may be warranted in patients who are taking immunomodulators or biologics. The primary care physician can play an important role in educating patients about the risk for skin cancer and counseling them on sun protection.

Colon Cancer Screening

With regard to colon cancer screening, patients with ulcerative colitis and Crohn disease of the colon have an increased risk of developing colorectal cancer. According to the AGA 2010 guideline, IBD patients should undergo a screening colonoscopy at a maximum of 8 years after onset of symptoms to obtain biopsies throughout the colon, to assess the microscopic extent of inflammation.[45,46] Patients who have ulcerative proctitis are not considered at increased risk for IBD-related colorectal cancer. Patients with extensive or left-sided colitis should begin surveillance within 1 to 2 years after initial screening colonoscopy. These same recommendations also apply to patients with Crohn colitis who have disease involving at least one-third of the colon.

The optimal surveillance interval has not been clearly defined, but after 2 negative examinations with no dysplasia, further surveillance colonoscopy should be performed every 1 to 3 years. Surveillance colonoscopy ideally should be performed when the colonic disease is in remission. Several special conditions deserve mention. Patients who have IBD and PSC should begin surveillance colonoscopy at the time when PSC is diagnosed, and undergo yearly colonoscopy thereafter. Patients who have a history of colorectal cancer in first-degree relatives, ongoing active inflammation, or anatomic abnormalities such as a foreshortened colon, stricture, or pseudopolyps may benefit from more frequent surveillance. A recent consensus statement outlines important technical considerations for the endoscopist who performs surveillance colonoscopies.[18,45–47]

Although the frequency of colon cancer screening and surveillance in IBD patients are often managed by the gastroenterologist, the primary care physician should be aware of the increased risk of colorectal neoplasia in the IBD population and the relevant guidelines based on disease duration. Patients with long-standing IBD who have minimal symptoms may have little contact with the subspecialist; hence, an awareness of risk can assure that patients are referred back to the gastroenterologist for timely colonoscopy.

Ophthalmologic Screening

Annual ophthalmologic screening is advisable for IBD patients. Patients who receive corticosteroids may develop cataracts, glaucoma, or other adverse eye effects.[48]

Furthermore, patients with IBD may have overt or subclinical extraintestinal manifestations involving the eye. One study by Felekis and colleagues[49] found ophthalmologic manifestations in 26 of 60 IBD patients (43%). As a general rule, any patient with IBD who complains of eye pain or vision changes should be referred for ophthalmologic evaluation immediately, as certain ophthalmologic complications can lead to permanent vision loss.

Depression Screening

Because of increased rates of depression in patients with IBD,[50] aggressive screening and support for depression should be pursued. Psychosocial factors play an important role in IBD. Depression is a common problem that may affect up to 15% to 35% of IBD patients.[51,52] Factors that may contribute to depression and psychological distress include the chronic and relapsing nature of IBD, the social ramifications of unpredictable bowel patterns, and the burden of medication and medical care. Steroid therapy is also associated with mood disorders.[53] One study reported that the lifetime risk for major depressive disorder was more than twice as high in IBD patients than in the general population.[50] Not only does depression adversely affect quality of life, it may also affect the patient's adherence to medication and other treatment recommendations. The primary care physician can play an important role in screening for and recognizing depression in IBD patients, and in initiating treatment or mental health referral as indicated.

Smoking Cessation

Smoking has a significant impact on IBD. Besides the known cardiopulmonary and cancer risks, smoking has a deleterious effect on the course of Crohn disease. The effects of smoking in ulcerative colitis and Crohn disease are divergent. Several studies have demonstrated that active smoking leads to a protective effect against ulcerative colitis. The exact mechanism behind smoking's protective effect remains unknown. Conversely, however, former smokers have a 70% increased risk of developing ulcerative colitis. Furthermore, studies have noted that active smokers have better controlled ulcerative colitis in comparison with former smokers and nonsmokers. Logically, nicotine replacement therapy trials have been completed but have not shown a benefit over conventional medical therapy.[54]

On the other hand, active and former smoking has clearly been demonstrated as a risk factor for developing Crohn disease. Smoking has also been linked to ileal involvement and complications in Crohn disease. Complications observed have included fistulizing or stenosing disease, recurrent disease, and repeated surgeries.[2] For the primary care physician, smoking cessation is one of the most clinically important and cost-effective methods of improving a patient's clinical course in Crohn disease.

Diet and Nutrition

Patients with IBD are at risk for malnutrition and specific micronutrient deficiencies.[55] Patients with Crohn disease, especially those who have fistulas, strictures, or prior small bowel resections, are more susceptible to micronutrient deficiencies that include vitamins, minerals, and trace elements. The mechanisms of nutritional deficiency vary and include decreased food intake, increased intestinal loss, malabsorption, and medication interference.

Several specific micronutrient deficiencies deserve mention. Iron deficiency is common in the IBD population.[55] Oral iron supplementation may be poorly tolerated because of gastrointestinal symptoms, thereby necessitating intravenous iron administration in a subset of patients. Folate deficiency may be less common given widespread supplementation in food products.[55] Vitamin B_{12} deficiency is an important consideration in Crohn disease because of its absorption in the terminal ileum. Patients who have had surgical resection of the terminal ileum are particularly at risk for the development of B_{12} deficiency. Other potential micronutrient deficiencies of particular note include calcium, vitamin D, magnesium, and zinc.

Traveling

When addressing travel with the IBD patient, there remains a dearth of studies and resources. The following information is derived from the second European evidence-based consensus on the prevention, diagnosis, and management of opportunistic infections in IBD.[35]

IBD patients should undergo recommended vaccinations for their destinations with special consideration given to avoidance of live vaccines if they are on immunosuppressants (this aspect is detailed further in the Vaccinations section). Serologic proof of successful seroconversion may be required in such cases as the hepatitis A vaccine. Patients should ensure their travel or health insurance also addresses emergent health concerns that include evacuation by air.

Regarding TB, if traveling for more than a month to a moderately or highly endemic area, IBD patients should be screened for latent TB before travel if the last screening was more than 1 year previously. IBD patients should have repeat latent TB screening tests completed 8 to 10 weeks after returning from their travels. IBD patients on immunomodulators require testing for latent TB regardless of duration of travel. If the tuberculin skin test is pursued, IBD patients on immunomodulators should complete a 2-step tuberculin skin test. Immunocompromised IBD patients should also take extra precautions in avoiding insect bites that could transmit infectious diseases, with regards to prevention of traveler's diarrhea, patients should avoid contaminated food and water sources. Bottled water with the seal intact is the safest form of hydration.

IBD patients require pretravel consultations with their primary care physician, gastroenterologist, and travel clinic before any excursions abroad. Patients can also refer to the Crohn and Colitis Foundation of America Web site for further information on travel (**Table 7**).

Table 7	
Suggested travel instructions for patients with inflammatory bowel disease	
Before travel	Explore potential medical providers at travel destinations
	Avoid live vaccines if immunosuppressed
	Ensure travel or health insurance provides for emergency health concerns including evacuation by air
During travel	Carry health history and home medical providers' information in carry-on baggage
	Carry prescription medications and copies of scripts in carry-on baggage
	Brush teeth with and only drink sterilized water (ideally bottled water with the seal intact)
	Avoid insect bites
After travel	Screen for latent tuberculosis if indicated

Data from Rahier JF, Magro F, Abreu C, et al. Second European evidence-based consensus on the prevention, diagnosis and management of opportunistic infections in inflammatory bowel disease. J Crohns Colitis 2014;8(6):443–68; and Crohn's & Colitis Foundation of America. Traveling with IBD. Available at: http://www.ccfa.org/resources/traveling-with-ibd.html. Accessed May 12, 2015.

SUMMARY

Treating IBD requires a comprehensive care team including the patient, primary care provider, and gastroenterologist. Patients often initially present to their primary providers with symptoms or complications of IBD. As such, this article reviews the clinical presentation, pathology, management, treatment-associated complications, and routine health maintenance of IBD. Primary care providers are instrumental in providing not only acute care but also individualized preventive care for the IBD patient.

REFERENCES

1. Abraham C, Cho JH. Inflammatory bowel disease. N Engl J Med 2009;361(21): 2066–78.
2. Loftus EV Jr. Clinical epidemiology of inflammatory bowel disease: incidence, prevalence, and environmental influences. Gastroenterology 2004;126(6): 1504–17.
3. Kappelman MD, Rifas-Shiman SL, Kleinman K, et al. The prevalence and geographic distribution of Crohn's disease and ulcerative colitis in the United States. Clin Gastroenterol Hepatol 2007;5(12):1424–9.
4. Shanahan F. Ulcerative colitis. In: Hawkey J, Richter JE, Garcia-Tsao G, et al, editors. Clinical gastroenterology and hepatology. Chichester (WS): Blackwell Publishing Ltd; 2012. p. 355–71.
5. Orholm M, Binder V, Sørensen TI, et al. Concordance of inflammatory bowel disease among Danish twins. Results of a nationwide study. Scand J Gastroenterol 2000;35(10):1075–81.
6. Orholm M, Munkholm P, Langholz E, et al. Familial occurrence of inflammatory bowel disease. N Engl J Med 1991;324(2):84–8.
7. Samuel S, Ingle SB, Dhillon S, et al. Cumulative incidence and risk factors for hospitalization and surgery in a population-based cohort of ulcerative colitis. Inflamm Bowel Dis 2013;19(9):1858–66.
8. Bernstein CN, Ng SC, Lakatos PL, et al. A review of mortality and surgery in ulcerative colitis: milestones of the seriousness of the disease. Inflamm Bowel Dis 2013;19(9):2001–10.
9. Reich KM, Chang HJ, Rezaie A, et al. The incidence rate of colectomy for medically refractory ulcerative colitis has declined in parallel with increasing anti-TNF use: a time-trend study. Aliment Pharmacol Ther 2014;40(6):629–38.
10. Freeman HJ. Granuloma-positive Crohn's disease. Can J Gastroenterol 2007; 21(9):583–7.
11. Vermeire SV, Gert Van Assche G, Rutgeers P. Crohn's disease. In: Hawkey J, Richter JE, Garcia-Tsao G, et al, editors. Clinical gastroenterology and hepatology. Chichester (WS): Blackwell Publishing Ltd; 2012. p. 372–93.
12. Lichtenstein GR, Hanauer SB, Sandborn WJ, et al. Management of Crohn's disease in adults. Am J Gastroenterol 2009;104(2):465–83 [quiz: 464, 484].
13. Munkholm P, Langholz E, Davidsen M, et al. Intestinal cancer risk and mortality in patients with Crohn's disease. Gastroenterology 1993;105(6):1716–23.
14. Sorrentino D, Fogel S, Van den Bogaerde J. Surgery for Crohn's disease and anti-TNF agents: the changing scenario. Expert Rev Gastroenterol Hepatol 2013;7(8): 689–700.
15. Monsen U, Sorstad J, Hellers G, et al. Extracolonic diagnoses in ulcerative colitis: an epidemiological study. Am J Gastroenterol 1990;85(6):711–6.
16. Williams H, Walker D, Orchard TR. Extraintestinal manifestations of inflammatory bowel disease. Curr Gastroenterol Rep 2008;10(6):597–605.

17. Grainge MJ, West J, Card TR. Venous thromboembolism during active disease and remission in inflammatory bowel disease: a cohort study. Lancet 2010; 375(9715):657–63.

18. Kornbluth A, Sachar DB, Practice Parameters Committee of the American College of Gastroenterology. Ulcerative colitis practice guidelines in adults: American College Of Gastroenterology, Practice Parameters Committee. Am J Gastroenterol 2010;105(3):501–23 [quiz: 524].

19. Wenzl HH. Diarrhea in chronic inflammatory bowel diseases. Gastroenterol Clin North Am 2012;41(3):651–75.

20. Berg AM, Kelly CP, Farraye FA. *Clostridium difficile* infection in the inflammatory bowel disease patient. Inflamm Bowel Dis 2013;19(1):194–204.

21. Dignass A, Van Assche G, Lindsay JO, et al. The second European evidence-based consensus on the diagnosis and management of Crohn's disease: current management. J Crohns Colitis 2010;4(1):28–62.

22. Best WR, Becktel JM, Singleton JW, et al. Development of a Crohn's disease activity index. National Cooperative Crohn's Disease Study. Gastroenterology 1976; 70(3):439–44.

23. Harvey RF, Bradshaw JM. A simple index of Crohn's-disease activity. Lancet 1980;1(8167):514.

24. Best WR. Predicting the Crohn's disease activity index from the Harvey-Bradshaw Index. Inflamm Bowel Dis 2006;12(4):304–10.

25. Burger D, Travis S. Conventional medical management of inflammatory bowel disease. Gastroenterology 2011;140(6):1827–37.e2.

26. D'Haens G, Baert F, van Assche G, et al. Early combined immunosuppression or conventional management in patients with newly diagnosed Crohn's disease: an open randomised trial. Lancet 2008;371(9613):660–7.

27. Lemann M, Mary JY, Duclos B, et al. Infliximab plus azathioprine for steroid-dependent Crohn's disease patients: a randomized placebo-controlled trial. Gastroenterology 2006;130(4):1054–61.

28. Lexicomp. 2014, Lexicomp. Available at: http://online.lexi.com. Accessed 14 June, 2015.

29. Selby L, Kane S, Wilson J, et al. Receipt of preventive health services by IBD patients is significantly lower than by primary care patients. Inflamm Bowel Dis 2008;14(2):253–8.

30. Selby L, Hoellein A, Wilson JF. Are primary care providers uncomfortable providing routine preventive care for inflammatory bowel disease patients? Dig Dis Sci 2011;56(3):819–24.

31. Sinclair JA, Wasan SK, Farraye FA. Health maintenance in the inflammatory bowel disease patient. Gastroenterol Clin North Am 2012;41(2):325–37.

32. Advisory Committee on Immunization Practices. Recommended adult immunization schedule, United States—2014. 2014; Available at: http://www.cdc.gov/vaccines/schedules/downloads/adult/adult-combined-schedule.pdf. Accessed 13 June, 2015.

33. National Center for Immunization and Respiratory Diseases. General recommendations on immunization—recommendations of the Advisory Committee on Immunization Practices (ACIP). MMWR Recomm Rep 2011;60(2):1–64.

34. Sands BE, Cuffari C, Katz J, et al. Guidelines for immunizations in patients with inflammatory bowel disease. Inflamm Bowel Dis 2004;10(5):677–92.

35. Rahier JF, Magro F, Abreu C, et al. Second European evidence-based consensus on the prevention, diagnosis and management of opportunistic infections in inflammatory bowel disease. J Crohns Colitis 2014;8(6):443–68.

36. Moscandrew M, Mahadevan U, Kane S. General health maintenance in IBD. Inflamm Bowel Dis 2009;15(9):1399–409.

37. Centers for Disease Control and Prevention. Tuberculosis associated with blocking agents against tumor necrosis factor-alpha—California, 2002-2003. MMWR Morb Mortal Wkly Rep 2004;53(30):683–6.

38. Bernstein CN. Osteoporosis in patients with inflammatory bowel disease. Clin Gastroenterol Hepatol 2006;4(2):152–6.

39. American Gastroenterological Association medical position statement: guidelines on osteoporosis in gastrointestinal diseases. Gastroenterology 2003;124(3):791–4.

40. Bernstein CN, Leslie WD, Leboff MS. AGA technical review on osteoporosis in gastrointestinal diseases. Gastroenterology 2003;124(3):795–841.

41. Rungoe C, Simonsen J, Riis L, et al. Inflammatory bowel disease and cervical neoplasia: a population-based nationwide cohort study. Clin Gastroenterol Hepatol 2015;13(4):693–700.e1.

42. Committee on Practice Bulletin-Gynecology. ACOG practice bulletin number 131: screening for cervical cancer. Obstet Gynecol 2012;120(5):1222–38.

43. Peyrin-Biroulet L, Khosrotehrani K, Carrat F, et al. Increased risk for nonmelanoma skin cancers in patients who receive thiopurines for inflammatory bowel disease. Gastroenterology 2011;141(5):1621–8.e1–5.

44. Long MD, Martin CF, Pipkin CA, et al. Risk of melanoma and nonmelanoma skin cancer among patients with inflammatory bowel disease. Gastroenterology 2012;143(2):390–9.e1.

45. Farraye FA, Odze RD, Eaden J, et al. AGA technical review on the diagnosis and management of colorectal neoplasia in inflammatory bowel disease. Gastroenterology 2010;138(2):746–74, 774.e1–4; [quiz e12–3].

46. Farraye FA, Odze RD, Eaden J, et al. AGA medical position statement on the diagnosis and management of colorectal neoplasia in inflammatory bowel disease. Gastroenterology 2010;138(2):738–45.

47. Laine L, Kaltenbach T, Barkun A, et al. SCENIC international consensus statement on surveillance and management of dysplasia in inflammatory bowel disease. Gastroenterology 2015;148(3):639–51.

48. Lichtenstein GR, Abreu MT, Cohen R, et al. American Gastroenterological Association Institute technical review on corticosteroids, immunomodulators, and infliximab in inflammatory bowel disease. Gastroenterology 2006;130(3):940–87.

49. Felekis T, Katsanos K, Kitsanou M, et al. Spectrum and frequency of ophthalmologic manifestations in patients with inflammatory bowel disease: a prospective single-center study. Inflamm Bowel Dis 2009;15(1):29–34.

50. Walker JR, Ediger JP, Graff LA, et al. The Manitoba IBD cohort study: a population-based study of the prevalence of lifetime and 12-month anxiety and mood disorders. Am J Gastroenterol 2008;103(8):1989–97.

51. Walker EA, Gelfand MD, Gelfand AN, et al. The relationship of current psychiatric disorder to functional disability and distress in patients with inflammatory bowel disease. Gen Hosp Psychiatry 1996;18(4):220–9.

52. Fuller-Thomson E, Sulman J. Depression and inflammatory bowel disease: findings from two nationally representative Canadian surveys. Inflamm Bowel Dis 2006;12(8):697–707.

53. Fardet L, Petersen I, Nazareth I. Suicidal behavior and severe neuropsychiatric disorders following glucocorticoid therapy in primary care. Am J Psychiatry 2012;169(5):491–7.

54. McGrath J, McDonald JW, Macdonald JK. Transdermal nicotine for induction of remission in ulcerative colitis. Cochrane Database Syst Rev 2004;(4): CD004722.
55. Hwang C, Ross V, Mahadevan U. Micronutrient deficiencies in inflammatory bowel disease: from A to zinc. Inflamm Bowel Dis 2012;18(10):1961–81.

Primary Care Management of Alcohol Misuse

Douglas Berger, MD, MLitt[a,b,]*, Katharine A. Bradley, MD, MPH[b,c,d,e]

KEYWORDS

- Alcohol misuse • Unhealthy alcohol use • Alcohol use disorder • Alcohol abuse
- Alcohol dependence • Alcohol screening • Brief intervention • Alcohol treatment

KEY POINTS

- More than 1 in 4 American adults consume alcohol above the recommended limits. One in 12 have an alcohol use disorder marked by harmful consequences.
- Both types of alcohol misuse contribute to acute injury and chronic disease, making alcohol the third largest cause of preventable death in the United States.
- Alcohol misuse alters the management of common conditions from insomnia to anemia.
- Primary care providers should be proactive, routinely screening adult patients with a tool validated to identify the full spectrum of alcohol misuse.
- A range of effective treatments are available for alcohol misuse, including brief counseling interventions, mutual-help groups, medications, and behavioral therapies.

INTRODUCTION

In the United States, alcohol is responsible for 3.5% of all deaths, the third largest preventable cause of death after tobacco use and being overweight.[1] Annual costs, including lost productivity, health care, legal, and other costs, are estimated at $223 billion per year or $746 per capita.[2] Despite this high prevalence and impact, alcohol-related care is inconsistent. Routine screening and behavioral intervention for alcohol misuse is recommended by the US Preventive Services Task Force (USPSTF)[3] and one of the most cost-effective clinical preventive services,[4,5] but only 16% of adults report ever discussing alcohol use with a health professional.[6] In a study assessing quality of care for 30 conditions across health systems, adherence

^a General Medicine Service, VA Puget Sound, Seattle, WA 98108, USA; ^b Department of Medicine, University of Washington, Seattle, WA 98101, USA; ^c Department of Health Services, University of Washington, Seattle, WA 98101, USA; ^d Group Health Research Institute, Seattle, WA, USA; ^e VA Health Services Research & Development (HSR&D) and Center of Excellence in Substance Abuse Treatment and Education (CESATE), Seattle, WA, USA
* Corresponding author. S-123 PCC, 1660 S. Columbian Way, Seattle WA 98108, USA.
E-mail address: douglas.berger@va.gov

Med Clin N Am 99 (2015) 989–1016
http://dx.doi.org/10.1016/j.mcna.2015.05.004
0025-7125/15/$ – see front matter Published by Elsevier Inc.

medical.theclinics.com

to quality indicators was worst for alcohol dependence.[7] Primary care providers have a critical role in improving identification and management of alcohol misuse.

DEFINITIONS, EPIDEMIOLOGY, AND CONSEQUENCES OF ALCOHOL MISUSE
Definitions

A host of terms are used to describe drinking (**Table 1**). Two concepts underlie the current nomenclature. First, although alcohol-related risks lie on a continuum and for some people any alcohol use poses significant risk (**Box 1**), it is useful to define a threshold below which alcohol use is generally of low risk. This threshold provides clear guidance to patients. Second, alcohol misuse encompasses a spectrum, from patients whose drinking puts them at risk for alcohol-related harm at one end to patients whose lives are overtaken by alcohol-related symptoms at the other. The 2 main types of alcohol misuse, risky drinking and alcohol use disorder (AUD), are defined by excessive consumption and impairment/consequences, respectively.

Alcohol misuse

In the United States, the threshold for risky drinking is defined by the National Institute of Alcoholism and Alcohol Abuse (NIAAA) and includes both daily and weekly limits (see **Table 1**).[8] Most patients who exceed weekly limits also exceed daily limits[8]; but there is heterogeneity, and chronic daily drinkers or binge drinkers may exceed one but not the other. Because of differences in body water/metabolism and clinical outcomes, limits are different for men and women.

Although the NIAAA limits were based primarily on the risk of having or developing an AUD,[8,9] Canadian, British, and Australian guidelines based on mortality and acute harms from alcohol misuse differ in only minor ways.[10–13] In discussing drinking limits with patients, it is critical to clarify the definition of a drink (**Fig. 1**). Whether poured at home or served in a bar, common portions include more, and sometimes much more, than a standard drink.[14,15] Definitions of a standard drink also vary internationally.

Alcohol use disorder

AUD is defined by the *Diagnostic and Statistical Manual of Mental Disorders* (*DSM*).[16] The most recent edition, *DSM-5*, replaced the diagnoses alcohol abuse and dependence with the single entity AUD graded mild, moderate, and severe. The revision emphasizes the continuity of use disorders while avoiding confusion around the term *dependence*, the unreliability of the abuse diagnosis, and "diagnostic orphans" meeting 2 dependence but no abuse criteria.[17] The new definition amalgamates criteria for abuse and dependence but replaces recurrent legal problems with the less context-dependent craving (**Table 2**). In the United States, rates of AUD as defined by the *DSM-IV* and *DSM-5* are similar, although there are slight differences in the populations included.[18]

Epidemiology

In US population surveys assessing past year drinking, 29% of adults meet the criteria for risky drinking,[19] of whom 8% to 11% meet the criteria for AUD and about 4% moderate to severe AUD (*DSM-IV* dependence).[18,20] Because of the vastly greater prevalence of risky drinking, most alcohol-related harms result from patients with more mild alcohol misuse, making it clinically important to address the full spectrum of misuse.[21–23]

Prevalence of alcohol misuse varies with age and sex (**Table 3**). Rates of AUD peak around 20 years of age.[20] Many people with AUD in adolescence or young adulthood go on to lives of low-risk use without any formal treatment, although their risk for AUD

Table 1
Alcohol terms

Key Terms	Definition	Synonyms
Low-risk drinking[a]	Drinking no more than Men: 4 drinks on any day AND 14 per week; Women: 3 drinks on any day AND 7 per week[b]	Lower risk use
Alcohol misuse	Drinking that risks or is accompanied by adverse consequences[c]	Unhealthy use
Risky drinking	Drinking quantities that exceed low risk daily OR weekly limits	Hazardous, at-risk use
Alcohol use disorder	Drinking that causes clinically significant impairment or distress meeting, in a 12-mo period, at least:	—
Mild	2 of 11 criteria	Abuse, harmful use
Moderate	4 of 11 criteria	Dependence, alcoholism
Severe	6 of 11 criteria	

Increasing consumption & consequences (↑) — *Decreasing prevalence* (↓)

Other Terms

- *Moderate drinking* is defined by US dietary guidelines as "up to 1 drink per day for women and up to 2 drinks per day for men," although it is sometimes used synonymously with low risk.[47]
- *Binge drinking* is a pattern of drinking that brings blood alcohol concentration levels to 0.08 g/dL. This pattern of drinking typically occurs after 4 drinks for women and 5 drinks for men, in about 2 h.

[a] For some patients, even quantities less than the National Institute on Alcohol Abuse and Alcoholism's limits pose significant risk (see **Box 1**).

[b] Many recommend[8,125] that patients older than 65 years drink no more than 3 drinks on any day and 7 per week, but this criterion has a less robust evidence base and is not included in all definitions or epidemiologic studies of risky drinking.

[c] Problem drinking, defined as drinking accompanied by adverse consequences not meeting the criteria for alcohol use disorder, is conceptually a part of alcohol misuse but is difficult to operationalize and, therefore, is less commonly used.

Data from Refs.[9,16,18,47,125,127]

Box 1
Patients for whom any alcohol use may be contraindicated

- Plan to drive, operate heavy machinery, or take part in other activities that require coordination and judgment
- Have a medical condition aggravated by drinking (eg, hepatitis C, pancreatitis, heart failure, atrial fibrillation)
- Take medications that interact with alcohol
- Are pregnant or trying to become pregnant
- Have a history of substance use disorder or strong family history of substance use disorder
- Are younger than legal drinking age

Data from Refs.[10,12,47,114,125]

---

later in life is elevated. Patients developing or still meeting the AUD criteria in middle age are more likely to have comorbidities and a chronic course, perhaps with periods of remission and relapse, with or without treatment.[21] Management of alcohol misuse in adolescents is reviewed elsewhere.[24]

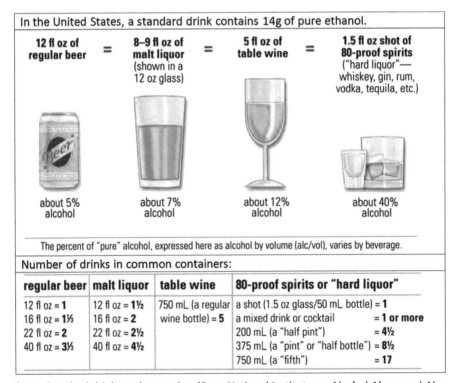

In the United States, a standard drink contains 14g of pure ethanol.

| 12 fl oz of regular beer | = | 8–9 fl oz of malt liquor (shown in a 12 oz glass) | = | 5 fl oz of table wine | = | 1.5 fl oz shot of 80-proof spirits ("hard liquor"— whiskey, gin, rum, vodka, tequila, etc.) |

| about 5% alcohol | about 7% alcohol | about 12% alcohol | about 40% alcohol |

The percent of "pure" alcohol, expressed here as alcohol by volume (alc/vol), varies by beverage.

Number of drinks in common containers:

regular beer	malt liquor	table wine	80-proof spirits or "hard liquor"
12 fl oz = 1	12 fl oz = 1½	750 mL (a regular wine bottle) = 5	a shot (1.5 oz glass/50 mL bottle) = 1
16 fl oz = 1⅓	16 fl oz = 2		a mixed drink or cocktail = 1 or more
22 fl oz = 2	22 fl oz = 2½		200 mL (a "half pint") = 4½
40 fl oz = 3⅓	40 fl oz = 4½		375 mL (a "pint" or "half bottle") = 8½
			750 mL (a "fifth") = 17

Fig. 1. Standard drinks and examples. (*From* National Institute on Alcohol Abuse and Alcoholism. Rethinking drinking alcohol and your health: research-based information from the National Institutes of Health. Bethesda (MD): US Department of Health and Human Services; 2010.)

Table 2
DSM-IV and DSM-5 criteria for AUD and suggestions for asking patients

Criterion	DSM-IV	DSM-5	How to Ask: In the Past Year Have You…
Hazardous situations	✓	✓	More than once gotten into situations while or after drinking that *increased your chances of getting hurt* (such as driving, swimming, using machinery, walking in a dangerous area, or having unsafe sex)?
Interpersonal problems	✓ (Abuse meets ≥1 criterion)	✓	Continued to drink even though it was causing *trouble* with your *family* or *friends*?
Role failure	✓	✓	Found that drinking, or being sick from drinking, often *interfered with taking care* of your *home* or *family* or caused *job* troubles or *school* problems?
Legal problems	✓	X	—
Withdrawal	✓	✓	Found that when the effects of alcohol were wearing off, you *had withdrawal symptoms,* such as trouble sleeping, shakiness, irritability, anxiety, depression, restlessness, nausea, or sweating or sensed things that were not there?
Tolerance	✓ (Dependence meets ≥3 criteria)	✓ (AUD meets ≥2 criteria)	Had to *drink much more* than you once did to *get the effect* you want or found that your *usual number* of drinks had *much less* effect than before?
Use more, longer	✓	✓	Had times when you ended up drinking *more or longer* than you intended?
Repeated attempts	✓	✓	More than once wanted to *cut down or stop drinking,* or tried to, but could not?
Time spent	✓	✓	Spent *a lot of time* drinking or being sick or getting over the aftereffects?
Health consequences	✓	✓	Continued to drink even though it was making you feel *depressed* or anxious or adding to *another health problem* or after having had a *memory blackout*?
Lost activities	✓	✓	*Given up or cut back on activities* that were important or interesting to you or gave you pleasure in order to drink?
Craving	X —	✓	Experienced *craving* (a strong need, or urge) to drink?

Note: For all diagnoses, symptoms must be present in a 12-month period and cause significant impairment or distress. In addition to the removal of legal problem and addition of craving, the *DSM-5* revision included minor phrasing changes in several criteria.
Data from Refs.[17,18,125]

Table 3
Past year prevalence of risky drinking and AUD

	Risky Drinking (%)	AUD (%)
Total	29	9
Sex		
Men	37	12
Women	23	5
Age (y)		
18–29	43	16
30–44	35	10
45–64	24	5
65+	10	2

Data from Dawson DA, Grant BF, Stinson FS, et al. Toward the attainment of low-risk drinking goals: a 10-year progress report. Alcohol Clin Exp Res 2004;28:1371–8; and Hasin DS, Stinson FS, Ogburn E, et al. Prevalence, correlates, disability, and comorbidity of DSM-IV alcohol abuse and dependence in the United States: results from the National Epidemiologic Survey on Alcohol and Related Conditions. Arch Gen Psychiatry 2007;64:830–42.

Family history is a powerful predictor of AUD, with 40% to 60% of risk thought to be genetic.[16] Heavy consumption is associated with having[25] and developing[26] AUD. Rates of risky drinking and AUD increase with income and education, but AUD-related treatment decreases.[19,20,27]

Harms of Alcohol Misuse

The harms of alcohol misuse include not only the effects of chronic alcohol consumption on individual drinkers but also acute harms that may affect others. Deaths from alcohol-related falls, drowning, fires, homicides, shootings, child maltreatment, and occupational injuries only hint at the full cost to lives, families, and society from exceeding daily limits.[28,29] Alcohol misuse increases risk of divorce and job loss.[30–32] Alcohol is involved in one-third of suicides,[33] motor vehicle fatalities,[34] and trauma more generally.[35]

Chronic alcohol consumption contributes to a range of cancers, including head and neck, esophagus, liver, colon, rectum, breast, and perhaps prostate.[36,37] Alcohol is a prominent cause of liver and pancreatic disease.[29,36] Although the relationship between alcohol and cardiovascular disease is complex, heavy use is associated with ischemic cardiovascular disease, ischemic and hemorrhagic stroke, cardiomyopathy, and arrhythmias, including atrial fibrillation.[36,37] Most of these risks are dose dependent (**Fig. 2**). Neurologic effects include cognitive deficits and peripheral neuropathy, most often a painful, axonal, distal symmetric polyneuropathy that may also include autonomic symptoms.[38] Reproductive effects include fetal alcohol syndrome and preterm birth.[29] Alcohol consumption is associated with dose-dependent increases in gout.[39] The most severe alcohol misuse causes a variety of electrolyte abnormalities, including hyponatremia, hypomagnesaemia, hypokalemia, hypocalcemia, and hypophosphatemia.[40,41]

Benefits of Alcohol

Low-risk alcohol use may be associated with reduced rates of diabetes, cardiovascular disease, and total mortality.[36,42] Cardiovascular benefits thought mediated by alterations in serum lipids and hemostatic factors remain controversial.[43] Unfortunately, chronic

Disease	Proportion of Deaths (Absolute Risk)	Relative Risk at different daily alcohol intake. -1% to -24%, -25% to -50%, 1% to 49%, 50% to 99%, 100% to 199%, 200% or more				
		1 Drink	2 Drinks	3–4 Drinks	5–6 Drinks	≥6 Drinks
Oral cavity, pharynx cancer	1 in 200	+42	+96	+197	+368	+697
Oral esophagus cancer	1 in 150	+20	+43	+87	+164	+367
Colon cancer	1 in 40	+3	+5	+9	+15	+26
Rectum cancer	1 in 200	+5	+10	+18	+30	+53
Liver cancer	1 in 200	+10	+21	+38	+60	+99
Larynx cancer	1 in 500	+21	+47	+95	+181	+399
Breast cancer (women)	1 in 45	+13	+27	+52	+93	+193
Liver cirrhosis (men)	1 in 90	+26	+59	+124	+254	+691
Liver cirrhosis (women)	1 in 160	+139	+242	+408	+666	+1251
Pancreatitis	1 in 750	+3	+12	+41	+133	+851
Epilepsy	1 in 1000	+19	+41	+81	+152	+353
Ischemic Heart Disease	1 in 13	−19	−19	−14	0	+31
Dysrhythmias	1 in 250	+8	+17	+32	+54	+102
Hypertension (men)	1 in 150	+13	+28	+54	+97	+203
Hypertension (women)	1 in 85	0	+48	+161	+417	+1414
Ischemic stroke (men)	1 in 80	−13	0	+8	+29	+70
Ischemic stroke (women)	1 in 65	−34	−25	0	+86	+497
Hemorrhagic stroke (men)	1 in 30	+10	+21	+39	+68	+133
Hemorrhagic stroke (women)	1 in 20	+22	+49	+101	+199	+502
Diabetes mellitus (men)	1 in 30	−12	0	0	0	+72
Diabetes mellitus (women)	1 in 30	−36	−40	0	+739	+1560

Fig. 2. Mortality risk for selected conditions by alcohol dose. Notes: Mortality data in the second column are drawn from deaths in Canada from 2002 to 2005. For most conditions, relative risks apply to those individuals less than 70 years of age. Relevant conditions for which data are not available include fetal alcohol syndrome, alcoholic hepatitis, alcoholic cardiomyopathy, and alcohol-related injury. (Adapted with permission from the Canadian Centre on Substance Abuse. Available at: http://www.ccsa.ca/Resource%20Library/2012-Communicating-Alcohol-Related-Health-Risks-en.pdf. Accessed May 8, 2015.)

benefits and harms of alcohol have been studied only observationally and often with data of limited quality and detail regarding consumption patterns.[44] Health benefits may, therefore, reflect confounding by behavioral, social, and economic advantages associated with low level drinking.[29,45,46] Putative differences between types of drinks (eg, red wine vs beer) are particularly subject to such confounding. Additionally, some of the apparent benefit of low-level drinking seems to be caused by misclassification of patients who stop drinking when they become ill.[42] Whatever the benefits of low-level alcohol use, guidelines suggest that known risks of alcohol preclude any recommendation of drinking alcohol as a means to improve health.[47,48]

MANAGEMENT OF SELECTED CONDITIONS IN PATIENTS WITH ALCOHOL MISUSE

Alcohol misuse has pervasive effects on medical care. Alcohol consumption is associated with a host of drug interactions[49,50] and is inversely associated with medication adherence.[51,52] Alcohol affects management of common medical conditions.

Insomnia

Alcohol misuse is strongly associated with insomnia. Low doses of alcohol reduce time to falling asleep in alcohol-naive patients, but tolerance to this effect usually occurs quickly.[53] Higher doses cause rebound wakefulness as alcohol is metabolized leading to worse sleep overall.[53] Alcohol exacerbates obstructive sleep apnea and restless legs syndrome.[53] Benzodiazepines and benzodiazepine receptor agonists (eg, zolpidem) are relatively contraindicated in alcohol misuse because of the risk of psychomotor impairment, respiratory depression, and addiction.[50,53,54] A small literature guides insomnia management in patients in recovery from AUD, but there is little solid evidence to guide treatment of insomnia in patients who are still drinking (**Box 2**).

Pain

In older adults, painful conditions do not clearly lead to alcohol consumption but do predict alcohol-related problems.[55] In the United States, labeling warns those who drink more than 3 drinks a day of increased hepatotoxicity from acetaminophen and gastrointestinal bleeding from nonsteroidal antiinflammatory drugs (NSAIDs). One expert deemed the acetaminophen warning a misconception, concluding that alcohol worsens acetaminophen overdose but does not increase the risk of therapeutic doses[56]; however, long-term use and unintentional overdose remain of concern.[57] The NSAID warning was also controversial.[58]

Alcohol is involved in one-fifth of opioid pain reliever–related overdoses and emergency department visits.[59] A history of AUD is a strong predictor of misuse of prescribed opioid medications[60,61] and a relative contraindication to chronic opioid therapy.[62] The opioid receptor agonist tramadol may be associated with a lower addictive risk than potent opioids, but it has been associated with overdose in combination with alcohol and remains subject to significant misuse.[59,63] Unfortunately, common alternative pharmacologic strategies (eg, selective norepinephrine reuptake inhibitors, antiepileptics, and muscle relaxants) are also thought to interact with

---

Box 2
Management of insomnia

- Educate patients about alcohol's effect on sleep (e.g. "At first people find alcohol helps them fall asleep faster, but this effect fades quickly with frequent drinking. Also, even if you fall asleep faster, sleep is shallow, fragmented, and worse overall. So, alcohol is usually a cause of sleep problems not good a solution.")

- Identify and treat co-occurring obstructive sleep apnea and restless legs syndrome (both are worsened by alcohol.)

- Identify and treat co-occurring mood and anxiety disorders.

- Avoid prescribing benzodiazepines or benzodiazepine receptor agonists (BzRAs) (eg, zolpidem, zaleplon, eszopiclone). Increased risk of misuse, cross-tolerance, and respiratory depression.

- Consider use of a sleep diary including alcohol and education about sleep hygiene.

- Offer referral for nonpharmacologic treatments, including stimulus control, relaxation therapy, and cognitive-behavior therapy (CBT). Limited evidence supports use of CBT in patients with both ongoing AUD and recent remission.[128] Although sleep restriction therapy is an effective behavioral treatment of insomnia, caution should be exercised with ongoing alcohol misuse.[129]

- Warn patients with AUD that sleep may take months to improve after alcohol cessation.

- For patients newly abstinent from alcohol, consider non-BzRA medications. Trazodone seems effective, but there are concerns about increased relapse.[130] Other options include antihistamines, other sedating antidepressants (eg, amitriptyline), alpha-2-delta ligands (eg, gabapentin), or the melatonin receptor agonist ramelteon.[130–132]

alcohol, primarily increasing the risk of sedation.[49] **Box 3** presents common-sense advice for managing pain in the setting of alcohol misuse.

Psychiatric Comorbidity

Rates of depression and anxiety disorders are 1.5 to 2.0 times higher in patients with AUD than the general population: approximately 19% and 17%, respectively.[64] (Rates of AUD among those with depression and anxiety are almost as high.[64]) Bipolar disorder, psychosis, posttraumatic stress disorder, personality disorders, and other substance use disorders are also more common in patients with AUD. Whether the psychiatric symptoms began before alcohol use and persist during abstinence can help distinguish between a distinct comorbid condition and symptoms caused by alcohol use, but the difference is not always obvious.[16] The traditional doctrine of *treat the alcohol problem first* (deferring management of mood/anxiety problems until after several weeks of abstinence)[65] is being replaced by a *treat the symptoms and sort it out later* approach.[66] Outcomes related to mood, anxiety, and alcohol use may all improve with cotreatment. Despite a recent positive trial combining sertraline and naltrexone,[67] evidence of benefit from selective serotonin reuptake inhibitors (SSRIs) has been more mixed than for tricyclic antidepressants (TCAs).[68,69] Nonetheless, SSRIs are considered first line because of the increased risk of sedation, overdose, and seizure with alternatives, such as TCAs, serotonin-norepinephrine reuptake inhibitors, and buproprion.[70]

Smoking is exceptionally common among drinkers. There remains debate about whether smoking cessation should be deferred during alcohol treatment.[71–73] A role for varenicline in reducing heavy drinking[74] might favor simultaneous treatment.

Hypertension

Observational studies[75,76] and intervention trials[77] consistently show dose-dependent increases in blood pressure with more-than-moderate alcohol consumption, and reductions in alcohol produce 2- to 3-mm decreases in systolic pressure similar to that seen with salt restriction.[78] It is less clear that moderate drinking causes

---

Box 3
Management of pain

- Although history of substance use disorder should not condemn patients to untreated pain, ongoing heavy drinking may limit effective pain management.

- Maximize nonpharmacologic treatments, including exercise, physical modalities, and behavioral therapies.

- Consider topical treatments (eg, capsaicin, lidocaine) and local procedures (eg, steroid injections) to further reduce the need for systemic treatment.

- Educate patients about the risk of acetaminophen overdose.

- If using NSAIDs, consider a proton-pump inhibitor for gastroduodenal protection.

- If using alpha-2-delta ligands (eg, gabapentin) or tricyclic antidepressants (eg, amitriptyline), start at low doses and increase cautiously.

- If using a muscle relaxant, avoid carisoprodol, whose primary metabolite is the barbiturate meprobamate.

- Avoid chronic opioid therapy in patients with active AUD. Cautious dosing and additional monitoring are prudent when opioids are necessary in the setting of acute pain or risky drinking.

hypertension, particularly in women.[76,79] Patients with mild hypertension willing to decrease drinking may sensibly defer antihypertensive medications, as with other lifestyle modifications. Those unwilling to decrease drinking or whose hypertension persists should be offered medication, although medication adherence is reduced with risky drinking.[52] No trials have specifically assessed antihypertensive medications in patients with heavy alcohol use. Alcohol can potentiate the effect of most antihypertensive medications other than beta-blockers, increasing the risk of tachycardia and dizziness. The risk is particularly acute for nitrates and alpha-blockers but may also occur with calcium channel blockers.[49,50]

Abdominal Pain and Alcoholic Liver Disease

Alcohol has varied effects on gastrointestinal function; abdominal pain, nausea, and diarrhea are common among patients with alcohol misuse. Despite an older literature on alcoholic gastritis, contemporary research linking alcohol intake to gastroesophageal reflux disease, gastritis, peptic ulcer disease, and Barrett esophagus is more mixed.[80–82] Acute and chronic pancreatitis are strongly linked with alcohol consumption. Acute pancreatitis usually presents with characteristic pain, vomiting, and elevations of amylase and/or lipase. Chronic pancreatitis has more varied symptoms and typically requires imaging for diagnosis. Although alcohol can cause diarrhea through direct changes in gut motility and absorption, providers should be alert to steatorrhea (in addition to pain and less commonly hyperglycemia) as signs of chronic pancreatitis. In patients with alcohol-related liver disease, decompensated cirrhosis, spontaneous bacterial peritonitis, and hepatocellular carcinoma would be ominous causes of abdominal pain. Providers should also be alert to acute alcoholic hepatitis in very heavy drinkers with or without cirrhosis. Patients with alcoholic hepatitis classically present with acute onset of jaundice, perhaps with fever, abdominal pain, anorexia, and encephalopathy, perhaps days to weeks after alcohol cessation or with a concomitant gastrointestinal bleed or spontaneous bacterial peritonitis.[83] Alcoholic ketoacidosis can also present with acute abdominal pain, nausea, and vomiting.[41]

Up to 90% of heavy drinkers develop alcoholic steatosis, a usually asymptomatic fatty infiltration that may regress with abstinence. Only 10% to 20% go on to develop fibrosis and cirrhosis; although there is a clear association between dose and risk, genetic predisposition also plays a significant role.[84] Chronic infection with hepatitis C so markedly increases the risk of cirrhosis and hepatocellular cancer in heavy drinkers that patients with chronic hepatitis C are advised to consume no alcohol.[84] Obesity also adds to risk.[84]

As patients with compensated cirrhosis may be asymptomatic and decompensation causes significant morbidity, early detection is a valuable goal. Jocelyn James reviews the symptoms, signs, and diagnostic test suggestive of cirrhosis elsewhere in this issue. Despite the development of several scoring systems as well as novel laboratory and imaging modalities, there are no guidelines for routine screening for cirrhosis in heavy drinkers.[85] An aggressive case-finding approach seems reasonable with routine physical examination for the stigmata of cirrhosis and routine evaluation of platelet count, liver function tests (LFTs), and international normalized ratio, although drinking alone may cause thrombocytopenia and transaminitis.

Osteoporosis

Risky drinking is associated with decreased bone mineral density, although in women the effect of moderate alcohol use is less clear. Alcohol use is associated with an increased risk of fracture, presumably related to bone health and falls.[86] Patients with risky drinking should be reminded of recommended calcium and vitamin D intake and the benefits of weight-bearing exercise. For those willing to consider additional therapy, screening dual-energy x-ray absorptiometry (DXA) may be appropriate. The National Osteoporosis Foundation recommends screening DXA for men and women aged 50 to 70 years with clinical risk factors for osteoporosis, including alcohol use more than 3 drinks per day.[87] The USPSTF recommends screening women (but not men) for osteoporosis when their calculated risk of fracture is similar to that of a 65-year-old women.[88] Alcohol is included in the recommended fracture risk assessment tool (FRAX) risk calculator as a binary measure. Because of different drink sizes, 2 standard US drinks are roughly equivalent to the 3 alcohol units in FRAX.

Although pathophysiologically distinct from osteoporosis, heavy drinkers are also at risk for osteonecrosis of the femoral head.[89]

Malnutrition, Wernicke Encephalopathy

Low-level alcohol use often adds calories and can contribute to obesity. At higher levels of consumption, alcohol may replace other foods and result in weight loss.[90,91] A range of micronutrient deficiencies result from reduced intake, absorption, and mobilization, although low socioeconomic status and social isolation also play important roles.[90,91]

Among complications of malnutrition in patients with AUD, providers should be particularly attentive to thiamine deficiency leading to acute Wernicke encephalopathy (WE). WE is defined by the classic triad of encephalopathy, oculomotor abnormalities (ophthalmoplegia, nystagmus), and cerebellar dysfunction (usually gait ataxia) or 2 features with history or testing suggestive of dietary deficiency.[92] Untreated WE can progress to coma and death or irreversible amnesia and confabulation (Korsakoff syndrome). Some recommend offering prophylactic oral thiamine to heavy drinkers if they are malnourished, have decompensated liver disease, or are entering alcohol withdrawal.[93] However, because of concern that alcohol use may reduce absorption of oral thiamine, intravenous thiamine is preferred for the treatment of WE.[92–94] Unfortunately there is no evidence to guide micronutrient supplementation in AUD.

Anemia

Anemia in patients with alcohol misuse requires careful evaluation. Even absent liver disease, alcohol can directly suppress hematopoiesis and cause megaloblastic, sideroblastic, and hemolytic anemias. Alcohol complicates evaluation of anemia by increasing mean corpuscular volume and ferritin levels. Although clinical cyanocobalamin (vitamin B_{12}) deficiency is less common, serum levels may be artificially preserved, making important to check metabolites, such as methylmalonic acid, when levels are equivocal.[95,96]

SCREENING FOR ALCOHOL MISUSE

Alcohol misuse is rarely apparent from routine evaluation. Clinicians suspect it in only a third of patients identified on programmatic screening.[97] Because of the benefits of alcohol counseling, the USPSTF recommends routine screening of patients aged 18 years and older.[3]

Routine Screening

From an array of validated screening tests,[98] the USPSTF recommends the 10-question Alcohol Use Disorders Identification Test (AUDIT), 3-question AUDIT-C, or single-question screening (**Table 4**).[3] Multi-question tools provide more detailed information

Table 4
Common screening instruments

Single Question Screen
(National Institute on Alcohol Abuse and Alcoholism, Variations Exist)

Question: How many times in the past year have you had X or more drinks in a day? (X is 5 for men, 4 for women.)

Scoring: One or more is considered a positive screen for alcohol misuse.

Score	Sensitivity (95% CI)	Specificity (95% CI)	+LR	−LR
≥1	82% (73%–89%)	79% (73%–84%)	3.9	0.2

AUDIT-C

Question	Points				
	0	1	2	3	4
1. How often do you have a drink containing alcohol?	Never	Monthly or less	2–4 times a month	2–3 times a week	4 or more times a week
2. How many drinks containing alcohol do you have on a typical day when you are drinking?	1 or 2	3 or 4	5 or 6	7–9	10 or more
3. How often do you have 6 or more drinks on one occasion?	Never	Less than monthly	Monthly	Weekly	Daily or almost daily

Scoring: Points from the 3 questions are summed for a total 0 to 12. A positive screen for alcohol misuse is usually considered ≥4 for men and ≥3 for women but may be adjusted for increased sensitivity or specificity. If patients answer *never* for the first question, scores of 0 can be entered for questions 2 and 3.

Score	Sensitivity	Specificity	+LR (95% CI)	−LR (95% CI)
Men ≥4	0.86	0.89	7.8 (5.5–11.1)	0.16 (0.1–0.2)
Women ≥3	0.73	0.91	7.9 (6.2–10)	0.29 (0.2–0.4)

The full AUDIT questions can be found at the World Health Organization. AUDIT, the alcohol use disorders identification test: guidelines for use in primary care. 2nd ed. Geneva, Switzerland: World Health Organization, Department of Mental Health and Substance Dependence; 2001.
Abbreviations: CI, confidence interval; LR, likelihood ratio.
Data from Refs.[98,140,141]

about drinking but can be cumbersome to administer without paper or electronic support, whereas single-question screening is more easily integrated into an interview.[98] As the traditional CAGE (cut down, annoyed, guilty, eye opener) questionnaire[99] does not identify risky drinking, it is not appropriate for screening, although it might be used as part of an assessment for AUD. All validated screening for alcohol misuse relies on patient report. Efforts should be made to invite honest responses by minimizing stigma and normalizing screening as relevant to and a routine part of medical care. This technique can be explicit (eg, Because it interacts with medications and affects health, I ask all my patients about alcohol use) or implicit (eg, by asking about alcohol after questions related to nicotine).

Unfortunately, no biomarker of alcohol misuse is sufficiently sensitive or specific to play a role in alcohol screening. However, several tests reflecting acute or chronic alcohol use might prompt evaluation or be used in monitoring/feedback (**Table 5**).

Table 5 Alcohol biomarkers		
Test	**Time to Normalize with Abstinence**	**Comments**
Acute alcohol use		
BAL	Hours	Reflects consumption in past few hours; BAL >150–200 mg/dL without intoxication is a good marker of physiologic tolerance
EtG EtS	1–2 d in urine	Highly sensitive, even alcohol hand gels may cause positive test
Chronic alcohol use		
GGT	2–4 wk	Elevated in patients drinking at least 5 drinks/day; false positives from liver, biliary disease, obesity, medications; suitable for monitoring/feedback
%CDT	2–3 wk	Elevated in patients drinking at least 5 drinks/day; more specific than GGT but still some hepatic and biliary false positives; suitable for monitoring/feedback
MCV	Months	Altered by hematologic and liver disease
AST, ALT	2–4 wk	Less sensitive than GGT or %CDT Classically, AST:ALT ratio >2:1 indicates alcoholic liver disease
PEth	2–4 wk	Elevated in patients drinking 3–4 drinks/day; emerging test with promising sensitivity and specificity

Abbreviations: ALT, alanine transaminase; AST, aspartate transaminase; BAL, blood alcohol level; CDT, carbohydrate deficient transferrin; EtG, ethyl glucuronide; EtS, ethyl sulfate; GGT, gamma-glutamyltransferase; MCV, mean corpuscular volume; PEth, phosphatidyl ethanol.
  Data from Refs.[16,133–136]

Alcohol Assessment

Screening identifies patients at risk for alcohol misuse; assessment is generally required to confirm risky drinking and identify any AUD. Assessment may also include alcohol-related complications, comorbidities (medical, psychiatric, other substance use), prior treatment and results, patient concerns, readiness for change, and need for medically supervised withdrawal. As high scores on AUDIT, AUDIT-C, and even single-question screens may demonstrate at least risky drinking and predict AUD[100,101] and brief intervention (BI) includes discussion of alcohol-related complications, primary care assessment may be intertwined with the screening that prompted it and the BI that likely follows (**Fig. 3**).

MANAGEMENT OF ALCOHOL MISUSE

In the past, in the United States, alcoholism was the only recognized form of alcohol misuse; abstinence was the only therapeutic goal; and treatment consisted of inpatient rehabilitation and outpatient mutual-help groups, such as Alcoholics Anonymous (AA). With increasing recognition of the spectrum of alcohol misuse has come a greater range of management goals and modalities.[21] For patients with risky drinking, the focus is on prevention; patients are generally advised to reduce consumption to less than the recommended limits. Alcohol counseling in primary care settings,

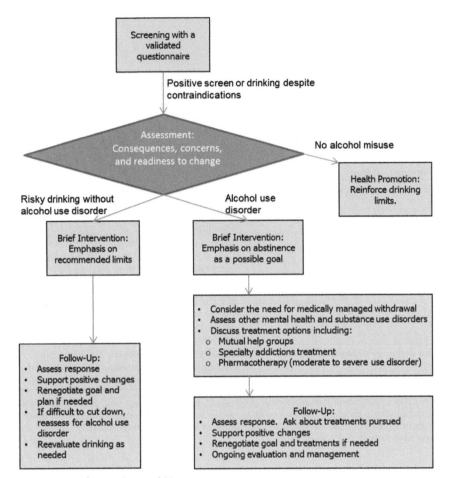

Fig. 3. Process of screening and BI.

traditionally called BI, is often adequate for patients with risky drinking. Patients with AUD are less likely to sustain low-risk drinking and, thus, are encouraged to abstain[8] but may choose different goals, for example, avoidance of drinking in dangerous situations. For patients with AUD, particularly moderate to severe AUD, treatment options include mutual-help groups, specialty behavioral treatments, and pharmacotherapy. Whatever the severity of alcohol misuse (risky drinking or AUD) the choice of management goal and strategy is an appropriate domain for shared decision making between patients and providers.

Brief Intervention: Alcohol Counseling in Primary Care

The evidence

Robust evidence supports alcohol counseling in primary care settings for patients with alcohol misuse.[102–105] One meta-analysis found an 11% increase in adherence to drinking limits at 12 months with BI compared with control interventions, with benefits lasting up to 4 years.[105] Although the earliest trials of BI included patients with alcohol dependence, the effects of screening and BI have been demonstrated primarily in patients with risky drinking and mild AUD rather than patients with moderate to severe AUD.[106]

Despite one meta-analysis showing reduced mortality with BI,[107] most trials evaluated self-reported drinking as the only outcome.[105] This limitation raises 2 opposing concerns: that BI does not reduce alcohol consumption but merely its report at follow-up[105] and conversely that repeated assessment of drinking in the control arms of BI trials is itself an intervention, masking the full effect size.[102] Taking trial data at face value, one meta-analysis concluded that providers would need to provide BI to 9.1 patients (6.7 patients for multi-contact interventions) to convert one from risky to low-risk drinking.[105] This number needed to treat is in addition to any benefit from identification and treatment of patients with more severe alcohol misuse.[105]

Conducting brief alcohol intervention

The heterogeneity of BI trials precludes evidence-based recommendation of a specific intervention method, duration, or content.[102] Specifically, analyses differ on whether longer, multi-contact interventions are meaningfully better than shorter, single-contact versions.[103,105] In general, BI includes

- Individualized feedback on risk, often based on results of screening or a more complete assessment
- Advice to change, with a menu of strategies
- Goal setting and plan for follow-up
- Delivery in an empathic rather than confrontational style that emphasizes patient autonomy and self-efficacy[108]

Clinicians may find it useful to distinguish between 2 strains of BI, brief advice and adaptations of motivational interviewing (**Box 4**).

Additional Treatments for Alcohol Use Disorder

Mutual-help groups and specialty behavioral treatment

Of patients seeking help for alcohol dependence, almost 80% reported using AA or similar 12-step programs.[109] Participation in AA is associated with a host of improved outcomes.[109] The few randomized trials of AA have not demonstrated benefit[110] leaving some question of whether AA participation causes or reflects improving outcomes. In addition to the 12-step principles of recovery, AA provides anonymity, an environment free of judgment, a focus on self-efficacy, and a sober social network. Providers should be comfortable referring patients to AA (**Box 5**).

Specialty behavioral addictions treatment in the United States variably includes evidence-based and non–evidence-based practices.[111] Evidence-based treatments include couples-based behavioral therapy, 12-step facilitation (support for participation in AA-type groups), motivation enhancement therapy (based on motivational interviewing), and cognitive behavioral therapy (identifying and changing thinking/behavior patterns).[65] Despite 2 prominent US trials[112,113] and numerous smaller studies, there is little evidence to support one psychosocial modality over another nor patient characteristics that predict a benefit from a specific modality.[21,65,114]

Pharmacotherapy

Strong evidence supports a modest benefit from pharmacotherapies for alcohol misuse when added to behavioral treatment.[115–117] In studies lasting up to a year, acamprosate increased rates of abstinence and naltrexone reduced the proportion of patients with heavy drinking, each with a number needed to treat between 9 and 12.[115–117] Both medications have a modest side effect profile. Disulfiram is an older, aversive therapy that causes unpleasant symptoms when alcohol is consumed. It

---

Box 4
Two approaches to Brief Intervention

Advice approach: Directive counseling is provided with an emphasis on personalized risk assessment and tailored recommendations.

For risky drinking:

- "You are drinking more than is medically safe. I strongly recommend that you cut down (or quit) and I am willing to help."

For alcohol use disorder:

- "Based on your report of (specify criteria), you have an AUD. I strongly recommend that you quit drinking and I am willing to help."
- "When people with AUDs try to reduce drinking rather than stop completely, they often return to heavy drinking."

Feedback on laboratory tests

- If GGT and CDT are in the normal range: "This is a positive sign that your liver has avoided harm so far and that now you have the opportunity to keep it that way by changing your drinking habits."
- If GGT and CDT are abnormal: "The test results are most likely a sign of unhealthy changes in your liver from heavy alcohol use. The longer you continue to drink, the harder it is to reverse the damage. But if you stop drinking, you may be able to get your liver tests back to normal."

Motivational interviewing/exploratory approach: This approach is a guided exploration of patients' ambivalence about behavior change highlighting discrepancies between priorities and current actions. Providers use reflective listening to reinforce talk of change. Goals are elicited from the patient.

- "What are the good things for you about using alcohol? What are the less good things?"
- "How important is it to you to cut down or stop drinking? On a scale of 0 to 10, where 0 is not at all important and 10 is extremely important, how would you rate yourself?" "Why are you at a (eg, 3) and not a 0?" "What would it take for you to go from a (eg, 3) to a (eg, 6)?"
- "No one can make you change or decide for you. What you do about your drinking is up to you."

Choosing an approach: The approaches are not mutually exclusive but can be challenging to combine in a single session. BI may occur over multiple visits and/or telephone follow-up. For patients unaware of alcohol's risks and unaffected by its harms, exploration of reasons for change may be premature and clear advice more appropriate. For patients with significant alcohol-related harm and extensive prior advice, further advice may turn ambivalence to resistance and an exploratory approach would be preferable.

Abbreviations: CDT, carbohydrate deficient transferrin; GGT, gamma-glutamyltransferase.
  Data from Refs.[8,108,142,143]

---

can be used only in abstinence and is increasingly reserved for situations in which family, friends, or a medical provider can monitor daily adherence (**Table 6**).[65,114,118] Additional medications may be used off-label for moderate to severe alcohol use disorder. Evidence is strongest for topiramate; others with less or mixed evidence include baclofen, varenicline, gabapentin, prazosin, and ondansetron.[117,118]

As with trials of BI, few pharmacotherapy trials included outcomes beyond self-reported consumption or symptoms of use disorder.[117] Most trials included patients with *DSM-IV* dependence,[117] but there is interest in using pharmacotherapy for patients with more moderate misuse.[65] Most trials, particularly of acamprosate, required

---

Box 5
Referral to mutual-help groups (eg, Alcoholics Anonymous)

Mutual-help basics

- Alcoholics Anonymous (AA, www.aa.org) is an anonymous, self-supporting fellowship open to anyone with a desire to stop drinking.

- Participation consists primarily of attendance at meetings and following the 12-steps but may also include having a home group and having or becoming a mentor/guide known as a sponsor.

- Meetings are widely available in time and location. Although they follow a similar structure, autonomous groups vary in style and demographics.

- Despite references to a higher power, many members are not religious and groups vary in their approach to spirituality.

- SMART Recovery (www.smartrecovery.org) offers a research-based alterative with both in-person and online meetings.

Making referrals

- Clinician referral increases AA participation.

- After asking what patients know about AA, providers can speak to any myths or concerns. (Current abstinence is not required to attend; patients with additional substance use problems or who take medications can be members; those concerned about anonymity can provide only a first name and might initially attend a meeting away from home/work.)

- Providers are encouraged to attend open meetings to become familiar with AA and the variety of local groups. AA service organizations can provide volunteer contacts willing to speak with patients and accompany them to their first meeting.

Data from Refs.[144–146]

---

abstinence before initiation of medication, although oral naltrexone and perhaps others may be initiated in patients with ongoing drinking.[117,119] There is a push to increase the use of alcohol pharmacotherapies in both primary and specialty care.[8,117,119,120]

Medical management of alcohol withdrawal

Starting 6 to 24 hours after cessation, patients with heavy alcohol use may develop symptoms of withdrawal, including agitation, anxiety, tremor, nausea, insomnia, diaphoresis, tachycardia, hypertension, hyperthermia, hallucinations/illusions, and seizures. Symptoms often remit over 24 to 48 hours but can progress to the potentially fatal syndrome of extreme disorientation called delirium tremens.

Although many patients withdraw from alcohol without medical supervision, detoxification or medical assistance with withdrawal is usually recommended for patients with alcohol dependence and other risk factors. Medical assistance can be provided in inpatient or outpatient settings (**Box 6**). Primary care providers must be able to identify alcohol withdrawal and patients at risk for severe withdrawal (see **Box 6**). For both inpatient and outpatient management, benzodiazepines are usually the first-line therapy, although alternatives may be considered, especially in outpatient settings. For inpatients, symptom-triggered management is usually preferred; but in the outpatient setting, fixed-dose or protocols may also be appropriate.[93,114] It is essential to link medical management of withdrawal to ongoing treatment.

Table 6
Alcohol pharmacotherapy

	Acamprosate	Naltrexone	Disulfiram
Mechanism of action	Reduces glutamate/ NMDA receptor hyperactivity, also acts at GABA receptors	Opioid receptor antagonist Decreases craving and reward	Inhibits aldehyde dehydrogenase causing unpleasant flushing, sweating, nausea, and tachycardia when alcohol is consumed
Typical dosing	666 mg oral 3 times daily	Oral: 50 mg daily IM: 380 mg every 4 wk, by medical staff	250 mg oral daily
Precautions	Dose reduction in renal impairment	• Avoid in acute hepatitis and liver failure; hepatotoxicity at higher doses • Verify free of prescribed and illicit opioid drugs before initiation • Avoid if anticipate need for opioid analgesia (eg, history of pancreatitis) Wallet card to alert emergency personnel recommended	• Contraindicated in severe cardiac disease, including coronary artery disease; hypersensitivity to rubber • Caution with history of liver disease, stroke, diabetes, epilepsy, and hypothyroidism • Must be free of alcohol at initiation
Side effects	Diarrhea, somnolence; often resolve with continued use	Nausea, vomiting, decreased appetite, headache, dizziness, fatigue, anxiety; local reactions for IM	Headache, fatigue, taste changes; rare hepatitis, optic and peripheral neuropathy, psychosis
Drug interactions	No known clinically relevant interactions	Blocks efficacy of opioid medications (analgesic, antidiarrheal, antitussive) and can precipitate opiod withdrawal	Include warfarin, metronidazole, amitriptyline, diazepam; alcohol-containing lotions, mouthwash, foods
Monitoring	Renal function	Liver function	Liver function

Abbreviations: GABA, γ-aminobutyric acid; IM, intramuscular; NMDA, N-methyl-d-aspartate.

Data from National Institute on Alcohol Abuse and Alcoholism. Helping patients who drink too much: a clinician's guide: October 2008 medications update. Available at: http://pubs.niaaa.nih. gov/publications/Practitioner/CliniciansGuide2005/PrescribingMeds.pdf. Accessed May 8, 2015; and SAMHSA. Incorporating alcohol pharmacotherapies into medical practice. Rockville (MD): Substance Abuse and Mental Health Services Administration; 2009.

Follow-up evaluation and managing patients in remission
For many patients, alcohol misuse should be treated as a chronic condition with long-term management and monitoring. Follow-up should include assessment of current drinking in relation to goals, adherence to planned therapy (eg, medication, AA meetings), and complications of drinking and treatment. Providers should support any positive changes or even further talk of change and, together with the patients, evaluate

---

Box 6
Common requirement for and contraindications to outpatient medically supervised withdrawal

Requirements

- Committed caregiver (family, friend) able to monitor patient, administer oral medications, and transport to visits
- Safe environment supportive of abstinence
- Provider available for daily visits and accessible by phone

Cautions and contraindications (risk factors for severe withdrawal)

- Greater than 60 years of age
- History of epileptic or withdrawal seizures, delirium tremens, head trauma, or structural brain lesion
- Moderate to severe withdrawal on a validated screening score (eg, CIWA-Ar)
- Medically unstable (eg, pregnancy, infection, bleeding, unstable heart disease, cirrhosis, marked renal insufficiency)
- Psychiatrically unstable (eg, suicidality, psychosis, cognitive impairment)
- Misuse of illicit or other drugs that can cause withdrawal (eg, benzodiazepines)
- BAL greater than 150, significant abnormalities of blood counts, electrolytes, LFTs, urine drug screen

Abbreviations: BAL, blood alcohol level; CIWA-Ar, clinical institute withdrawal assessment for alcohol, revised.
Data from Refs.[114,137–139]

---

the need for adjustment to the treatment goals or methods. For example, if patients with risky drinking have trouble cutting down, reevaluate for AUD. Providers can help patients identify and engage social support to help them achieve drinking goals. Gamma-glutamyltransferase and carbohydrate deficient transferrin can be used to monitor changes and provide positive feedback. Urine ethyl glucuronide or alcohol could be used to verify recent abstinence (see **Fig. 2**).

When patients achieve long-term stability or providers meet patients with a remote history of alcohol misuse, supportive discussion perhaps focused on the health benefits of reduced drinking or abstinence is appropriate. When such patients encounter major life stresses, discussion of strategies to prevent relapse (even pharmacotherapy) may be helpful.

SUMMARY: ALCOHOL CARE IN PRIMARY CARE

Barriers to alcohol care include lack of time, reimbursement, and training; concern that addressing alcohol misuse will offend patients; and beliefs that there are not effective interventions for alcohol misuse and patients must be ready to change.[102] Regarding time, there is interest in the use of team-based, telephone-based, and all-electronic screening and BI.[121] Even without these resources, identification of misuse with a single-question screen followed by interventions as brief as 5 minutes are effective.[105] Alcohol misuse screening and BI is a required service under current health care reform,[122] and counseling of at least 15 minutes' duration is increasingly reimbursed by insurers.[123]

For training, manuals for BI[8,124] and pharmacotherapy[8,118,119,142] are freely available, as are materials for patients.[10,120,125] As with other sensitive topics, a straightforward approach and measures to normalize screening (eg, I ask this of all my patients) can overcome most awkwardness and avoid offending patients. Patient report of alcohol screening is associated with high patient satisfaction.[126] Although the success of alcohol treatment remains modest, the effects of even small reductions in consumption can be profound. Risky drinking and mild AUD are far more common than more severe use disorder, cause significant morbidity, and may be particularly amenable to intervention, even for patients identified by screening rather than presenting with concerns about alcohol. Primary care providers are likely used to taking an active and optimistic approach to smoking cessation despite the low success rate of any single quit attempt and modest (but real) benefits of behavioral and pharmacologic aids to smoking cessation. Similarly, providers should be proactive with regard to alcohol, not necessarily waiting for patients to be fully ready to change or assuming that alcohol misuse is immutable.

Primary care providers have the advantage of addressing alcohol misuse in the context of other preventive health measures (eg, diet, exercise) and other symptoms (eg, insomnia, depressed mood). Ideally, primary care offers longitudinal, trusting relationships and ongoing follow-up. Such context can be important; trials in which BI was delivered by primary care providers showed greater benefit than trials in which BI was delivered by research staff.[105] Alcohol misuse is common, causes enormous morbidity and mortality, and impacts regular medical care. Primary care providers should routinely screen patients to identify the full spectrum of misuse. Management should be proactive, tailored to the severity of misuse, and chosen collaboratively with patients.

REFERENCES

1. Mokdad AH, Marks JS, Stroup DF, et al. Actual causes of death in the United States, 2000. JAMA 2004;291(10):1238–45.
2. Bouchery EE, Harwood HJ, Sacks JJ, et al. Economic costs of excessive alcohol consumption in the U.S., 2006. Am J Prev Med 2011;41(5):516–24.
3. Moyer VA. Screening and behavioral counseling interventions in primary care to reduce alcohol misuse: U.S. Preventive Services Task Force recommendation statement. Ann Intern Med 2013;159(3):210–8.
4. Maciosek MV, Coffield AB, Edwards NM, et al. Priorities among effective clinical preventive services: results of a systematic review and analysis. Am J Prev Med 2006;31(1):52–61.
5. Solberg LI, Maciosek MV, Edwards NM. Primary care intervention to reduce alcohol misuse ranking its health impact and cost effectiveness. Am J Prev Med 2008;34(2):143–52.
6. McKnight-Eily LR, Liu Y, Brewer RD, et al. Vital signs: communication between health professionals and their patients about alcohol use–44 states and the District of Columbia, 2011. MMWR Morb Mortal Wkly Rep 2014;63(1):16–22.
7. McGlynn EA, Asch SM, Adams J, et al. The quality of health care delivered to adults in the United States. N Engl J Med 2003;348(26):2635–45.
8. National Institute on Alcohol Abuse and Alcoholism. Helping patients who drink too much: a clinician's guide: updated 2005 edition. Rockville (MD): U.S. Dept. of Health and Human Services, National Institutes of Health; 2007.
9. National Institute on Alcohol Abuse and Alcoholism. Drinking levels defined. Available at: http://www.niaaa.nih.gov/alcohol-health/overview-alcohol-consumption/moderate-binge-drinking. Accessed December 14, 2014.

10. Canadian Centre on Substance Abuse. Canada's low-risk alcohol drinking guidelines. Available at: http://www.ccsa.ca. Accessed November 16, 2014.
11. Stockwell T, Butt P, Beirness D, et al. The basis for Canada's new low-risk drinking guidelines: a relative risk approach to estimating hazardous levels and patterns of alcohol use. Drug Alcohol Rev 2012;31(2):126–34.
12. National Health and Medical Research Council. Australian guidelines to reduce health risks from drinking alcohol. Canberra (Australia): National Health and Medical Research Council; 2009.
13. Great Britain., Department of Health. Lord President's report on action against alcohol misuse. London: HMSO; 1992.
14. Kerr WC, Stockwell T. Understanding standard drinks and drinking guidelines. Drug Alcohol Rev 2012;31(2):200–5.
15. Devos-Comby L, Lange JE. "My drink is larger than yours"? A literature review of self-defined drink sizes and standard drinks. Curr Drug Abuse Rev 2008;1(2): 162–76.
16. American Psychiatric Association. Diagnostic and statistical manual of mental disorders: DSM-5. 5th edition. Washington, DC: American Psychiatric Association; 2013.
17. Hasin DS, O'Brien CP, Auriacombe M, et al. DSM-5 criteria for substance use disorders: recommendations and rationale. Am J Psychiatry 2013;170(8): 834–51.
18. Dawson DA, Goldstein RB, Grant BF. Differences in the profiles of DSM-IV and DSM-5 alcohol use disorders: implications for clinicians. Alcohol Clin Exp Res 2013;37(Suppl 1):E305–13.
19. Dawson DA, Grant BF, Stinson FS, et al. Toward the attainment of low-risk drinking goals: a 10-year progress report. Alcohol Clin Exp Res 2004;28(9): 1371–8.
20. Hasin DS, Stinson FS, Ogburn E, et al. Prevalence, correlates, disability, and co-morbidity of DSM-IV alcohol abuse and dependence in the United States: results from the national epidemiologic survey on alcohol and related conditions. Arch Gen Psychiatry 2007;64(7):830–42.
21. Willenbring ML. Treatment of heavy drinking and alcohol use disorder. In: Ries R, Fiellin DA, Miller SC, et al, editors. The ASAM principles of addiction medicine. 5th edition. Philadelphia: Wolters Kluwer Health/Lippincott Williams & Wilkins; 2014. p. 375–88.
22. Rossow I, Romelsjö A. The extent of the "prevention paradox" in alcohol problems as a function of population drinking patterns. Addiction 2006;101(1): 84–90.
23. Stockwell T, Hawks D, Lang E, et al. Unravelling the preventive paradox for acute alcohol problems. Drug Alcohol Rev 1996;15(1):7–15.
24. National Institute on Alcohol Abuse and Alcoholism, American Academy of Pediatrics. Alcohol screening and brief intervention for youth a practitioner's guide. Rockville (MD): U.S. Dept. of Health and Human Services, National Institutes of Health; 2011.
25. Dawson DA, Grant BF, Li T-K. Quantifying the risks associated with exceeding recommended drinking limits. Alcohol Clin Exp Res 2005;29(5):902–8.
26. Dawson DA, Li T-K, Grant BF. A prospective study of risk drinking: at risk for what? Drug Alcohol Depend 2008;95(1–2):62–72.
27. Cohen E, Feinn R, Arias A, et al. Alcohol treatment utilization: findings from the National Epidemiologic Survey on Alcohol and Related Conditions. Drug Alcohol Depend 2007;86(2–3):214–21.

28. Stahre M, Roeber J, Kanny D, et al. Contribution of excessive alcohol consumption to deaths and years of potential life lost in the United States. Prev Chronic Dis 2014;11:E109.

29. World Health Organization, Management of Substance Abuse Unit. Global status report on alcohol and health, 2014. Geneva (Switzerland): World Health Organization; 2014.

30. Cranford JA. DSM-IV alcohol dependence and marital dissolution: evidence from the National Epidemiologic Survey on Alcohol and Related Conditions. J Stud Alcohol Drugs 2014;75(3):520–9.

31. Boden JM, Fergusson DM, Horwood LJ. Alcohol misuse and relationship breakdown: findings from a longitudinal birth cohort. Drug Alcohol Depend 2013; 133(1):115–20.

32. French MT, Maclean JC, Sindelar JL, et al. The morning after: alcohol misuse and employment problems. Appl Econ 2011;43(21):2705–20.

33. Centers for Disease Control and Prevention. Toxicology testing and results for suicide victims–13 states, 2004. MMWR Morb Mortal Wkly Rep 2006;55(46):1245–8.

34. National Highway Traffic Safety Administration. Traffic safety facts: 2012 data. Washington, DC: US Department of Transportation; 2013. Available online at: http://www-nrd.nhtsa.dot.gov/Pubs/812032.pdf.

35. MacLeod JBA, Hungerford DW. Alcohol-related injury visits: do we know the true prevalence in U.S. trauma centres? Injury 2011;42(9):922–6.

36. Rehm J, Baliunas D, Borges GLG, et al. The relation between different dimensions of alcohol consumption and burden of disease: an overview. Addiction 2010;105(5):817–43.

37. Shield KD, Parry C, Rehm J. Chronic diseases and conditions related to alcohol use. Alcohol Res 2013;35(2):155–73.

38. Koike H, Sobue G. Alcoholic neuropathy. Curr Opin Neurol 2006;19(5):481–6.

39. Wang M, Jiang X, Wu W, et al. A meta-analysis of alcohol consumption and the risk of gout. Clin Rheumatol 2013;32(11):1641–8.

40. Vamvakas S, Teschner M, Bahner U, et al. Alcohol abuse: potential role in electrolyte disturbances and kidney diseases. Clin Nephrol 1998;49(4):205–13.

41. Allison MG, McCurdy MT. Alcoholic metabolic emergencies. Emerg Med Clin North Am 2014;32(2):293–301.

42. Di Castelnuovo A, Costanzo S, Bagnardi V, et al. Alcohol dosing and total mortality in men and women: an updated meta-analysis of 34 prospective studies. Arch Intern Med 2006;166(22):2437–45.

43. Chikritzhs T, Stockwell T, Naimi T, et al. Has the leaning tower of presumed health benefits from "moderate" alcohol use finally collapsed? Addiction 2015; 110(5):726–7.

44. Dawson DA. Defining risk drinking. Alcohol Res Health 2011;34(2):144–56.

45. Naimi TS, Brown DW, Brewer RD, et al. Cardiovascular risk factors and confounders among nondrinking and moderate-drinking U.S. adults. Am J Prev Med 2005;28(4):369–73.

46. Holmes MV, Dale CE, Zuccolo L, et al. Association between alcohol and cardiovascular disease: Mendelian randomisation analysis based on individual participant data. BMJ 2014;349:g4164.

47. US Department of Health and Human Services, US Department of Agriculture. Dietary guidelines for Americans, 2010. Washington, DC: U.S. Dept. of Health and Human Services, U.S. Dept. of Agriculture; 2010.

48. American Heart Association Nutrition Committee, Lichtenstein AH, Appel LJ, et al. Diet and lifestyle recommendations revision 2006: a scientific statement

from the American Heart Association Nutrition Committee. Circulation 2006; 114(1):82–96.

49. National Institute on Alcohol Abuse and Alcoholism. Harmful interactions: mixing alcohol with medicines. Bethesda (MD): U.S. Dept. of Health and Human Services, National Institutes of Health; 2007.

50. Chan L-N, Anderson GD. Pharmacokinetic and pharmacodynamic drug interactions with ethanol (alcohol). Clin Pharmacokinet 2014;53(12):1115–36.

51. Grodensky CA, Golin CE, Ochtera RD, et al. Systematic review: effect of alcohol intake on adherence to outpatient medication regimens for chronic diseases. J Stud Alcohol Drugs 2012;73(6):899–910.

52. Bryson CL, Au DH, Sun H, et al. Alcohol screening scores and medication nonadherence. Ann Intern Med 2008;149(11):795–804.

53. Roehrs T, Roth T. Sleep, sleepiness, sleep disorders and alcohol use and abuse. Sleep Med Rev 2001;5(4):287–97.

54. Buysse DJ. Insomnia. JAMA 2013;309(7):706–16.

55. Brennan PL, Schutte KK, SooHoo S, et al. Painful medical conditions and alcohol use: a prospective study among older adults. Pain Med 2011;12(7):1049–59.

56. Rumack BH. Acetaminophen misconceptions. Hepatology 2004;40(1):10–5.

57. Food and Drug Administration. Organ-specific warnings; internal analgesic, antipyretic, and antirheumatic drug products for over-the-counter human use; final monograph. Fed Regist 2009;74(81):19385–409.

58. Food and Drug Administration. Internal analgesic, antipyretic, and antirheumatic drug products for over-the-counter human use; proposed amendment of the tentative final monograph; required warnings and other labeling. Fed Regist 2006;71(247):77314–52.

59. Jones CM, Paulozzi LJ, Mack KA. Alcohol involvement in opioid pain reliever and benzodiazepine drug abuse-related emergency department visits and drug-related deaths - United States, 2010. MMWR Morb Mortal Wkly Rep 2014;63(40):881–5.

60. Chou R, Fanciullo GJ, Fine PG, et al. Clinical guidelines for the use of chronic opioid therapy in chronic noncancer pain. J Pain 2009;10(2):113–30.

61. Turk DC, Swanson KS, Gatchel RJ. Predicting opioid misuse by chronic pain patients: a systematic review and literature synthesis. Clin J Pain 2008;24(6): 497–508.

62. Manchikanti L, Abdi S, Atluri S, et al. American Society of Interventional Pain Physicians (ASIPP) guidelines for responsible opioid prescribing in chronic non-cancer pain: part 2–guidance. Pain Physician 2012;15(3 Suppl):S67–116.

63. Department of Health and Human Services. Basis for the recommendation to schedule tramadol in schedule IV of the Controlled Substances Act. Available at: http://www.regulations.gov/#!docketDetail;D=DEA-2013-0010. Accessed January 25, 2015.

64. Grant BF, Stinson FS, Dawson DA, et al. Prevalence and co-occurrence of substance use disorders and independent mood and anxiety disorders: results from the National Epidemiologic Survey on Alcohol and Related Conditions. Arch Gen Psychiatry 2004;61(8):807–16.

65. National Collaborating Centre for Mental Health, Management of Harmful Drinking and Alcohol Dependence. National clinical practice guideline 115. London: National Institute for Health & Clinical Excellence; 2011.

66. Hobbs JDJ, Kushner MG, Lee SS, et al. Meta-analysis of supplemental treatment for depressive and anxiety disorders in patients being treated for alcohol dependence. Am J Addict 2011;20(4):319–29.

67. Pettinati HM, Oslin DW, Kampman KM, et al. A double-blind, placebo-controlled trial combining sertraline and naltrexone for treating co-occurring depression and alcohol dependence. Am J Psychiatry 2010;167(6):668–75.
68. Nunes EV, Levin FR. Treatment of depression in patients with alcohol or other drug dependence: a meta-analysis. JAMA 2004;291(15):1887–96.
69. Iovieno N, Tedeschini E, Bentley KH, et al. Antidepressants for major depressive disorder and dysthymic disorder in patients with comorbid alcohol use disorders: a meta-analysis of placebo-controlled randomized trials. J Clin Psychiatry 2011;72(8):1144–51.
70. Nunes EV, Weiss RD. Co-occurring addictive and mood disorders. In: Ries R, Fiellin DA, Miller SC, et al, editors. The ASAM principles of addiction medicine. 5th edition. Philadelphia: Wolters Kluwer Health/Lippincott Williams & Wilkins; 2014. p. 1300–32.
71. Kalman D, Kim S, DiGirolamo G, et al. Addressing tobacco use disorder in smokers in early remission from alcohol dependence: the case for integrating smoking cessation services in substance use disorder treatment programs. Clin Psychol Rev 2010;30(1):12–24.
72. Joseph AM, Willenbring ML, Nugent SM, et al. A randomized trial of concurrent versus delayed smoking intervention for patients in alcohol dependence treatment. J Stud Alcohol 2004;65(6):681–91.
73. Prochaska JJ, Delucchi K, Hall SM. A meta-analysis of smoking cessation interventions with individuals in substance abuse treatment or recovery. J Consult Clin Psychol 2004;72(6):1144–56.
74. Litten RZ, Ryan ML, Fertig JB, et al. A double-blind, placebo-controlled trial assessing the efficacy of varenicline tartrate for alcohol dependence. J Addict Med 2013;7(4):277–86.
75. Beilin LJ, Puddey IB. Alcohol and hypertension: an update. Hypertension 2006; 47(6):1035–8.
76. Briasoulis A, Agarwal V, Messerli FH. Alcohol consumption and the risk of hypertension in men and women: a systematic review and meta-analysis. J Clin Hypertens 2012;14(11):792–8.
77. McFadden CB, Brensinger CM, Berlin JA, et al. Systematic review of the effect of daily alcohol intake on blood pressure. Am J Hypertens 2005;18(2 Pt 1): 276–86.
78. Xin X, He J, Frontini MG, et al. Effects of alcohol reduction on blood pressure: a meta-analysis of randomized controlled trials. Hypertension 2001;38(5):1112–7.
79. Sesso HD, Cook NR, Buring JE, et al. Alcohol consumption and the risk of hypertension in women and men. Hypertension 2008;51(4):1080–7.
80. Teyssen S, Singer MV. Alcohol-related diseases of the oesophagus and stomach. Best Pract Res Clin Gastroenterol 2003;17(4):557–73.
81. Taylor B, Rehm J, Gmel G. Moderate alcohol consumption and the gastrointestinal tract. Dig Dis 2005;23(3–4):170–6.
82. Kaltenbach T, Crockett S, Gerson LB. Are lifestyle measures effective in patients with gastroesophageal reflux disease? An evidence-based approach. Arch Intern Med 2006;166(9):965–71.
83. Lucey MR, Mathurin P, Morgan TR. Alcoholic hepatitis. N Engl J Med 2009; 360(26):2758–69.
84. O'Shea RS, Dasarathy S, McCullough AJ, et al. Alcoholic liver disease. Hepatology 2010;51(1):307–28.
85. Tsochatzis EA, Bosch J, Burroughs AK. Liver cirrhosis. Lancet 2014;383(9930): 1749–61.

86. Nieves JW. Chapter 34-Nonskeletal risk factors for osteoporosis and fractures. In: Marcus R, Feldman D, Dempster D, et al, editors. Osteoporosis. 4th edition. San Diego (CA): Academic Press; 2013. p. 817–39.
87. Cosman F, de Beur SJ, LeBoff MS, et al. Clinician's guide to prevention and treatment of osteoporosis. Osteoporos Int 2014;25(10):2359–81.
88. U.S. Preventive Services Task Force. Screening for osteoporosis: U.S. Preventive Services Task Force recommendation statement. Ann Intern Med 2011; 154(5):356–64.
89. Zalavras CG, Lieberman JR. Osteonecrosis of the femoral head: evaluation and treatment. J Am Acad Orthop Surg 2014;22(7):455–64.
90. Markowitz JS, McRae AL, Sonne SC. Oral nutritional supplementation for the alcoholic patient: a brief overview. Ann Clin Psychiatry 2000;12(3):153–8.
91. Santolaria F, González-Reimers E. Alcohol and nutrition: an overview. In: Watson RR, Preedy VR, Zibadi S, editors. Alcohol, nutrition, and health consequences. New York: Humana Press; 2013. p. 3–14.
92. Galvin R, Bråthen G, Ivashynka A, et al. EFNS guidelines for diagnosis, therapy and prevention of Wernicke encephalopathy. Eur J Neurol 2010;17(12):1408–18.
93. National Clinical Guideline Centre (UK). Alcohol use disorders: diagnosis and clinical management of alcohol-related physical complications. London: Royal College of Physicians; 2010.
94. Day E, Bentham PW, Callaghan R, et al. Thiamine for prevention and treatment of Wernicke-Korsakoff Syndrome in people who abuse alcohol. Cochrane Database Syst Rev 2013;(7):CD004033.
95. Girard DE, Kumar KL, McAfee JH. Hematologic effects of acute and chronic alcohol abuse. Hematol Oncol Clin North Am 1987;1(2):321–34.
96. Fragasso A, Mannarella C, Ciancio A, et al. Functional vitamin B12 deficiency in alcoholics: an intriguing finding in a retrospective study of megaloblastic anemic patients. Eur J Intern Med 2010;21(2):97–100.
97. Vinson DC, Turner BJ, Manning BK, et al. Clinician suspicion of an alcohol problem: an observational study from the AAFP National Research Network. Ann Fam Med 2013;11(1):53–9.
98. Bradley K, Berger D. Screening for unhealthy alcohol use. In: Saitz R, editor. Addressing unhealthy alcohol use in primary care. New York: Springer; 2013. p. 7–27.
99. Ewing JA. Detecting alcoholism. The CAGE questionnaire. JAMA 1984;252(14): 1905–7.
100. Rubinsky AD, Kivlahan DR, Volk RJ, et al. Estimating risk of alcohol dependence using alcohol screening scores. Drug Alcohol Depend 2010;108(1–2): 29–36.
101. Saitz R, Cheng DM, Allensworth-Davies D, et al. The ability of single screening questions for unhealthy alcohol and other drug use to identify substance dependence in primary care. J Stud Alcohol Drugs 2014;75(1):153–7.
102. O'Donnell A, Anderson P, Newbury-Birch D, et al. The impact of brief alcohol interventions in primary healthcare: a systematic review of reviews. Alcohol Alcohol 2014;49(1):66–78.
103. Kaner EFS, Beyer F, Dickinson HO, et al. Effectiveness of brief alcohol interventions in primary care populations. Cochrane Database Syst Rev 2007;(2):CD004148.
104. Kaner EFS, Dickinson HO, Beyer F, et al. The effectiveness of brief alcohol interventions in primary care settings: a systematic review. Drug Alcohol Rev 2009; 28(3):301–23.

105. Jonas DE, Garbutt JC, Amick HR, et al. Behavioral counseling after screening for alcohol misuse in primary care: a systematic review and meta-analysis for the U.S. preventive services task force. Ann Intern Med 2012;157(9):645–54.

106. Saitz R. Alcohol screening and brief intervention in primary care: absence of evidence for efficacy in people with dependence or very heavy drinking. Drug Alcohol Rev 2010;29(6):631–40.

107. Cuijpers P, Riper H, Lemmers L. The effects on mortality of brief interventions for problem drinking: a meta-analysis. Addiction 2004;99(7):839–45.

108. Bien TH, Miller WR, Tonigan JS. Brief interventions for alcohol problems: a review. Addiction 1993;88(3):315–35.

109. McCrady BS, Tonigan JS. Recent research into twelve-step programs. In: Ries R, Fiellin DA, Miller SC, et al, editors. The ASAM principles of addiction medicine. 5th edition. Philadelphia: Wolters Kluwer Health/Lippincott Williams & Wilkins; 2014. p. 1043–59.

110. Ferri M, Amato L, Davoli M. Alcoholics Anonymous and other 12-step programmes for alcohol dependence. Cochrane Database Syst Rev 2006;(3):CD005032.

111. Carroll KM. Dissemination of evidence-based practices: how far we've come, and how much further we've got to go. Addiction 2012;107(6):1031–3.

112. Project Match Research Group. Matching alcoholism treatments to client heterogeneity: project MATCH posttreatment drinking outcomes. J Stud Alcohol 1997; 58(1):7–29.

113. Anton RF, O'Malley SS, Ciraulo DA, et al. Combined pharmacotherapies and behavioral interventions for alcohol dependence: the COMBINE study: a randomized controlled trial. JAMA 2006;295(17):2003–17.

114. Department of Veterans Affairs, Department of Defense. VA/DOD clinical guideline for management of substance use disorders. Washington, DC: Dept. of Veterans Affairs, Dept. of Defense; 2009.

115. Rösner S, Hackl-Herrwerth A, Leucht S, et al. Acamprosate for alcohol dependence. Cochrane Database Syst Rev 2010;(9):CD004332.

116. Rösner S, Hackl-Herrwerth A, Leucht S, et al. Opioid antagonists for alcohol dependence. Cochrane Database Syst Rev 2010;(12):CD001867.

117. Jonas DE, Amick HR, Feltner C, et al. Pharmacotherapy for adults with alcohol-use disorders in outpatient settings. Rockville (MD): Agency for Healthcare Research and Quality; 2014.

118. National Institute on Alcohol Abuse and Alcoholism. Helping patients who drink too much: a clinician's guide: October 2008 medications update. Available at: http://pubs.niaaa.nih.gov/publications/Practitioner/CliniciansGuide2005/PrescribingMeds.pdf. Accessed November 22, 2014.

119. SAMHSA. Incorporating alcohol pharmacotherapies into medical practice. Rockville (MD): Substance Abuse and Mental Health Services Administration; 2009.

120. National Institute on Alcohol Abuse and Alcoholism. Treatment for alcohol problems: finding and getting help. Bethesda (MD): National Institute on Alcohol Abuse and Alcoholism; 2014.

121. Saitz R. Brief intervention for unhealthy alcohol use. In: Saitz R, editor. Addressing unhealthy alcohol use in primary care. New York: Springer; 2013. p. 41–8.

122. Preventive care benefits. HealthCare.gov. Available at: https://www.healthcare.gov/preventive-care-benefits/#part=1. Accessed November 16, 2014.

123. Coding for Reimbursement. Available at: http://www.samhsa.gov/sbirt/coding-reimbursement. Accessed November 16, 2014.

124. Babor T, World Health Organization. Brief intervention for hazardous and harmful drinking: a manual for use in primary care. Geneva (Switzerland): World Health Organization, Dept. of Mental Health and Substance Dependence; 2001.
125. National Institute on Alcohol Abuse and Alcoholism. Rethinking drinking alcohol and your health: research-based information from the National Institutes of Health, U.S. Department of Health and Human Services. Bethesda (MD): U.S. Dept. of Health and Human Services, National Institutes of Health; 2010.
126. Saitz R, Horton NJ, Cheng DM, et al. Alcohol counseling reflects higher quality of primary care. J Gen Intern Med 2008;23(9):1482–6.
127. Saitz R. Clinical practice. Unhealthy alcohol use. N Engl J Med 2005;352(6):596–607.
128. Brooks AT, Wallen GR. Sleep disturbances in individuals with alcohol-related disorders: a review of cognitive-behavioral therapy for insomnia (CBT-I) and associated non-pharmacological therapies. Subst Abuse 2014;8:55–62.
129. Schutte-Rodin S, Broch L, Buysse D, et al. Clinical guideline for the evaluation and management of chronic insomnia in adults. J Clin Sleep Med 2008;4(5):487–504.
130. Kolla BP, Mansukhani MP, Schneekloth T. Pharmacological treatment of insomnia in alcohol recovery: a systematic review. Alcohol Alcohol 2011;46(5):578–85.
131. Friedmann PD, Herman DS, Freedman S, et al. Treatment of sleep disturbance in alcohol recovery: a national survey of addiction medicine physicians. J Addict Dis 2003;22(2):91–103.
132. Brower KJ, Conroy DA, Kurth ME, et al. Ramelteon and improved insomnia in alcohol-dependent patients: a case series. J Clin Sleep Med 2011;7(3):274–5.
133. Neumann T, Spies C. Use of biomarkers for alcohol use disorders in clinical practice. Addiction 2003;98(Suppl 2):81–91.
134. Substance Abuse and Mental Health Services Administration. The role of biomarkers in the treatment of alcohol use disorders, 2012 Revision. Advisory 2012;11(2):1–8. Available online at: http://store.samhsa.gov/shin/content//SMA12-4686/SMA12-4686.pdf.
135. Hashimoto E, Riederer PF, Hesselbrock VM, et al. Consensus paper of the WFSBP task force on biological markers: biological markers for alcoholism. World J Biol Psychiatry 2013;14(8):549–64.
136. Ingall GB. Alcohol biomarkers. Clin Lab Med 2012;32(3):391–406.
137. Muncie HL, Yasinian Y, Oge' L. Outpatient management of alcohol withdrawal syndrome. Am Fam Physician 2013;88(9):589–95.
138. Bierer MF, Saitz R. Unhealthy alcohol and drug use in primary care. In: Johnson BA, editor. Addiction medicine. New York: Springer; 2010. p. 847–74.
139. Alcohol-use disorders: diagnosis, assessment and management of harmful drinking and alcohol dependence | Guidance and guidelines | NICE. Available at: http://www.nice.org.uk/guidance/cg115. Accessed November 22, 2014.
140. Smith PC, Schmidt SM, Allensworth-Davies D, et al. Primary care validation of a single-question alcohol screening test. J Gen Intern Med 2009;24(7):783–8.
141. Bradley KA, DeBenedetti AF, Volk RJ, et al. AUDIT-C as a brief screen for alcohol misuse in primary care. Alcohol Clin Exp Res 2007;31(7):1208–17.
142. Pettinati HM, Mattson ME, National Institute on Alcohol Abuse and Alcoholism (U.S.). Medical management treatment manual: a clinical research guide for medically trained clinicians providing pharmacotherapy as part of the treatment for alcohol dependence. Bethesda (MD): U.S. Dept. of Health and Human Services, National Institutes of Health, National Institute on Alcohol Abuse and Alcoholism; 2010.

143. Humeniuk R, Henry-Edwards S, Ali R, et al. The ASSIST-linked brief intervention for hazardous and harmful substance use: manual for use in primary care. Geneva (Switzerland): World Health Organization; 2010.
144. Nace EP. Twelve-step programs in addiction recovery. In: Ries R, Fiellin DA, Miller SC, et al, editors. The ASAM principles of addiction medicine. 5th edition. Philadelphia: Wolters Kluwer Health/Lippincott Williams & Wilkins; 2014. p. 1033–42.
145. Amodeo M, López LM. Making effective referrals to Alcoholics Anonymous and other 12-step programs. In: Saitz R, editor. Addressing unhealthy alcohol use in primary care. New York: Springer; 2013. p. 73–83.
146. Alcoholics Anonymous World Services. AA as a resource for the health care professional. Available at: http://www.aa.org/pages/en_US/information-for-professionals. Accessed November 22, 2014.

Care of the Homeless Patient

Jared Wilson Klein, MD, MPH[a],*, Simha Reddy, MD[b]

KEYWORDS

- Homelessness • Harm reduction • Housing first • Respite

KEY POINTS

- Homelessness is common and has devastating health consequences.
- Medical providers should devote significant attention to building rapport with homeless patients by expressing compassion through empathetic listening.
- It may be useful to tailor care for common chronic medical conditions to homeless persons' physical settings.
- Linking homeless patients to appropriate services, in particular housing, can help mitigate some adverse health effects.
- There are many vulnerable subpopulations of homeless persons who may require targeted interventions.

INTRODUCTION

Housing is one of the most fundamental human needs. Unfortunately, homelessness in the United States is a pervasive and persistent problem. The most recently available point estimate from January 2013 counted more than 600,000 Americans experiencing homelessness.[1] Still, this count likely underestimates the impact of homelessness in this country. Although many individuals are chronically homeless, many more have unstable housing and are at risk of homelessness, struggling with poverty and high housing costs as a percentage of total income. The acutely homeless may sleep in cars, double-up with friends or family, or fall in and out of shelters or other temporary living situations. Some of the most vulnerable homeless persons are so-called rough sleepers, who sleep outside and may eschew the assistance offered by shelters or other service providers (**Fig. 1**).

Disclosures: None.
[a] Division of General Internal Medicine, Department of Medicine, Harborview Medical Center, University of Washington, 325 Ninth Avenue, Box 359780, Seattle, WA 98104, USA; [b] Division of General Internal Medicine, Department of Medicine, VA Puget Sound Health Care System, University of Washington, 1660 South Columbian Way, Seattle, WA 98108, USA
* Corresponding author.
E-mail address: jaredwk@uw.edu

Med Clin N Am 99 (2015) 1017–1038
http://dx.doi.org/10.1016/j.mcna.2015.05.011   medical.theclinics.com

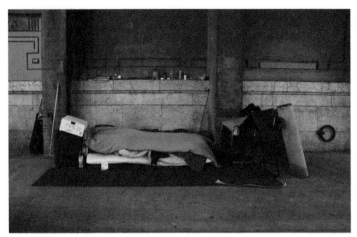

Fig. 1. Homeless man sleeping under bridge. (*From* Paris: Pixabay; 2011. Available at: http://pixabay.com/en/paris-france-city-cities-urban-187872/. Accessed December 5, 2014.)

There are complex interactions between homelessness and health.[2] Persons without adequate housing experience continuous threats to their health, whether from diseases, complications, or environmental dangers. This milieu leads to disturbingly poor health outcomes. Homeless persons have a mortality rates 3 to 4 times higher than the general population.[3] This means a young homeless man in the United States may expect to live only into his late 40s compared with a housed man who expects to live nearly until the age of 80.[4]

Simultaneously these individuals are generally less equipped to cope with various insults due to mental illness, cognitive impairment, substance use, or simply lack of adequate resources. A continual struggle between competing demands may prevent homeless persons from accessing services or following through on medical recommendations. Even if they are able to access health care services, homeless individuals may suffer discrimination or maltreatment as a result of their situations or associated comorbid conditions. This article aims to discuss general strategies when caring for homeless patients, highlight practical tips for addressing common clinical syndromes, and discuss the unique needs of vulnerable homeless subpopulations.

CLINIC VISIT

A remark from a receptionist, looks from nurses, or a provider's reluctance to shake hands—the most important moment in a clinic visit with homeless patients may occur before they ever enter the examination room. Homeless patients often report suffering discrimination in health care settings because of their homelessness[5] and are less likely to follow-up as a result. Warmth, respect, and a welcoming atmosphere are essential to building a therapeutic relationship. In addition to explicitly welcoming a patient to clinic, this is also accomplished at a systems level by accommodating walk-in appointments whenever possible. Key components of the history and physical examination are outlined in **Tables 1** and **2**, respectively (**Figs. 2** and **3**). As the visit draws to an end, it is important to carefully review the plan, which should address medical issues, how to connect to social resources, and follow-up. Because it is impossible to predict the myriad potential barriers, the plan should be created collaboratively (eg, "Do you see any obstacles to getting and taking this medication?"). Providing written instructions and an updated medication list (consider use of a

Table 1
Key components of medical history for homeless patients

Component	Examples
To build rapport, address acute concerns.	"What do you want to make sure we talk about today?"
Update personal and emergency contact information.	"How can I get in touch with you between now and your next visit?" "How do you get your mail?" "Do you accept text messages? Do you have enough minutes on your cell phone to receive calls?"[a]
Ask about specific refuge details.	"Where did you sleep last night?" "What shelter do you usually use?"
Inquire directly about common asymptomatic conditions.	"Have you ever been diagnosed with hypertension, or high blood pressure?" "Has a doctor ever told you that you have hepatitis C?"
Ask about stress and mood before directly questioning about mental health conditions.	"How have you been sleeping?" "How has your mood been lately?" "It sounds like you have been under a lot of stress recently."
Probe about food insecurity	"Where do you usually eat your meals?" "Tell me about what meals you ate yesterday?"
Inquire about personal safety.	"Do you feel safe where you are staying?" "Have you ever been harmed by someone else?"

[a] Avoid sending personal health information via texts but they can be helpful in reminding about appointments and coordinating care.

wallet-sized health card) may help improve adherence and mitigate difficulties from fragmentation of care. Neither literacy nor health literacy should be assumed ("Do you ever have trouble with reading health forms?" or "To make sure I explained it properly, can you tell me your understanding of the plan?"). The primary goal is not necessarily to gather all possible information but to provide empathetic, active listening for patients who often struggle with social isolation and to build a relationship so they are willing to return. Follow-up is essential to the plan: if a suitable way to contact a patient is unavailable, plan on having the patient return after a short interval, even if just to review laboratory results.

Table 2
Key components of the physical examination for homeless patients

Component	Examples
Skin examination	Acanthosis nigricans (insulin resistance) Spider angiomas and palmar erythema (chronic liver disease) Scars (prior surgeries or injuries)
Dental examination	Dental caries Gingivitis
Foot examination	Tinea pedis (see **Fig. 2**) Venous insufficiency and chronic edema (see **Fig. 3**) Exposure (immersion foot, trench foot, frostbite) Infection (cellulitis and abscess) Stress fractures and overuse injuries

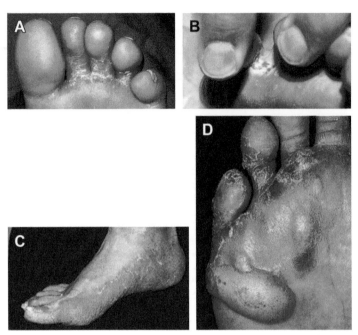

Fig. 2. Tinea pedis. (*A*) Interdigital tinea pedis. (*B*) White macerated web between fourth and fifth toes. (*C*) Moccasin distribution of tinea pedis. (*D*) Bullous tinea. (*From* White G, Cox N. Diseases of the skin. 2nd edition. St Louis (MO): Mosby; 2006; with permission.)

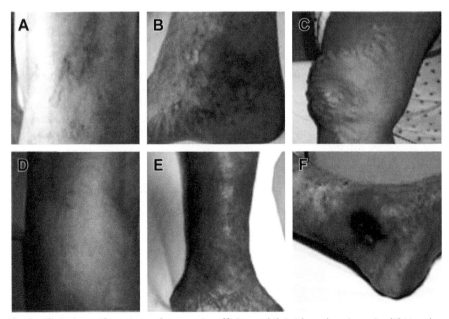

Fig. 3. Clinical manifestations of venous insufficiency. (*A*) Spider telangiectasia. (*B*) Venulectasia in a corona phlebectatica distribution. (*C*) Tributary varicose vein. (*D*) Reticular varicose vein. (*E*) Lipodermatosclerosis. (*F*) Venous ulceration. (*From* Fan C. Venous insufficiency. In: Abbara S, Kalva SP, editors. Problem solving in cardiovascular imaging. Philadelphia: Saunders; 2013. p. 800–12; with permission.)

SPECIFIC MANAGEMENT
Diabetes Mellitus

Homeless diabetics typically suffer from poor glycemic control and several barriers to adequate disease management.[6] The treatment of diabetes in this population should focus on simplifying regimens, patient education, and avoiding extremes of blood glucose. If using insulin, it is preferable to use insulin pens whenever possible, because they lead to greater adherence and improved control and may be less likely to be stolen than standard needles and syringes.[7] Although insulin lasts longer if refrigerated, it should generally last a full month if kept at reasonable temperatures; patients can minimize heat degradation by not keeping the insulin right next to their skin. Food insecurity is clearly a major barrier to good diabetes control, and efforts should be made to ensure patients have access to all available food resources in their community. They should also be advised about better and worse food choices, even when selection is limited. If using prandial insulin or a sulfonylurea, patients should be reminded that it should not be used if food is unavailable, a situation that tends to arise more frequently toward the end of each month. Patients should also receive extensive education on the symptoms of hypo- and hyperglycemia. Being on one's feet all day, along with a lack of sufficient clean, dry socks or access to well-fitting shoes all increase the risk of diabetic foot complications. Careful attention should be paid to the feet and, whenever possible, patients should be provided with new socks during clinic visits.

Hypertension

The rate of poorly controlled hypertension is greater in the homeless community than among domiciled patients.[8] Chronic stress, smoking, drug and alcohol use, and lack of healthy food all contribute to elevated pressures. Interviews with homeless hypertensive patients demonstrate the importance of clear education around the topic.[9] Because health literacy varies dramatically, it is important to clearly state that "hypertension" means "high blood pressure," and to ensure that patients understand it as a long-term, typically silent problem. For those who do experience symptomatic hypertension, they may be under the impression that when the headache or dyspnea has gone away, so has the problem. This has implications for whether patients use their medications on a regular basis or only as needed, when symptoms arise.

With only half of homeless smokers reporting having been advised to quit, there is room for greater counseling on therapeutic lifestyle changes, albeit with sensitivity to the numerous barriers homeless patients may face.[10] These may include a lack of control over available food, a lack of understanding of specific recommendations, the influence of family or friends, lack of access to exercise equipment, or even habit and enjoyment of the unhealthy activity.[11] Counseling in these situations likely requires creative problem solving with patients, such as finding safe places to walk or minimizing sodium in shelter food by foregoing items like gravy. If available at a subsidized cost, nicotine replacement therapy can be proffered as both a safer and potentially more cost-effective solution than cigarettes. A special emphasis should be placed on avoidance of the highest risk activities, such as cocaine use. Even if a patient does not quit, a reduction in frequency or amount used may diminish the risk of stroke, and this connection can be made explicit to the patient.

In choosing an antihypertensive regimen, the likelihood of follow-up should be taken into account. If there is concern that a patient will not be able to come in for follow-up laboratory tests, a patient should be steered toward a calcium channel blocker rather than angiotensin-converting enzyme inhibitor, angiotensin-receptor blocker, or diuretic. Diuretics have an added downside of increased urination in a population with limited access to bathrooms, although in some settings they may be the most cost-effective option.

Cardiovascular Disease

A common cause of death in this marginalized population is cardiovascular disease, with cardiovascular disease 3 times more common in homeless aged 25 to 44 compared with their age-matched peers.[11] The homeless are more likely to have underdiagnosed and undertreated predisposing conditions, such as hypertension and diabetes.[2] This is in addition to a higher rate of smoking, higher rate of substance abuse, and chronic stress. All of these lead inexorably to earlier death and greater morbidity due to myocardial infarction and stroke.

When focused on secondary prevention, medication counseling is paramount. A patient with a prior history of myocardial infarction and heart failure may be prescribed a dizzying number of medications, all of which have a potential benefit. Even though several pharmacies have low-cost plans, patients may not be able to afford the copays, or the cost of replacing stolen medications. Ideally, patients can be connected to assistance programs or charity care. At times, it may be necessary to prioritize medications for patients (eg, emphasizing the need for aspirin and clopidogrel in a patient with a recent stent). Additionally, discussion of how to use medications may be beneficial, such as reminding patients to use diuretics whenever is most convenient for them in terms of bathroom access, rather than at fixed times.

Lung Disease

With the rate of smoking reaching 4 times that of the general population, it is no surprise that chronic obstructive pulmonary disease (COPD) is also more common.[2,12] In addition, the greater exposure to sick contacts and close quarters increases the risk of COPD exacerbations, and patients should be strongly encouraged to get vaccinated against influenza and *Streptococcus pneumoniae*. In addition to simplifying medication regimens as much as possible (eg, daily dosing with long-acting agents), attention should be paid to inhaler technique to optimize effectiveness.

The provision of medical equipment for COPD and obstructive sleep apnea offers unique logistical challenges. In patients with a need for supplemental oxygen, some shelters may be willing to accept delivery of tanks, but this should not be assumed and should be arranged prior to discharge if patients are in the hospital. Those in need of continuous positive airway pressure/bilevel positive airway pressure machines may not have regular access to electricity, especially at night, so battery-operated machines may be beneficial if available. Alternatively, a dental appliance may be a reasonable alternative.

Hepatitis and Chronic Liver Disease

Nowhere is the complex interaction between housing, mental health, and physical health better exemplified than in the care of a homeless patient with liver disease. Compared with the general population, the rates of hepatitis B, hepatitis C, and alcohol dependence are all significantly higher.[2] Complications of liver disease are a common cause of death among the homeless.[13]

The prevention of liver disease begins with counseling on risk reduction, which may involve discussion of alcohol or intravenous substance use, referral to a needle exchange program, or provision of condoms to promote safer sex. Screening at least once for hepatitis C is recommended, but more frequent screening should be considered for those at increased risk.[14] The recent development of rapid hepatitis C antibody screening allows for the testing of individuals who otherwise may not return for laboratory results. With regard to the physical examination, attention should be paid to traditional stigmata of liver disease but also more disease-specific findings, such as porphyria cutanea tarda (**Fig. 4**) or leukocytoclastic vasculitis (**Fig. 5**).

Once chronic liver disease is discovered, through laboratory tests, imaging, or physical examination, strategies for treatment should be carefully considered. Despite the recent development of shorter, more effective treatment regimens for hepatitis C, it may be reasonable to delay treatment of most homeless patients until housing is achieved to achieve optimal efficacy. Although almost all treatments now spare interferon, the regimens remain expensive and require frequent follow-up.

Regarding treating the complications of end-stage liver disease, adjustment in the approach to medications may improve compliance. In treating hepatic encephalopathy, the use of rifaximin rather than lactulose has the advantage of not requiring easy access to a toilet, although it can be prohibitively expensive. When lactulose or diuretics are needed to treat complications of end-stage liver disease, patients can be counseled to use them whenever they believe they will have bathroom access rather than insisting on fixed times.

Human Immunodeficiency Virus

HIV testing is recommended for all patients at least once and more often when at increased risk. As discussed previously, counseling on safe needle and sex practices may aid in prevention. The use of rapid HIV testing is more practical and less invasive than the traditional venipunctur and has been used in several outreach settings.[15]

Current guidelines suggest all HIV infected patients begin treatment as soon as possible. Although lack of housing is associated with decreased medication adherence, homelessness should not by itself be considered a contraindication to begin treatment with antiretrovirals.[16] Rather, the goal should be to choose an appropriate regimen and provide support around taking it regularly. Generally, in choosing a regimen, the major considerations are resistance patterns, prior treatment regimens, side effects, and convenience. When adherence is a concern, some providers choose regimens with a higher barrier to resistance, such as protease inhibitors, even at the expense of convenience. Yet, one study among seropositive homeless patients found

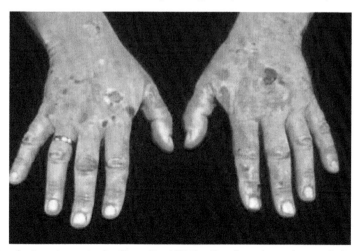

Fig. 4. Porphyria cutanea tarda. (*From* Ferri FF. Ferri's color atlas and text of clinical medicine. Philadelphia: Saunders; 2009. p. 44–5; with permission.)

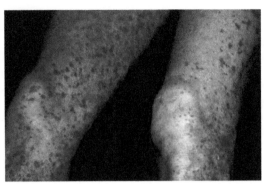

Fig. 5. Hepatitis C–associated vasculitis. (*From* Shinkai K, Fox LP. Cutaneous vasculitis. In: Bolognia JL, Jorizzo JL, Schaffer JV, editors. Dermatology. Amsterdam: Elsevier Limited; 2012. p. 385–410.e2; with permission.)

that the use of once daily combination efavirenz/tenofovir/emtricitabine (Atripla) was associated with greater adherence and virologic control than a multiple pill protease inhibitor–based regimen.[17] The potential psychiatric effects of efavirenz, however, should be carefully considered before prescribing it for anyone struggling with mental illness. Other currently approved once-daily combinations include emtricitabine/rilpivirine/tenofovir (Complera), abacavir/dolutegravir/lamivudine (Triumeq), and elvitegravir, cobicistat, emtricitabine, tenofovir (Stribild), each of which has its own particular considerations but does not have significant neuropsychiatric effects.

Finally, due to both federal funding and several charitable organizations, HIV-infected patients may be eligible for unique housing and other local social support resources. They should be connected to local HIV/AIDS organizations to help facilitate such referrals.

Outbreaks and Infestations

Contagious infectious diseases have long been a concern among homeless patients, particularly those using shelters given the close contact that typically occurs in this setting. Contact tracing can be particularly challenging and the numbers of exposures are typically high among homeless populations, complicating management during outbreaks.[18] General hygiene measures are highly recommended for homeless patients in shelters, including hand hygiene, covering coughs or sneezes, and avoiding contact with bodily fluids.

The most widely studied infectious agents among homeless populations are tuberculosis and influenza. There are regularly outbreaks of tuberculosis among homeless persons living in shelters, and homelessness remains a risk factor for tuberculosis, particularly among patients with comorbid HIV infection.[19] That said, the majority of tuberculosis cases diagnosed in the United States occurs in foreign-born patients. Options for tuberculosis control include screening staff and clients, improved ventilation, and utilization of UV lights for decontamination.[20] Influenza is similarly likely to spread in the close quarters found in most homeless shelters.[21] In addition to the routine hygiene measures discussed previously, vaccination can be particularly effective for controlling the spread of flu.[22]

The homeless population is at increased risk of exposure to cutaneous parasites, and the index of suspicion should be high for homeless patients presenting with pruritic papules or vesicles.[23] The distribution of lesions and physical examination should help differentiate between scabies (**Figs. 6** and **7**), bedbugs (**Fig. 8**), body lice (**Figs. 9**

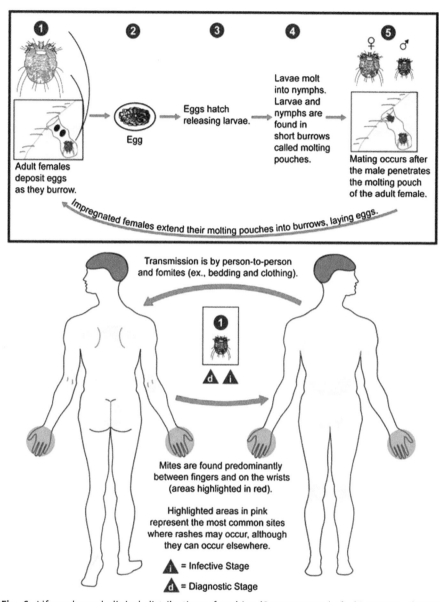

Fig. 6. Life-cycle and clinical distribution of scabies (*Sarcoptes scabei*). (*Courtesy of* CDC/ Alexander J. da Silva, PhD/Melanie Moser, BS, Atlanta, GA; with permission.)

and **10**), and fleas (**Table 3**). Complications can arise from secondary bacterial infections. The treatment of bedbugs and fleas is focused on symptom relief of the hypersensitivity reaction and attempting to control exposure to the parasites. In the treatment of scabies, permethrin cream is ideal, but oral ivermectin may also be used if a patient is unable to apply the cream. Permethrin may also be used in the treatment of body and head lice, but the more effective treatment is effective removal

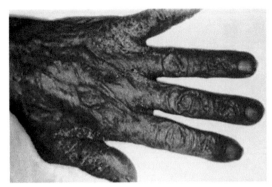

Fig. 7. Scabies rash. Dorsal view of an older patient's hand demonstrating a crusted scabies infestation by the scabies mite, *Sarcoptes scabiei*. Note the localized crusting in the interdigital web spaces. (*Courtesy of* Reed and Carnrich Pharmaceuticals/CDC, 1975.)

of the parasite through laundering clothes and bedding at high temperature as well as shaving if needed.

Mental Health

An estimated 25% to 50% of people with serious mental illness suffer from homelessness at some point in their life.[24] In turn, homelessness often exacerbates underlying mental illness as well as precipitating depression and anxiety. The most successful interventions for homeless patients with serious mental illness have revolved around case management and permanent supportive housing, and patients should be referred to such programs whenever possible. Such programs have been shown to

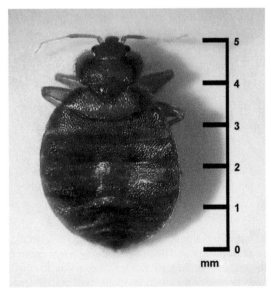

Fig. 8. Adult bedbug, *Cimex lectularius*. (*Courtesy of* CDC/CDC-DPDx; Blaine Mathison, BS, Atlanta, GA; with permission.)

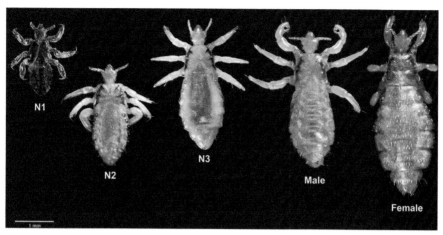

Fig. 9. Body lice. Nymphal-staged lice (stage 1, stage 2, and stage 3) and adult lice (male and female). (*Courtesy of* CDC/Joseph Strycharz, PhD, Kyong Sup Yoon, PhD, Frank Collins, PhD, Atlanta, GA; James Gathany, BS; with permission.)

lead to better quality of life, reduction in substance use, and decreased need for intensive support services.[25,26]

With regard to pharmacologic treatment, patients with significant difficulty holding onto and taking medications may benefit from depot preparations of antipsychotics. Otherwise, it is important to discuss with patients how they want medications dispensed. Because of theft, some patients may wish to have more frequent fills of smaller amounts.

Trauma and Injuries

Trauma, defined as actual or threatened danger to the physical integrity of self or another person, can be an almost daily experience for many homeless persons. Even after adjusting for comorbidities, homeless patients are more likely to suffer unintentional and intentional injuries, including assaults and self-inflicted wounds.[27] Particularly common injuries include pedestrian versus motor vehicle collisions,

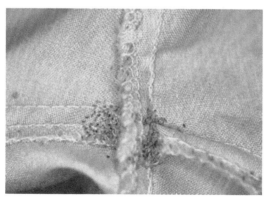

Fig. 10. Body lice eggs in the seams of clothing. (*From* Bolognia JL, Schaffer JV, Duncan KO, et al. Infestations. In: Dermatology essentials. Amsterdam: Elsevier; 2014. p. 701–9; with permission.)

Table 3
Characteristics of cutaneous parasites

Diagnosis	Clinical Presentation
Scabies	Burrows and excoriations in the hands, axilla, and inguinal regions
Bedbugs	Small red papules in areas not covered by bedclothes
Body lice	Distribution can vary; lice or eggs can often be found on clothing
Fleas	Hemorrhagic papules typically over ankles

traumatic brain injuries, falls, stab wounds, and other penetrating trauma. Certain vulnerable populations might be particularly at risk for domestic and interpersonal violence (discussed previously).[28] Many argue that the state of homelessness is itself a traumatic experience with profound loss and sense of neglect. Patients are often left with significant physical impairments, including amputations, cognitive impairment, and chronic pain.

These various insults and injuries take an emotional as well as physical toll on patients. To appropriately and sensitively broach the subject of trauma, clinicians caring for homeless patients should be aware of the principles of trauma-informed care (**Table 4**).[29] Training of providers and staff is important and integration or linkage to appropriate mental health services is crucial. Clinicians should recognize the cardinal symptoms of posttraumatic stress disorder (PTSD), including hypervigilance, intrusive thoughts (flashbacksand nightmares), and dissociation. Multidisciplinary teams can be helpful in managing patients' PTSD symptoms by using techniques such as cognitive behavioral therapy and exposure therapy.[30] The cornerstone of pharmacotherapy is the selective serotonin reuptake inhibitor class of medications (**Table 5**), but prazosin can be particularly helpful if there are predominant nightmare symptoms.

Substance Use Disorders

Addiction is a particularly challenging, yet all too common, condition among homeless persons. Unfortunately it can be challenging to treat when patients remain unhoused.[31] A multidisciplinary model with strong case management is recommended. The most important role of the clinician when caring for an addicted homeless patient is to address the substance use directly while maintaining empathy. In addition to providing encouragement, clinicians should be prepared to prescribe pharmacotherapy for homeless persons with substance use disorders.

Table 4
Trauma-informed care principles

Domain	Examples
Trauma awareness	• Screening for trauma • Staff education and training • Patient education
Safety	• Physically and emotionally safe environment • Respectful, culturally competent • Avoid retraumatization
Empowerment	• Supporting patient choice and autonomy • Shared decision making • Patient engagement
Resiliency	• Instill hope • Highlight strengths and opportunities

Table 5			
Commonly used selective serotonin reuptake inhibitors			
Medication	**Brand Name**	**Dosing**	**Side Effects**
Fluoxetine	Prozac	20–80 mg Daily	Gastrointestinal upset, headache,
Sertraline	Zoloft	50–200 mg Daily	xerostomia, sexual dysfunction,
Paroxetine	Paxil	20–50 mg Daily	tremor, suicidality
Citalopram	Celexa	20–40 mg Daily	

For patients with alcohol use disorders, there are 3 Food and Drug Administration–approved medications that can be considered (**Table 6**). Patients with opioid use disorders who are interested in treatment should either be referred to methadone maintenance programs or treated with buprenorphine.[32,33] The more structured and supportive environment of methadone maintenance programs may be important, especially for patients who have comorbid mental health diagnoses or polysubstance use disorders. There is a dearth of evidence supporting pharmacotherapy for other illicit substances, in particular stimulants, such as cocaine and methamphetamines. In these situations, behavioral interventions are recommended, including 12-step programs, cognitive behavioral therapy, and motivational interviewing.[34,35]

Chronic Pain

Chronic pain is more prevalent among homeless patients than the general population, with up to two-thirds of patients reporting pain lasting greater than 3 months.[36] A surprisingly high proportion of physicians are entirely unaware of pain complaints among their homeless patients, making it is especially important for clinicians to inquire about pain when seeing unhoused patients.[37]

As with housed patients, homeless patients with chronic pain are best served by a multidisciplinary approach (**Box 1**). Behavioral health interventions might be useful in a motivated patient. Targeted physical therapy and manual approaches should be offered, but acceptance could be limited by cost or competing demands. Similarly,

Table 6					
Medications for alcohol use disorder					
Medication	**Brand Name**	**Dosing**	**Cost**	**Efficacy**	**Side Effects**
Naltrexone	Revia (oral), Vivitrol (IM)	50 mg Daily (oral), 380 mg Monthly (IM)	$$ (oral), $$$ (IM)	Reduces cravings and consumption, not good for abstinence	Hepatotoxicity, suicidality, cannot use if taking opioids
Acamprosate	Campral	333–666 mg TID	$	Modestly effective, adherence difficult	Gastrointestinal upset, depression or anxiety
Disulfiram	Antabuse	250–500 mg Daily	$	Best with motivated patient in monitored program	Hepatotoxicity, neuropathy

Abbreviations: $, least expensive; $$$, most expensive; IM, intramuscular.

Box 1
Nonopioid strategies for managing chronic pain

Behavioral interventions
- Cognitive behavioral therapy
- Biofeedback

Manual interventions
- Physical therapy
- Massage
- Acupuncture
- Ice or heat
- Transcutaneous electrical nerve stimulation unit

Nonopioid pharmacotherapy
- Acetaminophen
- NSAIDs
- Neuropathic agents (gabapentin, TCAs, etc.)
- Topical agents (lidocaine, capsaicin, methyl salicylate, menthol, etc.)

Procedural interventions
- Steroid injections (intra-articular, epidural, etc.)
- Hyaluronan injections

---

thermal modalities and electrical neuromodulation often are difficult for homeless patients lacking access to refrigeration, electricity, or secure storage.

Nonopioid medications are first line for the management of chronic pain. Acetaminophen in low to moderate doses is almost always safe. For select patients, nonsteroidal anti-inflammatory drugs (NSAIDs) are an acceptable option. Agents targeting neuropathic pain, such as gabapentin and tricyclic antidepressants (TCAs), are often helpful and typically have a safer side-effect profile than opioids, although there is a small risk of intentional or unintentional overdose with TCAs. Some patients find relief from topical analgesics. Injections have the benefit of immediate administration, without the need for ongoing monitoring by the clinician or a pill burden for the patient.

Understandably, there is often reluctance to prescribe opioid medications to homeless patients in the setting of comorbid substance use disorders, concern about follow-up and monitoring requirements, or uncertainty about the security of medications. As with all patients, opioids should be used with extreme caution and only at low to moderate doses when prescribed for chronic noncancer pain. If prescribed, a small supply with more frequent refills might reduce the chance of having opioids misplaced or stolen.

Preventive Services

Preventive care for homeless patients often loses priority in light of more pressing health concerns. That said, vaccines are excellent interventions that require no follow-up. Standard vaccine schedules should be followed, as recommended by the Advisory Committee on Immunization Practices (**Fig. 11**).[38] Special attention should be paid to indications for administration of the 13-valent conjugate pneumococcal

Recommended adult immunization schedule, by vaccine and age group[1]

VACCINE ▼	AGE GROUP ►	19–21 years	22–26 years	27–49 years	50–59 years	60–64 years	≥65 years
Influenza [2,*]		1 dose annually					
Tetanus, diphtheria, pertussis (Td/Tdap) [3,*]		Substitute 1-time dose of Tdap for Td booster; then boost with Td every 10 yrs					
Varicella [4,*]		2 doses					
Human papillomavirus (HPV) Female [5,*]		3 doses					
Human papillomavirus (HPV) Male [5,*]		3 doses					
Zoster [6]						1 dose	
Measles, mumps, rubella (MMR) [7,*]		1 or 2 doses					
Pneumococcal 13-valent conjugate (PCV13) [8,*]		1 dose					
Pneumococcal polysaccharide (PPSV23) [9,10]		1 or 2 doses					1 dose
Meningococcal [11,*]		1 or more doses					
Hepatitis A [12,*]		2 doses					
Hepatitis B [13,*]		3 doses					
Haemophilus influenzae type b (Hib) [14,*]		1 or 3 doses					

For all persons in this category who meet the age requirements and who lack documentation of vaccination or have no evidence of previous infection; zoster vaccine recommended regardless of prior episode of zoster

Recommended if some other risk factor is present (e.g., on the basis of medical, occupational, lifestyle, or other indication)

No recommendation

Report all clinically significant postvaccination reactions to the Vaccine Adverse Event Reporting System (VAERS). Reporting forms and instructions on filing a VAERS report are available at www.vaers.hhs.gov or by telephone, 800-822-7967.

Information on how to file a Vaccine Injury Compensation Program claim is available at www.hrsa.gov/vaccinecompensation or by telephone, 800-338-2382. To file a claim for vaccine injury, contact the U.S. Court of Federal Claims, 717 Madison Place, N.W., Washington, D.C. 20005; telephone, 202-357-6400.

Additional information about the vaccines in this schedule, extent of available data, and contraindications for vaccination is also available at www.cdc.gov/vaccines or from the CDC-INFO Contact Center at 800-CDC-INFO (800-232-4636) in English and Spanish, 8:00 a.m.–8:00 p.m. Eastern Time, Monday - Friday, excluding holidays.

Use of trade names and commercial sources is for identification only and does not imply endorsement by the U.S. Department of Health and Human Services.

The recommendations in this schedule were approved by the Centers for Disease Control and Prevention's (CDC) Advisory Committee on Immunization Practices (ACIP), the American Academy of Family Physicians (AAFP), the American College of Physicians (ACP), American College of Obstetricians and Gynecologists (ACOG) and American College of Nurse-Midwives (ACNM).

Vaccines that might be indicated for adults based on medical and other indications[1]

VACCINE ▼	INDICATION ►	Pregnancy	Immuno-compromising conditions (excluding human immunodeficiency virus [HIV]) [4,6,7,8,15]	HIV infection CD4 + T lymphocyte count [4,6,7,8,15] <200 cells/μL	≥200 cells/μL	Men who have sex with men (MSM)	Kidney failure, end-stage renal disease, receipt of hemodialysis	Heart disease, chronic lung disease, chronic alcoholism	Asplenia (including elective splenectomy and persistent complement component deficiencies) [8,14]	Chronic liver disease	Diabetes	Healthcare personnel
Influenza [2,*]		1 dose IIV annually		1 dose IIV or LAIV annually		1 dose IIV annually						1 dose IIV or LAIV annually
Tetanus, diphtheria, pertussis (Td/Tdap) [3,*]		1 dose Tdap each pregnancy	Substitute 1-time dose of Tdap for Td booster; then boost with Td every 10 yrs									
Varicella [4,*]		Contraindicated			2 doses							
Human papillomavirus (HPV) Female [5,*]		3 doses through age 26 yrs			3 doses through age 26 yrs							
Human papillomavirus (HPV) Male [5,*]		3 doses through age 26 yrs			3 doses through age 21 yrs							
Zoster [6]		Contraindicated			1 dose							
Measles, mumps, rubella (MMR) [7,*]		Contraindicated			1 or 2 doses							
Pneumococcal 13-valent conjugate (PCV13) [8,*]		1 dose										
Pneumococcal polysaccharide (PPSV23) [9,10]		1 or 2 doses										
Meningococcal [11,*]		1 or more doses										
Hepatitis A [12,*]		2 doses										
Hepatitis B [13,*]		3 doses										
Haemophilus influenzae type b (Hib) [14,*]		post-HSCT recipients only	1 or 3 doses									

For all persons in this category who meet the age requirements and who lack documentation of vaccination or have no evidence of previous infection; zoster vaccine recommended regardless of prior episode of zoster

Recommended if some other risk factor is present (e.g., on the basis of medical, occupational, lifestyle, or other indications)

No recommendation

These schedules indicate the recommended age groups and medical indications for which administration of currently licensed vaccines is commonly indicated for adults ages 19 years and older, as of February 1, 2014. For all vaccines being recommended on the Adult Immunization Schedule: a vaccine series does not need to be restarted, regardless of the time that has elapsed between doses. Licensed combination vaccines may be used whenever any components of the combination are indicated and when the vaccine's other components are not contraindicated. For detailed recommendations on all vaccines, including those used primarily for travelers or that are issued during the year, consult the manufacturers' package inserts and the complete statements from the Advisory Committee on Immunization Practices (www.cdc.gov/vaccines/hcp/acip-recs/index.html). Use of trade names and commercial sources is for identification only and does not imply endorsement by the U.S. Department of Health and Human Services.

Fig. 11. Adult immunization schedules, United States, 2014. Note: These recommendations must be read with the footnotes that follow containing number of doses, intervals between doses, and other important information. (*From* Centers for Disease Control and Prevention, Advisory Committee on Immunization Practices (ACIP). Adult immunization schedules, United States, 2014. Available at: http://www.cdc.gov/vaccines/schedules/hcp/adult.html. Accessed October 30, 2014.)

vaccine and the 23-valent polysaccharide pneumococcal vaccine (**Box 2**). It is crucial to vaccinate patients for influenza. Given higher rates of injuries and trauma, vaccination with the tetanus diphtheria vaccine is important. Current recommendations call for 1-time use of the adult tetanus, diphtheria, acellular pertussis vaccine, which also provides protection against the causative organism for whooping cough.

Box 2
Major indications for pneumococcal vaccination in adults

13-Valent Conjugate Vaccine	23-Valent Polysaccharide Vaccine
Age over 65 y	Age over 65 y
Immunocompromise	Immunocompromise
• HIV infection	• HIV infection
• Solid organ transplantation	• Solid organ transplantation
• Generalized malignancy	• Generalized malignancy
• Leukemia, lymphoma, or multiple myeloma	• Leukemia, lymphoma, or multiple myeloma
• Iatrogenic immunosuppression (including chronic steroids)	• Iatrogenic immunosuppression (including chronic steroids)
Functional or anatomic asplenia	Functional or anatomic asplenia
Chronic kidney disease	Chronic kidney disease
—	Cigarette smoking
—	Alcoholism
—	Diabetes mellitus
—	Chronic lung disease
—	Chronic liver disease
—	Chronic heart disease

Administer pneumococcal conjugate vaccine 13, first, then pneumococcal polysaccharide vaccine 23, 12 months later.

Other preventive services should be offered, but clinicians must give careful consideration to a patient's living situation (**Box 3**). For example, collection of stool sample for occult blood testing or colonoscopy preparation may be difficult or impossible while living in a shelter or on the streets.[39] Providers should collect contact information and try to ensure a reliable follow-up plan when performing cancer screening so that abnormal Papanicolaou smear or mammogram results will lead to appropriate subsequent testing and treatment.

SPECIFIC POPULATIONS
Women and Children

Upwards of 40% of the homeless population is composed of families, frequently single mothers with young children. Domestic or interpersonal violence is common and may even contribute to homelessness among women.[40]

Box 3
Homeless diagnostic panel

• Basic metabolic panel

• Lipid panel

• Hemoglobin A_{1c}

• HIV testing

• Viral hepatitis panel (A, B, C)

• Interferon gamma release assay (or tuberculin skin test)

Lack of adequate housing has multiple consequences for a family unit. A majority of families are broken up to obtain emergency housing, because most shelters are segregated by gender.[41] School-age children may fall behind educational milestones and often experience significant psychological distress as a result of homelessness. Parents are also at increased risk of mental health problems, including depression and even suicide attempt.[42] It is important to connect these patients with social services, including adequate housing and employment opportunities.

Teens

Approximately one-half million adolescents and young adults are homeless in the United States any given year.[43] Although many leave home only temporarily, some become chronically homeless. Many of these youths have experienced physical or sexual abuse in their previous living situation. They are less likely to complete high school and have high rates of HIV infection, substance use, and mental health disorders compared with housed peers.[44] Connecting these vulnerable patients with care can be challenging given mistrust of authority figures and lack of social skills. Targeted programs that have been adapted for adolescent needs and preferences may be helpful as are efforts to reconnect youths to functional families.[45]

Older Adults and Elders

In general, homelessness is uncommon among people over 65 years of age. This is likely due to a combination of social supports available to this age cohort (subsidized housing programs, Social Security income, Medicare, and so forth) as well as decreased life expectancy among homeless persons.[46] Despite these factors, there is a growing cohort of homeless over age 50, which is at least partially due to the aging baby boomers. These older adults are more likely than younger homeless persons to have health problems and cognitive deficits and require more intensive services.[47] Multidisciplinary teams with an emphasis on acquiring stable housing and addressing chronic illness have been proposed as key steps to caring for this highly vulnerable subset of homeless patients.[48]

Veterans

Veterans are overrepresented among the homeless population, accounting for just over 12% of all homeless adults.[49] Veterans have often suffered physical and emotional wounds during their time in service, even if they did not serve on a battlefield, increasing their risk of homelessness. In response to this crisis, however, the Department of Veterans Affairs embarked on an audacious goal at the beginning of 2010 to end veteran homelessness within 5 years. Although this has not been achieved, veteran homelessness has dropped by 33% in that time frame.[50] This can be attributed to comprehensive services for homeless veterans that include job training, short-term housing support, transitional housing, permanent supportive housing, and specialized primary care and outreach efforts. Homeless veterans and their families should be connected to local Veterans Affairs resources whenever possible. Even veterans not typically eligible for health care may have some housing options available to them.

Lesbian, Gay, Bisexual, and Transgender

Studies have shown that lesbian, gay, bisexual, and transgender (LGBT) homeless persons are highly vulnerable. They are more frequently victimized and have higher rates of substance use and mental health disorders compared with heterosexual homeless persons.[51] Many are adolescents whose sexual orientation has been rejected by their families.[52] Key strategies in caring for homeless LGBT patients involve creation of a safe and inclusive environment, asking about sexual orientation and gender identity in an open and nonjudgmental manner, encouraging nondiscrimination among staff, and using appropriate pronouns.[53]

FUTURE DIRECTIONS
Housing

The past several decades have seen 2 major innovations in housing. In rapid rehousing, homeless clients are provided with short-term relief, such as move-in costs and first month's rent, to help people get back on their feet. The hope is to prevent an acute homeless episode from becoming chronic homelessness. Retention in housing at 1 year is typically greater than 85%.[54]

Permanent supportive housing, on the other hand, focuses on chronically homeless clients, getting them into either individual apartments or into project-based housing. Typically the client pays some proportion of their income in rent rather than a fixed amount. This is coupled with ongoing case management to prevent relapse into homelessness. These interventions have demonstrated significant success, with greater retention in housing and dramatically lower costs to the system.[31]

Medical Respite

Over the past decade there has been growing recognition that many homeless patients with acute medical issues are too sick to recover on the streets but do not meet criteria for hospital admission. In response, medical respite facilities have been expanding nationwide to provide acute and postacute care for homeless patients. Medical respites provide a diverse array of services, including wound care, intravenous antibiotics, and short-term medication monitoring.[55] These programs also link patients with necessary services, such as addiction treatment, mental health care, and transitional housing. Services are delivered in a variety of settings: on-site at emergency shelters, in freestanding facilities, or within nursing homes. Several studies have shown a reduction in hospital length of stay and readmission among homeless patients treated at medical respites, making this a promising intervention.[56,57]

Palliative Care

One particularly difficult issue is providing palliative care to the homeless, an area of ongoing research. Palliative care providers or teams focused on the terminally ill homeless can bring significant relief to an extraordinarily vulnerable group of patients.[58]

Alternative Approaches to Primary Care for Homeless Patients

Because of the unique challenges posed by this population, some primary care clinics and providers have come to specialize in homeless health. Health Care for the Homeless is a network of federally funded providers and clinics that has been functioning since the mid-1980s. They use a variety of approaches, often incorporating outreach and case management, as well as offering excellent practical resources to other providers.[59] The Veterans Health Administration has also recently begun to offer medical homes focused on homeless veterans, demonstrating reductions in emergency department use with high-intensity services.[60]

SUMMARY

Providing medical care to homeless patients can be both challenging and extremely rewarding. Many of the principles discussed in this article are applicable to all patients but may be particularly effective in engaging and building trust with homeless persons. This article includes multiple practical suggestions for how to approach specific clinical dilemmas that are commonly seen in homeless patients and attempts to provide insight regarding specific vulnerable homeless populations. In addition to providing outstanding clinical care to homeless patients, clinicians have a role in advocating for systemic change to address structural and societal factors that contribute to homelessness.[61]

REFERENCES

1. The State of Homelessness in America. National alliance to end homelessness. 2014. Available at: http://www.endhomelessness.org/library/entry/the-state-of-homelessness-2014. Accessed October 9, 2014.
2. Fazel S, Geddes JR, Kushel M. The health of homeless people in high-income countries: descriptive epidemiology, health consequences, and clinical and policy recommendations. Lancet 2014;384:1529–40.
3. O'Connell JJ. Premature mortality in homeless populations: a review of the literature. Nashville (TN): National Health Care for the Homeless Council, Inc; 2005. Available at: http://www.nhchc.org/wp-content/uploads/2011/10/Premature-Mortality.pdf.
4. World Health Organization Global Health Observatory Data Repository. Available at: http://apps.who.int/gho/data/node.main.688?lang=en. Accessed October 16, 2014.
5. Wen CK, Hudak PL, Hwang SW. Homeless people's perceptions of welcomeness and unwelcomeness in healthcare encounters. J Gen Intern Med 2007;22:1011–7.
6. Hwang SW, Bugeja AL. Barriers to appropriate diabetes management among homeless people in Toronto. CMAJ 2000;163(2):161–5.
7. Wilk T, Mora PF, Chaney S, et al. Use of an insulin pen by homeless patients with diabetes mellitus. J Am Acad Nurse Pract 2002;14(8):372–80.
8. Lee TC, Hanlon JG, Ben-David J, et al. Risk factors for cardiovascular disease in homeless adults. Circulation 2005;111:2629–35.
9. Moczygemba LR, Kennedy AK, Marks SA, et al. A qualitative analysis of perceptions and barriers to therapeutic lifestyle changes among homeless hypertensive patients. Res Social Adm Pharm 2013;9:467–81.
10. Baggett TP. Cigarette smoking and advice to quit in a national sample of homeless adults. Am J Prev Med 2010;39:164–72.
11. Jones CA, Perera A, Chow M, et al. Cardiovascular disease risk among the poor and homeless – what we know so far. Curr Cardiol Rev 2009;5:69–77.
12. Snyder LD, Eisner MD. Obstructive lung disease among the urban homeless. Chest 2004;125(5):1719–25.
13. Hibbs JR, Benner L, Klugman L, et al. Mortality in a cohort of homeless adults in Philadelphia. N Engl J Med 1994;331(5):304–9.
14. Bharel M, Creaven B, Morris G, et al. Health care delivery strategies: addressing key preventive health measures in homeless health care settings. Nashville (TN): Health Care for the Homeless Clinicians' Network, National Health Care for the Homeless Council, Inc; 2011.
15. Bucher JB, Thomas KM, Guzman D, et al. Community-based rapid HIV testing in homeless and marginally housed adults in San Francisco. HIV Med 2007;8(1):28–31.

16. Kidder DP, Wolitski RJ, Campsmith ML, et al. Health status, health care use, medication use, and medication adherence among homeless and housed people living with HIV/AIDS. Am J Public Health 2007;97(12):2238–45.
17. Bansberg DR. A single tablet regimen is associated with higher adherence and viral suppression than multiple tablet regimens in HIV+ homeless and marginally housed people. AIDS 2010;24(18):2835–40.
18. Hwang SW, Kiss A, Ho MM, et al. Infectious disease exposures and contact tracing in homeless shelters. J Health Care Poor Underserved 2008;19(4): 1163–7.
19. Centers for Disease Control and Prevention. Homelessness is a risk-factor for TB. 2014. Available at: http://www.cdc.gov/features/dstb2011data/. Accessed November 10, 2014.
20. Gore B, Smith K. Tuberculosis infection control: a practical manual for preventing TB, 2011. San Francisco (CA): Curry International Tuberculosis Center; 2011. Available at: http://www.currytbcenter.ucsf.edu/TB_IC/docs/IC_book_2011.pdf. Accessed November 10, 2014.
21. Bucher SJ, Brickner PW, Vincent RL. Influenzalike illness among homeless persons. Emerg Infect Dis 2006;12(7):1162–3.
22. Scott M. Pandemic influenza guidance for homeless shelters and homeless service providers. Nashville (TN): National Health Care for the Homeless Council, Inc; 2009. Available at: http://www.nhchc.org/wp-content/uploads/2011/10/flumanual.pdf. Accessed November 10, 2014.
23. Markova A, Kam SA, Miller DD, et al. In the clinic: common cutaneous parasites. Ann Intern Med 2014;161(5). ITC3-1.
24. Bauer LK, Baggett TP, Stern TA, et al. Caring for homeless persons with serious mental illness in general hospitals. Psychosomatics 2013;54:14–21.
25. Padgett DK, Stanhope V, Henwood BF, et al. Substance use outcomes among homeless clients with serious mental illness: comparing housing first with treatment first programs. Community Ment Health J 2011;47:227–32.
26. Tsemberis S, Kent D, Respress C. Housing stability and recovery among chronically homeless persons with co-occurring disorders in Washington, DC. Am J Public Health 2012;102(1):13–6.
27. Hammig B, Jozkowski K, Jones C. Injury-related visits and comorbid conditions among homeless persons presenting to emergency departments. Acad Emerg Med 2014;21:449–55.
28. Browne A, Bassuk SS. Intimate violence in the lives of homeless and poor housed women: prevalence and patterns in an ethnically diverse sample. Am J Orthopsychiatry 1997;67(2):261–78.
29. Hopper EK, Bassuk EL, Olivet J. Shelter from the storm: trauma-informed care in homelessness services settings. Open Health Serv Pol J 2010;3:80–100.
30. Institutes of Medicine. Treatment of posttraumatic stress disorder: an assessment of the evidence. Washington, DC: National Academies Press; 2008.
31. Larimer ME, Malone DK, Garner MD, et al. Health care and public service use and costs before and after provision of housing for chronically homeless persons with severe alcohol problems. JAMA 2009;301(13):1349–57.
32. Mattick RP, Breen C, Kimber J, et al. Methadone maintenance therapy versus no opioid replacement therapy for opioid dependence. Cochrane Database Syst Rev 2009;(3):CD002209.
33. Mattick RP, Breen C, Kimber J, et al. Buprenorphine maintenance versus placebo or methadone maintenance for opioid dependence. Cochrane Database Syst Rev 2014;(2):CD002207.

34. Carroll K, Rounsaville B, Keller D. Relapse prevention strategies for the treatment of cocaine abuse. Am J Drug Alcohol Abuse 1991;17(3):249–65.
35. Stotts AM, Schmitz JM, Rhoades HM, et al. Motivational interviewing with cocaine-dependent patients: a pilot study. J Consult Clin Psychol 2001;69:858–62.
36. Fisher R, Ewing J, Garrett A, et al. The nature and prevalence of chronic pain in homeless persons: an observational study. F1000Res 2013;2:164.
37. Hwang SW, Wilkins E, Chambers C, et al. Chronic pain among homeless persons: characteristics, treatment, and barriers to management. BMC Fam Pract 2011;12:73.
38. Adult Immunization Schedules, United States. Advisory committee on immunization practices (ACIP). 2014. Available at: http://www.cdc.gov/vaccines/schedules/hcp/adult.html. Accessed November 30, 2014.
39. Asgary R, Garland V, Jakubowski A, et al. Colorectal cancer screening among the homeless population of new york city shelter-based clinics. Am J Public Health 2014;104(7):1307–13.
40. National Coalition for the Homeless. Fact sheet #7: domestic violence and homelessness. Available at: http://nationalhomeless.org/wp-content/uploads/2014/06/Domestic-Violence-Fact-Sheet.pdf. Accessed November 16, 2014.
41. U.S. Conference of Mayors. A status report on hunger and homelessness in America's cities: 2004 and 2005. Available at: http://usmayors.org/hungersurvey/2004/onlinereport/HungerAndHomelessnessReport2004.pdf. Accessed November 16, 2014.
42. Bassuk EL, Weinreb LF, Buckner JC, et al. The characteristics and needs of sheltered homeless and low-income housed mothers. JAMA 1996;276(8):640–6.
43. National Alliance to End Homelessness. An emerging framework for ending unaccompanied youth homelessness. 2012. Available at: http://www.endhomelessness.org/library/entry/an-emerging-framework-for-ending-unaccompanied-youth-homelessness. Accessed November 16, 2014.
44. Robertson MJ, Toro PA. Homeless youth: research, intervention, and policy. In: Fosburg LB, Dennis DL, editors. Practical lessons: the 1998 national symposium on homelessness research. Washington, DC: Department of Housing and Urban Development; 1999. p. 77–108.
45. Health Care for the Homeless Branch, Bureau of Primary Care Research, Health Services and Research Administration. Understanding the health care needs of homeless youth. Program Assistance Letter 2001–10. 2001. Available at: http://bphc.hrsa.gov/policiesregulations/policies/pal200110.html. Accessed November 16, 2014.
46. Culhane DP, Metraux S, Byrne T, et al. The aging of contemporary homelessness. Contexts 2013. Available at: http://works.bepress.com/dennis_culhane/119. Accessed November 16, 2014.
47. Gelberg L, Linn LS, Mayer-Oakes SA. Differences in health status between older and younger homeless adults. J Am Geriatr Soc 1990;38(11):1220–9.
48. HCH Clinicians Network. Aging on the streets. Healing Hands 2008;12(2):1–6. Available at: http://www.nhchc.org/wp-content/uploads/2011/09/Apr08Healing Hands.pdf. Accessed November 16, 2014.
49. Henry M, Cortes A, Morris S. The 2013 annual homeless assessment report (AHAR) to congress. Washington, DC: US Dept of Housing and Urban Development; 2013. Available at. https://www.hudexchange.info/resources/documents/ahar-2013-part1.pdf.
50. HUD, VA, and USICH announce 33% drop in veteran homelessness since 2010. US Department of Housing and Urban Development. HUDNo_14–103. Available at: http://portal.hud.gov/hudportal/HUD?src=/press/press_releases_media_advisories/2014/HUDNo_14-103. Accessed December 14, 2014.

51. Cochran BN, Stewart AJ, Ginzler JA, et al. Challenges faced by homeless sexual minorities: comparison of gay, lesbian, bisexual, and transgender homeless adolescents with their heterosexual counterparts. Am J Public Health 2002;92: 773–7.

52. Durso LE, Gates GJ. Serving our youth: findings from a national survey of service providers working with lesbian, gay, bisexual, and transgender youth who are homeless or at risk of becoming homeless. Los Angeles, CA: The Williams Institute with True Colors Fund and The Palette Fund; 2012. Available at: http://fortytonone.org/wp-content/uploads/2012/06/LGBT-Homeless-Youth-Survey-Final-Report-7-11-12.pdf. Accessed December 8, 2014.

53. Ray N. Lesbian, gay, bisexual and transgender youth: an epidemic of homelessness. New York, NY: National Gay and Lesbian Task Force Policy Institute and the National Coalition for the Homeless; 2006. Available at: http://www.thetaskforce.org/static_html/downloads/reports/reports/HomelessYouth.pdf.   Accessed December 8, 2014.

54. Byrne T, Kuhn J, Culhane DP, et al. Impact and performance of the supportive services for veteran families (SSVF) program: results from the FY 2013 program year. Philadelphia, PA: VA National Center on Homelessness among Veterans Research Briefs; 2014. Available at: http://www.endveteranhomelessness.org/content/impact-and-performance-ssvf-program-results-fy-2013-program-year.

55. Ciambrone S, Edgington S. Medical respite services for homeless people: practical planning. Nashville (TN): Respite Care Providers Network, National Health Care for the Homeless Council, Inc; 2009.

56. Doran KM, Ragins KT, Gross CP, et al. Medical respite programs for homeless patients: a systematic review. J Health Care Poor Underserved 2013;24(2):499–524.

57. Buchanan D, Doblin B, Sai T, et al. The effects of respite care for homeless patients: a cohort study. Am J Public Health 2006;96:1278–81.

58. Podymow T, Turnbull J, Coyle D. Shelter-based palliative care for the homeless terminally ill. Palliat Med 2006;20(2):81–6.

59. Zlotnick C, Zerger S, Wolfe PB. Health care for the homeless: what we have learned in the past 30 years and what's next. Am J Public Health 2013; 103(Suppl 2):S199–205.

60. O'Toole TP, Bourgault C, Johnson EE, et al. New to care: demands on a health system when homeless veterans are enrolled in a medical home model. Am J Public Health 2013;103(S2):S374–9.

61. Hwang SW, Burns T. Health interventions for people who are homeless. Lancet 2014;384:1541–7.

Care of Adult Refugees with Chronic Conditions

Genji Terasaki, MD*, Nicole Chow Ahrenholz, MD, Mahri Z. Haider, MD, MPH

KEYWORDS

- Refugee • Immigrant • Asylee • Primary care • Mental health • Chronic disease
- Cross-cultural medicine • Language

KEY POINTS

- Refugees make up a subset of immigrants who have been forcibly displaced from their homes by persecution, generalized violence, rape, and human rights abuses.
- Use of a professional medical interpreter is essential for patients with limited English proficiency.
- Primary care providers should be vigilant for latent infectious conditions such as tuberculosis and hepatitis B virus infection.
- Mental health conditions such as depression, anxiety, and posttraumatic stress disorder are very common in traumatized populations. Screening for these is necessary.
- Multiple barriers to managing chronic conditions in refugee patients exist, including transportation, language, challenges in navigating pharmacies, and insurance. Providers should recognize competing agendas or explanatory models related to their patients' conditions.

Video of 82-year-old man's description of how torture relates to chronic leg pain accompanies this article at http://www.medical.theclinics.com/

INTRODUCTION

Fleeing from generalized violence, rape, and torture, more than 17 million people worldwide are unable to return to their home countries. Civil conflicts and systematic persecutions, some of which have persisted for years, have forced millions into a state of protracted exile in neighboring countries. Many live and wait in overcrowded refugee camps hoping for restoration of political stability, acceptance, and safety in their home countries. The goal of the United Nations High Commissioner for Refugees

Disclosures: We have no commercial or financial conflicts of interest, or any funding sources.
Section of General Internal Medicine, Department of Medicine, Harborview Medical Center, University of Washington, Box 359780, 325 Ninth Avenue, Seattle, WA 98104, USA
* Corresponding author.
E-mail address: terasaki@uw.edu

Med Clin N Am 99 (2015) 1039–1058
http://dx.doi.org/10.1016/j.mcna.2015.05.006
0025-7125/15/$ – see front matter © 2015 Elsevier Inc. All rights reserved.

(UNHCR) is to work toward long-term solutions of either voluntary repatriation or local integration into their host country. However, in some cases, the UNHCR has no other option than to permanently resettle refugees to a third country such as the United States, Australia, or Canada.[1]

The United States uses a legal definition of a refugee that is similar to the 1951 United Nations' Convention: a person outside of the United States who demonstrates a history of "persecution or fear of persecution due to race, religion, nationality, political opinion, or membership in a particular social group.[2]" In 2014, the United States admitted almost 70,000 refugees, with the largest numbers originating from Iraq, Burma (Myanmar), Somalia, and Bhutan (**Fig. 1**). As a subset of the total immigrant population, refugees have been resettled in all but 2 states, with a large proportion going to Texas, California, New York, and Michigan (**Fig. 2**).[3] In addition to the refugees who are accepted for admission before their departure from overseas, asylum seekers make up an important group of potential immigrants who apply for asylum after arrival to the United States. To receive asylum, an immigration court must determine whether the asylum seeker meets the same legal definition as a refugee. In 2013, the US Citizenship and Immigration Services granted asylum to 25,199 individuals with the largest proportion being from the People's Republic of China (34%).[4]

The legal status of refugee or asylee is important because, in addition to receiving asylum, it confers several short-term government assistance programs, not available to other immigrants. Refugees receive 8 months of medical coverage, representing a window period to complete an initial health evaluation and obtain subspecialty consultation if necessary. They are also eligible to apply for health insurance through the Affordable Care Act; other immigrants must wait 5 years. The government has partnered with private voluntary agencies to assists refugees in their resettlement process with services such as orientation, food and clothing, initial housing, and sponsor programs. Voluntary agencies may also provide case management, English language

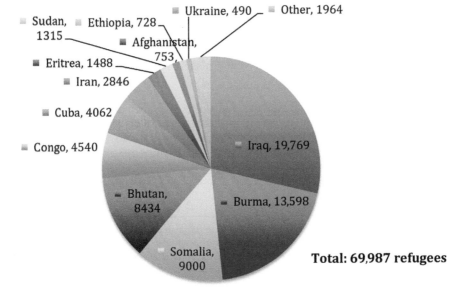

Fig. 1. Countries of origin of refugees resettled to the United States during fiscal year 2014. (*Data from* Refugee Processing Center. Reports. Available at: http://www.wrapsnet.org/Reports/AdmissionsArrivals/tabid/211/Default.aspx. Accessed October 29, 2014.)

All Nationalities

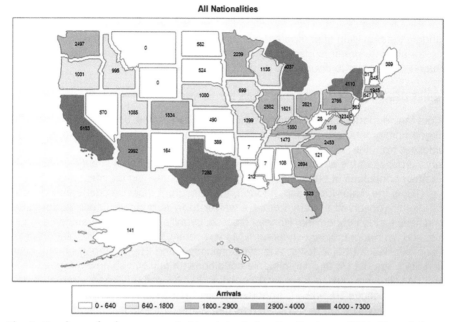

Fig. 2. Numbers of refugees accepted by state during the fiscal year 2014. (*From* Refugee Processing Center. Reports. Available at: http://www.wrapsnet.org/Reports/AdmissionsArrivals/tabid/211/Default.aspx. Accessed October 29, 2014; with permission.)

classes, and vocational training. Also, in contrast to other immigrants, refugees and asylees are entitled to an accelerated path to citizenship. They can apply for a green card after the first year and for citizenship at 5 years.

Whereas much of the published literature on refugees and asylees has addressed the medical care during first year after resettlement, this article primarily focuses on the long-term management of adults in primary care. The first section briefly covers the overseas and domestic evaluation, which is an opportunity to detect and treat latent infectious conditions before they emerge later with dire consequences. Additionally, mental health issues are prevalent in refugee and asylee populations and need to be recognized and managed in a culturally appropriate manner. The final section focuses on chronic disease management in this vulnerable population.

THE IMPORTANCE OF USING A TRAINED INTERPRETER

The impact of language barriers on health care is well documented in the literature. When compared with fluent English speakers, communication problems contribute to adverse events at a higher rate for patients with limited English proficiency.[5] These patients have lower rates of preventive screening and services and higher rates of hospitalization and drug complications.[6] Additionally, language barriers are associated with lower patient satisfaction and a lower rate of adherence to medication regimens.[7–9] Given the high stakes of medical interpretation and its inherent difficulties of accurately conveying meaning across language and culture, using a trained interpreter is essential. One study compared trained interpreters to ad hoc interpreters (ie, family members, hospital staff, untrained volunteers, and friends) and found significant higher error rates among ad hoc interpreters.[10] In particular, using family members is problematic when it comes to discussing sensitive topics. Moreover, Title VI of the Civil Rights Act of 1964 and the Department of Health and Human Services mandate the provision of competent interpreters in all health care settings.[11] Having a face-to-face interpreter is ideal but medical telephonic services are widely available, cheaper, and easier to coordinate without scheduling ahead of time.

A BRIEF DESCRIPTION OF THE OVERSEAS EVALUATION

Before their departure, all immigrants bound for United States, both refugees and non-refugee immigrants, are required to have a medical evaluation in accordance with guidelines from the Centers for Disease Control and Prevention (CDC). One of the primary purposes of the evaluation is to "prevent the importation of infectious diseases and other conditions of public health significance.[2]" Screening for infectious tuberculosis (TB) is the major focus and, if found, the immigrant must be adequately treated with directly observed therapy before a waiver to fly is granted. Other inadmissible conditions include gonorrhea, Hansen disease, syphilis, chancroid, granuloma inguinale, and lymphogranuloma venereum. More recently, severe acute respiratory syndrome, viral hemorrhagic fever, and avian influenza, and Ebola, among others, have been added to the list of quarantinable conditions. In reality, very few refugees have been denied entry due to a medical condition (0.4%) and, of those, almost all had untreated infectious TB (93%).[12] Importantly, as of 2010, human immunodeficiency virus (HIV) testing is no longer performed as part of the overseas evaluation and the HIV status is often unknown at the time of arrival.[13]

In most cases, refugees are exposed to harsh living conditions with inadequate health care, sanitation, and access to safe water. Due to their increased risk, the CDC recommends presumptive treatment of parasitic infections for many groups. For example, sub-Saharan Africans living in endemic countries receive artemisinin-based combination therapy directed at *Plasmodium falciparum* malaria before departure.[14] Many refugees also are administered presumptive antihelminthic agents directed at *Strongyloides stercoralis* and *Schistosoma* species, both of which can persist subclinically for years after immigration and lead to complications.[15]

Age-appropriate vaccinations, such as measles-mumps-rubella, tetanus, and pertussis, are required of refugees, the same as for persons born in the United States. There is an effort overseas to provide as many of the vaccines that are available, even though refugees are technically not required to have any before their departure.[16] However, in order to apply for a green card at 1 year after arrival, refugees must complete all vaccination series (except human papillomavirus vaccine, zoster vaccine, and the new 13-valent pneumococcal conjugate vaccine). In the cases of hepatitis A and varicella, demonstrating serologic evidence of immunity before vaccination is cost-effective.[16] Hepatitis B virus (HBV) testing should also be done before vaccinating to identify those with current infection.

THE DOMESTIC EVALUATION OF ADULTS

All refugees are recommended to have a domestic medical evaluation. Ideally, this should occur soon after arrival and includes rescreening for TB, mental health screening, and testing for HBV, anemia, and sexually transmitted infections such as HIV, syphilis, chlamydia, and gonorrhea. It should also confirm, either through the overseas documentation or testing, that the appropriate presumptive anthelminthic therapies were administered. Finally, this evaluation is meant to identify chronic diseases such as diabetes and hypertension and update vaccinations. In many regions of the United States, the local health departments have assumed the responsibility for following-up newly arrived persons with TB within 30 days. However, for non-TB conditions, there is a wide range of models at the state and county levels, and many parts of the country rely on primary care physicians to perform the domestic evaluation. In reality, it is likely that a large proportion of refugees do not receive the recommended evaluation.[17] Even for TB, the actual rates of follow-up after arrival ranged from zero (Montana) to 100% (Delaware) with a median rate of 75% in 2009.[12]

Unless there is clear documentation of prior screening and treatment, primary care providers may consider a conservative approach and not assume that any part of the domestic evaluation was previously performed. In the authors' experience, relying on the patient's memory of prior treatments can be fraught with recall errors and the authors tend to err on the side of retesting, even years after immigration. The following discussion is a brief overview of infections with a long latency period that may be less familiar to North American providers: TB, parasites, and HBV. More detailed instructions of diagnosis and treatment can found at the CDC website: http://www.cdc.gov/immigrantrefugeehealth/guidelines/domestic/domestic-guidelines.html.

Tuberculosis

In 2013, there were almost 10,000 new cases of active TB in the United States with 64% occurring in foreign-born persons.[18] It is recommended that all immigrants from regions where TB is endemic be screened. The evaluation starts with eliciting symptoms of active TB, such as a cough, fever, hemoptysis, weight loss, and night sweats, usually of several weeks or months duration. If negative, the clinician should proceed to screen for latent TB infection with a tuberculin skin test or interferon-gamma release assay followed by a 2-view chest radiograph. All patients diagnosed with TB must have their HIV status evaluated. The decision to offer treatment of latent TB infection is based on weighing the risks of reactivation with the risks of treatment. Estimates of these risks can be found using an online calculator, such as www.tstin3d.com from McGill University. Ample time for a clear discussion of the risks and benefits of treatment is important, as well as a 1-month follow-up appointment to check for medication side effects and to confirm an understanding of the pharmacy refill process.

Chronic Parasitic Worm Infections

Refugees may have been exposed to a multitude of helminthes, depending on the region and living conditions before emigration. However, when in North America without a means to complete its life cycle, most worms (eg, ascaris, *Trichuris*, hookworm) will gradually decrease in number and be excreted uneventfully from their adult host within a year or 2. There are, however, 2 important exceptions: *S stercoralis* and *Schistosoma* species.

Strongyloides is a soil-transmitted round worm that can complete its life-cycle entirely within a human host. This unique property of autoinfection allows *Strongyloides* to persist indefinitely in the human carrier even in the absence of recurrent exposure. The dreaded complication is hyperinfection, which is a process of massive dissemination of *Strongyloides* larvae and presents dramatically with gram-negative sepsis and carries a high mortality rate. Those who become immunosuppressed (eg, high-dose corticosteroid therapy) are at the greatest risk even many years after leaving the endemic area. Standard stool examination is insensitive for detection (<50% sensitivity).[19] Therefore, all refugees and immigrants from endemic areas should either receive empiric treatment or be screened with serology.

Schistosomiasis is extremely prevalent with an estimated 200 million infected persons worldwide.[20] Chronic disease is caused by the host's immune response to migration and entrapment of eggs through tissues, thereby causing inflammation and fibrosis.[21] Infection with *S mansoni*, *S japonicum*, and *S mekongi* typically results in egg deposition in microvasculature of the liver or intestines, causing hepatomegaly, portal hypertension, and polyposis of the small and large bowels. The classic manifestation of *S haematobium* is within the genitourinary tract and is a major risk factor for renal disease and bladder carcinoma. Diagnostic screening is indicated for individuals from endemic regions, even in the absence of symptoms. Screening tools include serology and stool studies. Hematuria found on urinalysis without other explanation may warrant an evaluation for *S haemotobium*.[22]

Hepatitis B Infection

Almost all chronic HBV infections are acquired at birth or early childhood. Chronic infection substantially increases the risk of cirrhosis, fulminant hepatitis, liver transplant, and liver cancer. Whereas the overall prevalence is relatively low in United States (0.4%), refugees have a significantly high rate of infection ranging from 5% to 14%.[23,24] The highest rates were observed in refugees from sub-Saharan Africa (10.5%) and East Asia (13%).[25] The CDC recommends routine screening with serologic testing of immigrants from endemic areas.[26] HBV surface antigen is the marker of on-going viral replication and warrants further evaluation to determine whether treatment is needed. Even for inactive carrier state, life-long serial monitoring for liver function and screening for hepatocellular carcinoma (HCC) are necessary. HBV infection is distinct from other hepatitides such as hepatitis C virus infection in that it can lead to the development of HCC in the absence of cirrhosis. Therefore, experts recommend that patients receive a screening liver ultrasound or non–maternal alpha fetoprotein test every 6 to 12 months.[27] **Box 1** shows the recommended age to begin HCC screening. It is also recommended that patients be counseled regarding transmission (eg, sexual contact and sharing razors and toothbrushes). Household contacts who are not already infected and nonimmune should be vaccinated.[27]

MENTAL HEALTH

Being from all regions of the world, refugees, and asylees are diverse, representing a multitude of language groups, levels of education, socioeconomic backgrounds, and belief systems. However, they share a life-changing experience of having been violently displaced from their home and either personally experienced or witnessed

---

Box 1
Surveillance ultrasound every 6 to 12 months for HCC screening is recommended for the following groups of patients

Asian men older than 40 years

Asian women older greater than 50 years

All cirrhotic HBV carriers

Family history of HCC

Africans older than 20 years

Any carrier older than 40 years with alanine aminotransferase elevation and/or HBV DNA greater than 2000 IU/mL

Data from Lok AS, McMahon BJ. Chronic hepatitis B: update 2009. Hepatology 2009;50:661–2.

significant trauma. During their migration, they often experience a transitional period in an intermediate country or refugee camp, where they are often exposed to more violence, deprivation, and uncertainty about the future. Though meant to be temporary, many live in refugee camps for years and even decades while awaiting permanent resettlement.

After their arrival to the United States, the postmigration stresses of rebuilding a new life without the benefit of social capital, credentials, or money are underestimated. For most who lack English proficiency on arrival, the difficulty of communicating and navigating through complex systems such as hospitals, banks, and schools is a constant reminder of their loss of power. Many accept minimal wage jobs and, from what little earnings they receive, are expected to send a proportion to family members abroad. The stress of day-to-day survival is compounded because many continue to bear the chronic pains of past physical and psychological injuries. They remember friends and family members who were killed, tortured, injured, or left behind. Often, not knowing the whereabouts of their love ones is most distressing and inhibits the healing process (**Table 1**).

Given the stresses before, during, and after migration, refugees have high rates of posttraumatic stress disorder (PTSD), depression, anxiety, and somatization.[28] One systematic review and meta-analysis estimated a prevalence of PTSD of 30.6% and depression of 30.8% among 81,866 refugees and conflict-affected populations.[29] However, rates vary widely based on the country of origin, with prevalence ranging from 3% to 86% for PTSD and 3% to 80% for major depression.[30] Many also meet criteria for more than one mental health disorder: 86% of those with major depression met criteria for PTSD.[31] Risk factors for PTSD and depression included cumulative exposure to potentially traumatic events, time since conflict, and a history of torture.[29] In terms of disability and mortality, the exact toll is unknown but a recent report of newly resettled Bhutanese refugees between 2009 and 2012 estimated the annual suicide rate at 24.4 per 100,000 persons, almost twice that of the overall US population. In the same report, a survey of adult Bhutanese refugees found that 3% of participants had contemplated suicide at some point.[32]

Detection and Treatment

Various screening tools for mental health disorders exist but differ in terms of language availability, domain of interest (depression, anxiety, and PTSD), and feasibility. Commonly used tools that have been validated in multiple languages include the Harvard Trauma Questionnaire (HTQ) for PTSD and the Hopkins Symptom Checklist

| Table 1 | | |
The "triple trauma" of common stressors affecting refugees across the major periods of migration		
Premigration	**Migration and Refugee Camp**	**Postmigration and Resettlement**
Persecution	Violence	Discrimination
Violence	Deprivation	Social isolation
Torture	Uncertainty about future	Financial problems
Loss of possessions	Separation from loved ones	Housing
Loss of loved ones		Employment
		Transportation
		Language barrier
		Generational acculturation
		Loss of social status

(HSCL-25) for depression.[33,34] Developed more recently, the Refugee Health Screener-15 (RHS-15) is a relatively short instrument used to detect depression, PTSD, and anxiety. Validated in new arrivals from Iraq, Bhutan, and Burma (Myanmar), the RHS-15 is open-access and can be found through the Pathways to Wellness program at www.lcsnw.org/pathways/.[35]

Barriers to discussing psychiatric disorders are several. On the part of the provider, there may be a discomfort with dealing with mental health issues, lack of time, and scarcity of mental health resources to refer patients. Patients' views of mental illness vary widely based on previous experience and one's medical and cultural beliefs. Although some may readily accept and openly talk about their depression, others may strongly resist any mention of a psychiatric diagnosis. Providers should be sensitive to the fact that mental health disorders are highly stigmatized in many countries (more so than our own) and the label of "being crazy" can lead to severe marginalization or detention.

Some patients may prefer to discuss symptoms such as fatigue, abdominal pain, headaches, and dizziness rather than diagnoses. In the authors' experience, inquiring about sleep can be a nonthreatening way to broach the topic and may open the door to further questions about nightmares, worries, and sadness. Clinicians can also look for opportunities to acknowledge and validate patients' on-going daily struggles, including concerns about unsafe neighborhoods, worries about their children, finances, and physical ailments, as a lead-in to discussing mental health. Communication can be tricky at times when an unintended linguistic nuance can lead to a misunderstanding, even with a professional interpreter. Providers should also accept that encounters with non-English speaking refugees require more time and it may take multiple visits to fully discuss a topic as complex as mental health. A patient-centered approach, as stated by Rhema and colleagues,[36] can help to overcome barriers, "the refugee experience is one of disempowerment. Refugees are best served when provided with education about procedures and services that include opportunities of choice... explanations and instructions that allow refugees to have control over choices are more effective." In the rush of seeing patients, it is easy to forget that supportive listening can be therapeutic and build trust.

Ideally, treatment should be multidisciplinary and involve the efforts of primary care providers, social workers, psychiatrists, psychologists, and community organizations. However, it may be the case that a patient will view their problem outside of the realm of what western medicine can offer and seek a solution through their church or mosque, friends and family, or traditional healers.[37] Several studies have shown improvement with psychological interventions, including cognitive behavioral therapy and narrative exposure therapy (extinction conditioning) and, if available, these should be offered.[38,39] The prescribing of medicines, such as an antidepressant or α-adrenergic antagonist (eg, prazosin) for PTSD, may be met with resistance and often requires extensive education. Patients, familiar with immediate-acting medications such as antibiotics, may agree to start an antidepressant but discontinue it after a few days due to lack of effect. The authors have found that the willingness to take a medication increases with anticipatory guidance about potential side effects, onset of action, and treatment duration.

Survivors of Torture

Despite international declarations and conventions prohibiting its practice, torture is common worldwide. Broadly defined, torture is an act of inflicting psychological or physical pain on another person with the intention of coercing information or action, or as punishment, or purely for sadistic purposes. In many cases the objective behind torture is political and meant to terrorize a population and "stifle dissent, intimidate opposition, and strengthen the forces of tyranny."[40] For the individual, it serves to humiliate the person and destroy their faith in themselves. Examples include rape, beatings, amputations, suspension, confinement, asphyxiation, and mock executions. Witnessing and forcing one to perpetrate the torture of others are also common[41] (**Table 2**).

As of 2000, it was estimated that approximately 400,000 torture survivors lived in the United States[42] and the number is certainly much higher now. The Amnesty International Report of 2012 found torture and ill treatment in 112 countries, including most countries from which the United States receives refugees.[43] Prevalence of torture varies widely by the population studied; however, a meta-analysis including 42,626 refugees and other conflict-affected groups showed an overall prevalence of 21%.[29] A study of 1134 Somali and Oromo refugees living in the United States showed a prevalence of 44%.[28] Another report found that 56% of Iraqi refugees had been tortured.[44]

The psychological and physical impact of torture can be long lasting. Mental health disorders occur frequently in survivors of torture, with rates as high as 81.1% with clinically significant anxiety, 84.5% with clinically significant depression, and 45.7% with symptoms of PTSD.[45] Chronic pain is extremely common. One study reported that 78% reported persistent multiple pains, mainly in the head and low back.[46] Falanga, or beating the soles of the feet, can result in subcutaneous fibrosis or compartment

Table 2
Common methods of torture

Physical Methods	Psychological Methods
Blunt trauma eg, beatings all over; falanga, beating the soles of the feet; telefono, striking the ears	Humiliation eg, mocking, sexual humiliation, forced breaking of religious taboos
Penetrating trauma eg, cutting, amputations	Threats
Crushing trauma	Mock executions
Positional torture eg, suspension, confinement in small spaces, fixation by ropes or chains	Deprivation of: Light and sound Food and drink Access to toilet facilities Sleep Company Access to medicine and medical care
Shaking	Witnessing or perpetrating the torture of others
Asphyxiation	—
Chemical torture	—
Burns eg, electrical, acid, cigarettes	—
Pharmacologic or microbiologic torture eg, forced ingestion of medications, inoculation of pathogens such as HIV	—
Sexual torture	—

Adapted from Wenzel T, Kastrup MC, Eisenman DP. Survivors of torture: a hidden population. In: Walker PF, Barnett ED, editors. Immigrant medicine. China: Saunders-Elsevier; 2007. p. 657; with permission.

syndrome in the feet, as well as severe pain lasting for years. Sexual dysfunction and chronic pain are common sequelae of genital torture and female genital cutting. Head trauma can result in traumatic brain injury with effects on memory, attention, and behavior.[47]

Clinicians should have a high degree of suspicion for a history of torture in refugees, particularly those with symptoms of depression, anxiety, PTSD, or those with chronic physical complaints. The topic should be broached gently to prevent patients from feeling interrogated. Often, a history of torture is revealed over several visits, some- times over the course of years, as a patient becomes comfortable with their physician. Awareness of a torture history can help prevent traumatization because tests such as phlebotomy, electrocardiograms, gynecologic examinations, and imaging studies may have the unintended effect of triggering negative memories from the past. Asking about a patient's history of torture is also important so that providers can support their process of self-healing. Moreover, it serves as a reminder for us as health providers to remain patient and compassionate while providing necessary medical care.

Somatization and Chronic Pain

Somatization is described as "a tendency to experience and communicate somatic distress in response to psychosocial stress to seek medical help for it."[48] Somatic symptoms vary and take on different expressions based on cultural syndromes, such as those described in Asian populations. For example, the palpitations produced by anxiety can be thought of as a weak heart in China and the resulting fear of cardiac arrest or infarction can predispose the sufferer to be hypervigilant of any cardiac symptom. Among Cambodian patients, symptoms of anxiety and PTSD can present as a sore neck and fear of death due to rupture of the neck vessels can lead patients report any symptom involving the head and neck, including headache, dizziness, and tinnitus.[49]

Although chronic pain is often attributed to somatization, organic causes such as osteoarthritis, rheumatologic disorders, and osteomalacia must not be overlooked. When compared with other immigrants, refugees are more likely to have arthritis and activity-limitation due to pain.[50] Treatment of chronic pain and somatization should include evaluation for coexisting mental health disorders and a history of trauma, including torture (Video 1; available online at http://www.medical.theclinics.com/). Current social stressors can be a contributor to somatization and should be addressed.[51] Explaining the limitations of allopathic medicine can help in negotiating what constitutes an appropriate workup of pain complaints, such as in the patients who request multiple tests or procedures. Treatment modalities include acupuncture, trigger point injection, therapeutic massage, antidepressant medications, cognitive behavioral therapy, and relaxation techniques. Providers and patients are encouraged to openly discuss the use of traditional treatments.[52–54]

CHRONIC NONCOMMUNICABLE DISEASES

The healthy migrant bias argues that first-generation migrants are often healthier than those in the host population because they are self-selecting for the process of migra- tion.[55,56] However, this advantage may be temporary because refugees are at high risk of developing chronic disease through the process of acculturation.[57,58] Therefore, whereas the burden of chronic noncommunicable disease may differ among refugees on arrival to the United States, age-appropriate guidelines for screening of chronic dis- ease still applies.[59]

Many factors can affect a patient's ability to manage their chronic medical conditions. Proactive management of chronic disease is similar to other preventive health services in that it requires an element of forward thinking and purpose in life.[60] Often an improvement in finances or housing, or stabilization of a mental health condition, can provide the motivation to engage in the management of chronic disease. Rather than discuss the treatment guidelines for these chronic diseases, management principles in refugees are highlighted.

Hypertension

Hypertension is prevalent and sometimes challenging to manage in refugees. Of those adult refugees and asylees, who arrived in Massachusetts from 2001 to 2005, 22% had hypertension.[61] This ranged from 9% (East and Southeast Asia) to 32% (Europe and Central Asia).[61] Although some refugees from urban areas may be familiar with chronic disease, others may have limited experience with the idea of an asymptomatic disease, which has a waxing and waning course and is incurable.

Making patients aware of their diagnosis is often a prerequisite to medication adherence and behavioral modifications. One study found that foreign-born participants were less likely to be aware of their hypertension and overweight status than participants born in the United States.[62] Having awareness of a diagnosis allows patients to make meaning of their new illness, thereby providing motivation for behavioral change.

A patient-centered approach to managing hypertension includes eliciting the patient's explanatory model of disease.[63] Understanding the patient's beliefs around the causes, course of illness, and treatment of hypertension will guide their management. Although the literature is limited in refugees, a recent article provided examples of how explanatory models can lead to certain self-management behaviors, outlined in **Table 3**.[64]

Finally, it is worthwhile to consider the patient's motivation for disease management. The desire to control hypertension will likely be met with some obstacles, whether it is other health conditions, financial issues, or competing life stressors. This will be balanced by respect for the provider and the belief that controlled blood pressure will be of benefit. The role of hypertension in cardiovascular disease and the notion of risk-factor modification are often unfamiliar to refugees and deserve explicit explanation. **Table 4** provides recommendations for common areas of miscommunication around medications.

Diabetes

Refugees from Bhutan, Iraq, and Burma make up greater than 60% of all incoming refugees to the United States.[65] Estimates of diabetes in Bhutanese refugees ranges from 11% to 14% and data on Iraqi refugees revealed that 35% had at least 1 of 3 chronic medical conditions, including hypertension, diabetes, or obesity.[66–68] One study looking at Hmong refugees put the blame for diabetes on the refugee movement itself, placing the individual with little control over their ill health.[69] In addition to understanding explanatory models of disease, the management of diabetes often requires an understanding of traditional foods, history of food deprivation, and religious fasting.

Food and diet are inherently tied up in culture and religion. The discussion of nutrition and diet is much more relevant if it includes traditional foods. Culturally appropriate meal planning handouts are available in many languages (http://www.kingcounty.gov/healthservices/health/chronic/reach/diabetes.aspx). Furthermore, patients who have had a history of food deprivation or starvation should be approached with sensitivity. One study noted a relationship in Cambodian refugee

Table 3
Explanatory models and corresponding hypertension self-management behaviors

Explanatory Model	Hypertension Self-management Behavior
Cause	
Stress as primary cause	Stays calm, avoids stressful situations; takes antidepressant as treatment
Exercise causes increased BP	Avoids exercise to keep BP low
Pain causes increased BP	Managing pain, taking pain medications will control hypertension
Course of illness	
Hypertension comes and goes	Takes medications when BP goes up
BP cannot be controlled	Will not exercise and forgets medications
Little concern about hypertension; it does not affect my life	Avoids going to the doctor; forgets medications
Own definition of what is considered high	Only takes medication when BP is >190/100 mm Hg
Symptoms	
I can tell when my BP is high; I get headaches and dizziness	Takes medications only when symptoms occur
I have no symptoms of high BP, therefore it is not a problem	Does not take medications
Eating bacon does not make me feel bad, so it does not affect my BP	Eats bacon as desired
Treatment	
Only exercise can help me control my high BP	Exercises and, therefore, allows himself to smoke, drink, and not take medication
Garlic and vinegar can help me control my high BP	Focuses on these remedies while not taking medications or altering diet or sodium intake

Abbreviation: BP, blood pressure.
Data from Bokhour BG, Cohn ES, Cortes DE, et al. The role of patients' explanatory models and daily-lived experience in hypertension self-management. J Gen Intern Med 2012;27:1626–34.

women with a past experience of food deprivation and current overweight or obesity[70] (**Box 2** for patient case).

Many of the world's religions practice fasting. Much of the research on fasting and diabetes management focuses on fasting during the holy month of Ramadan. The Epidemiology of Diabetes and Ramadan (EPIDIAR) study found that 79% of patients with type 2 diabetes reported fasting during Ramadan.[71] Another study showed that patients in a Ramadan education program had a decrease in hypoglycemic events whereas a comparison group had a 4-fold increase in hypoglycemic events compared with their baseline.[72] Interventions included in the study are summarized in **Table 5**. The American Diabetes Association recommends individual management plans and close follow-up around Ramadan. **Table 6** summarizes recommendations for adjusting medications for type 2 diabetes during Ramadan.[73] Many patients forego clinic appointments during the month of Ramadan and, therefore, these conversations should ideally occur in advance.

Finally, there is an increase in awareness of the genetic variability in the pharmacokinetic and pharmacodynamics effects between different ethnic groups. When prescribing medications for a heterogeneous group of patients, a one-size-fits-all

Table 4
Common areas of miscommunication around medications

Interpreters	Always use an interpreter during every visit but particularly when making medication changes
Adherence	Ask patients to bring in all medications to each visit (including inhalers and glucometer)
	Use objective evidence to assess adherence (date of last refill, number of pills left)
	Remind patients that it is unsafe for you to increase medications if they are not taking them, so it is better if they are transparent
Timeline	Give patients a sense of the timeline for which to expect results so they do not discontinue a medication after a few doses
Refills	Often the pharmacy refill system is not well understood
	Remind patients that it is preferable to use one pharmacy and that they do not need to wait until an appointment to get medications refills
Side effects	Stating expected side effects can help warn the patient but if a patient associates a medication with a certain side effect it is unlikely that they will continue to take it (even if think it is unlikely to be the cause)
Daily vs as-needed	Be clear about which medications are daily despite symptoms and which are used for symptoms (inhalers, as-needed pain medications).
Tools	Identify barriers to compliance and use tools when appropriate
	Pill organizers are great to help organize but will not remind a patient to take medications
Sharing	Explicitly remind patients not to share their medications or to use medications prescribed for others
Teach back	Ask them to tell you how they take the medications
Team-based	Clinical pharmacists are a great resource for medication reconciliation and inhaler teaching
Traditional medicine	Ask about traditional or herbal medications

Adapted from Avery K. Medication non-adherence issues with refugee and immigrant patients. EthnoMed. Available at: https://ethnomed.org/clinical/pharmacy/medication-non-adherence-issues-with-refugee-and-immigrant-patients. Accessed May 11, 2015.

Box 2
Case example of negotiating the management of diabetes in a Cambodian woman

Case example

A 67-year-old Cambodian woman with poorly controlled diabetes and obesity returned to clinic to review her laboratory results. The hemoglobin A1c was 14%. Her primary care provider was frustrated because during the past year, she tried multiple times to engage the patient to reduce her portion size and lose weight.

However, at an appointment with a nutritionist, the patient revealed that she lost several children to starvation during the Pol Pot era. She herself nearly starved and she recalled her desperate attempts to find food. Even now, feelings of hunger invariably bring back these painful memories.

After learning this, her primary care physician and nutritionist were able to adjust their counseling approach, putting more emphasis on exercise and eating nonstarchy vegetables rather than on limiting portion sizes. During the next 2 years, the patient eventually reduced her body mass index from 30 to 28 and decreased her hemoglobin A1c to 7.8%.

Table 5
Educational interventions for patients with diabetes during Ramadan

Risk Assessment	Advise patients to seek medical advice from a physician before Ramadan to assess their risk of fasting and make recommendations.
Advise patient	Consider discussing the option of not fasting if appropriate but be prepared to hear "no."
Exercise	Avoid rigorous exercise.
Diet	Encourage slow energy release foods (wheat, beans), not food high in fat. Iftar food is, by nature, fried. Limit dates, which are used to break fast. Limit sugar in tea. Avoid eating sweet dessert nightly; save it for Eid.
Hydration	Increase fluids, specifically water. Water is healthier than soda, juice, or sugary tea. Remember to drink water throughout the night.
Glucose monitoring	Advise patient that checking blood glucose does not constitute breaking fast.
When to break fast	Remind patients that they need to break fast if hypoglycemia does occur.

Data from Bravis V, Hui E, Salih S, et al. Ramadan Education and Awareness in Diabetes (READ) programme for Muslims with Type 2 diabetes who fast during Ramadan. Diabet Med 2010;27:327–31.

approach may not be the best approach. For example, studies have demonstrated that Asians (East Asian, Malay, and Indian) can achieve the same therapeutic effects using a lower dose of a statin (HMG-coenzyme A reductase inhibitor) compared with patients of European descent. As more knowledge is gained, providers may consider a lower starting dose in their Asian immigrant patients.[74,75]

Table 6
Recommended changes to treatment regimen in patients with Type 2 diabetes who fast during Ramadan

Before Ramadan	During Ramadan
Patients on diet and exercise control	Consider modifying the time and intensity of physical activity.
Patients on oral metformin	Consider adjusting timing of dose (ie, metformin 500 mg tid; during Ramadan change to metformin 1000 mg at sunset meal and 500 mg at predawn meal).
Patients on sulfonylureas	If once per day, adjust dose based on risk of hypoglycemia and give at sunset meal. If twice per day, use half the usual morning dose at the predawn meal and usual dose at the sunset meal.
Patients on premixed or intermediate acting insulin twice daily	Take usual dose at sunset meal and half usual dose at predawn meal. Also consider changing to long-acting in the evening and short-acting with meals.
Patients on long-acting insulin in the evening and short-acting with meals	Consider adjusting if at high risk of hypoglycemia or hyperglycemia, or continue with careful monitoring of blood glucose and adjust as necessary.

Adapted from Al-Arouj M, Assaad-Khalil S, Buse J, et al. Recommendations for management of diabetes during Ramadan: update 2010. Diabetes Care 2010;33:1901.

SUMMARY

More than 3 million refugees have been admitted to the United States since the 1970s and almost all have become citizens, raised families, and work as productive members of society.[76] On the surface, their story seems typical, resembling that of any other American immigrant. However, deeper down, refugee patients carry the scars of a violent past, which can continue to affect their health even years later. Although many are resilient and are able to heal themselves, others continue to struggle with depression, anxiety, and PTSD, which can flare up with emotional stress or physical pain. Primary care providers can forge a strong, therapeutic partnership with their refugee patients but it requires patience, compassion, and willingness to educate them about their health. By knowing aspects of their histories, clinicians can better support them through their healing process while managing chronic conditions, palliating pain, and offering preventive services.

ACKNOWLEDGMENTS

The authors would like to thank Dr Carey Jackson for his help and support with this article, as well as Rozie Erlewine and Yetta Levine, who filmed and edited the video clip.

SUPPLEMENTARY DATA

Supplementary data related to this article can be found online at http://dx.doi.org/10.1016/j.mcna.2015.05.006.

REFERENCES

1. United Nations High Commissioner for Refugee. UNHCR: Global Trends 2013: United Nations; 2014 June 20, 2014. Available online at: http://www.unhcr.org/5399a14f9.html. Accessed November 1, 2014.
2. United States Citizenship and Immigration Services (USCIS), Department of Homeland Security. Available online at: http://www.uscis.gov/humanitarian/refugees-asylum/refugees. Accessed June 12, 2015.
3. Summary of Refugee Admissions. 2014. Available at: http://www.wrapsnet.org. Accessed November 1, 2014.
4. Martin DC, Yankay JE. Annual flow report: Refugees and Asylees: 2013. Homeland Security OIS; 2014. Available online at: http://www.dhs.gov/sites/default/files/publications/ois_rfa_fr_2013.pdf.
5. Divi C, Koss RG, Schmaltz SP, et al. Language proficiency and adverse events in US hospitals: a pilot study. Int J Qual Health Care 2007;19:60–7.
6. Jackson JC, Nguyen D, Hu N, et al. Alterations in medical interpretation during routine primary care. J Gen Intern Med 2011;26:259–64.
7. Carmona RH. Improving language access: a personal and national agenda. J Gen Intern Med 2007;22(Suppl 2):277–8.
8. David RA, Rhee M. The impact of language as a barrier to effective health care in an underserved urban Hispanic community. Mt Sinai J Med 1998;65:393–7.
9. Flores G. The impact of medical interpreter services on the quality of health care: a systematic review. Med Care Res Rev 2005;62:255–99.
10. Flores G, Laws MB, Mayo SJ, et al. Errors in medical interpretation and their potential clinical consequences in pediatric encounters. Pediatrics 2003;111:6–14.

11. Department of Health and Human Services. Guidance to federal financial assistance recipients regarding title VI prohibition. Against national origin discrimination affecting limited English proficient persons: Policy guidance document. Available online at: http://www.hhs.gov/ocr/civilrights/resources/specialtopics/lep/hhslepguidancepdf.pdf. Accessed November 26, 2014.

12. Lee D, Philen R, Wang Z, et al. Disease surveillance among newly arriving refugees and immigrants—Electronic Disease Notification System, United States, 2009. MMWR Surveill Summ 2013;62:1–20.

13. Division of Global Migration and Quarantine, Technical Instructions for Panel Physicians. 2014. Available at: http://www.cdc.gov/immigrantrefugeehealth/exams/ti/panel/technical-instructions-panel-physicians.html. Accessed November 12, 2014.

14. Division of Global Migration and Quarantine, Center for Disease Control and Prevention. Guidelines for Pre-departure Presumptive Treatment and Directed Treatment for Malaria for all Refugees from Sub Saharan Africa. Available online at: http://www.cdc.gov/immigrantrefugeehealth/pdf/malaria-overseas.pdf. Accessed November 12, 2014.

15. Division of Global Migration and Quarantine, Centers for Disease Control and Prevention. Guidelines for overseas presumptive treatment of strongyloidiasis, schistosomiasis, and soil-transmitted helminth infections. 2012. Available online at: http://www.cdc.gov/immigrantrefugeehealth/guidelines/overseas/intestinal-parasites-overseas.html. Accessed November 12, 2014.

16. Division of Global Migration and Quarantine, Evaluating and Updating Immunizations during the Domestic Medical Examination for Newly Arrived Refugees. 2012. Available at: http://www.cdc.gov/immigrantrefugeehealth/guidelines/domestic/immunizations-guidelines.html. Accessed November 12, 2014.

17. Waldorf B, Gill C, Crosby SS. Assessing adherence to accepted national guidelines for immigrant and refugee screening and vaccines in an urban primary care practice: a retrospective chart review. J Immigr Minor Health 2014;16:839–45.

18. Alami NN, Yuen CM, Miramontes R, et al. Trends in tuberculosis - United States, 2013. MMWR Morb Mortal Wkly Rep 2014;63:229–33.

19. Boulware DR, Stauffer WM 3rd, Walker PF. Hypereosinophilic syndrome and mepolizumab. N Engl J Med 2008;358:2839 [author reply: 2839–40].

20. King CH, Dickman K, Tisch DJ. Reassessment of the cost of chronic helmintic infection: a meta-analysis of disability-related outcomes in endemic schistosomiasis. Lancet 2005;365:1561–9.

21. Gryseels B, Polman K, Clerinx J, et al. Human schistosomiasis. Lancet 2006;368:1106–18.

22. Strickland GT, Ramirez BL. Schistosomiasis. In: Strickland GT, editor. Hunter's tropical medicine and emerging infectious diseases. 8th edition. Philadelphia: W.B. Saunders Company; 2000. p. 802–32.

23. Pottie K, Janakiram P, Topp P, et al. Prevalence of selected preventable and treatable diseases among government-assisted refugees: implications for primary care providers. Can Fam Physician 2007;53:1928–34.

24. Lifson AR, Thai D, O'Fallon A, et al. Prevalence of tuberculosis, hepatitis B virus, and intestinal parasitic infections among refugees to Minnesota. Public Health Rep 2002;117:69–77.

25. Rossi C, Shrier I, Marshall L, et al. Seroprevalence of chronic hepatitis B virus infection and prior immunity in immigrants and refugees: a systematic review and meta-analysis. PLoS One 2012;7:e44611.

26. Weinbaum CM, Williams I, Mast EE, et al. Recommendations for identification and public health management of persons with chronic hepatitis B virus infection. MMWR Recomm Rep 2008;57:1–20.

27. Lok AS, McMahon BJ. Chronic hepatitis B: update 2009. Hepatology 2009;50: 661–2.

28. Jaranson JM, Butcher J, Halcon L, et al. Somali and Oromo refugees: correlates of torture and trauma history. Am J Public Health 2004;94:591–8.

29. Steel Z, Chey T, Silove D, et al. Association of torture and other potentially traumatic events with mental health outcomes among populations exposed to mass conflict and displacement: a systematic review and meta-analysis. JAMA 2009;302:537–49.

30. Fazel M, Wheeler J, Danesh J. Prevalence of serious mental disorder in 7000 refugees resettled in western countries: a systematic review. Lancet 2005;365: 1309–14.

31. Marshall GN, Schell TL, Elliott MN, et al. Mental health of Cambodian refugees 2 decades after resettlement in the United States. JAMA 2005;294:571–9.

32. Centers for Disease Control and Prevention (CDC). Suicide and suicidal ideation among Bhutanese refugees–United States, 2009-2012. MMWR Morb Mortal Wkly Rep 2013;62:533–6.

33. Mollica RF, Caspi-Yavin Y, Bollini P, et al. The Harvard Trauma Questionnaire. Validating a cross-cultural instrument for measuring torture, trauma, and post-traumatic stress disorder in Indochinese refugees. J Nerv Ment Dis 1992;180: 111–6.

34. Derogatis LR, Lipman RS, Rickels K, et al. The Hopkins Symptom Checklist (HSCL): a self-report symptom inventory. Behav Sci 1974;19:1–15.

35. Hollifield M, Verbillis-Kolp S, Farmer B, et al. The Refugee Health Screener-15 (RHS-15): development and validation of an instrument for anxiety, depression, and PTSD in refugees. Gen Hosp Psychiatry 2013;35:202–9.

36. Rhema SH, Gray A, Verbillis-Kolp S, et al. Mental health screening. In: Annamalai A, editor. Refugee health care. New York: Springer; 2014. p. 166.

37. Piwowarczyk L, Bishop H, Yusuf A, et al. Congolese and Somali beliefs about mental health services. J Nerv Ment Dis 2014;202:209–16.

38. McFarlane CA, Kaplan I. Evidence-based psychological interventions for adult survivors of torture and trauma: a 30-year review. Transcult Psychiatry 2012;49: 539–67.

39. Stenmark H, Catani C, Neuner F, et al. Treating PTSD in refugees and asylum seekers within the general health care system. A randomized controlled multi-center study. Behav Res Ther 2013;51:641–7.

40. Gorman R. Refugee survivors of torture: trauma and treatment. Prof Psychol Res Pract 2011;32:443–51.

41. Wenzel T, Kastrup MC, Eisenman DP. Survivors of torture: a hidden population. In: Walker PF, Barnett ED, editors. Immigrant medicine. Beijing (china): Saunders-Elsevier; 2007. p. 657.

42. Dross P. Survivors of politically motivated torture: a large, growing, and invisible population of crime victims. Washington, DC: U.S. Department of Justice OfVoC; 2000.

43. Amnesty International Annual Report 2011: The State of the World's Human Rights. 2011. Available at: http://files.amnesty.org/air11/air_2011_full_en.pdf. Accessed October 16, 2014.

44. Willard CL, Rabin M, Lawless M. The prevalence of torture and associated symptoms in United States iraqi refugees. J Immigr Minor Health 2014;16:1069–76.

45. Keller A, Lhewa D, Rosenfeld B, et al. Traumatic experiences and psychological distress in an urban refugee population seeking treatment services. J Nerv Ment Dis 2006;194:188–94.
46. Williams AC, Pena CR, Rice AS. Persistent pain in survivors of torture: a cohort study. J Pain Symptom Manage 2010;40:715–22.
47. Healing the Hurt. Available at: http://www.cvt.org/resources/publications. Accessed November 8, 2014.
48. Lipowski ZJ. Somatization: the concept and its clinical application. Am J Psychiatry 1988;145:1358–68.
49. Hinton DE, Park L, Hsia C, et al. Anxiety disorder presentations in Asian populations: a review. CNS Neurosci Ther 2009;15:295–303.
50. Yun K, Fuentes-Afflick E, Desai MM. Prevalence of chronic disease and insurance coverage among refugees in the United States. J Immigr Minor Health 2012;14: 933–40.
51. Schweitzer RD, Brough M, Vromans L, et al. Mental health of newly arrived Burmese refugees in Australia: contributions of pre-migration and post-migration experience. Aust N Z J Psychiatry 2011;45:299–307.
52. Annamalai A. Somatization in refugees: an overview. Rochester (NY): 2014 North American Refugee Health Conference; 2014.
53. Kroenke K. Patients presenting with somatic complaints: epidemiology, psychiatric comorbidity and management. Int J Methods Psychiatr Res 2003;12: 34–43.
54. Allen LA, Woolfolk RL, Escobar JI, et al. Cognitive-behavioral therapy for somatization disorder: a randomized controlled trial. Arch Intern Med 2006;166: 1512–8.
55. Thomas SL, Thomas SD. Displacement and health. Br Med Bull 2004;69:115–27.
56. Buja A, Gini R, Visca M, et al. Prevalence of chronic diseases by immigrant status and disparities in chronic disease management in immigrants: a population-based cohort study, Valore Project. BMC Public Health 2013;13:504.
57. Palinkas LA, Pickwell SM. Acculturation as a risk factor for chronic disease among Cambodian refugees in the United States. Soc Sci Med 1995;40:1643–53.
58. Huh J, Prause JA, Dooley CD. The impact of nativity on chronic diseases, self-rated health and comorbidity status of Asian and Hispanic immigrants. J Immigr Minor Health 2008;10:103–18.
59. Amara AH, Aljunid SM. Noncommunicable diseases among urban refugees and asylum-seekers in developing countries: a neglected health care need. Global Health 2014;10:24.
60. Kim ES, Strecher VJ, Ryff CD. Purpose in life and use of preventive health care services. Proc Natl Acad Sci U S A 2014;111:16331–6.
61. Geltman PL, Dookeran NM, Battaglia T, et al. Chronic disease and its risk factors among refugees and asylees in Massachusetts, 2001-2005. Prev Chronic Dis 2010;7:A51.
62. Langellier BA, Garza JR, Glik D, et al. Immigration disparities in cardiovascular disease risk factor awareness. J Immigr Minor Health 2012;14:918–25.
63. Kleinman A, Eisenberg L, Good B. Culture, illness, and care: clinical lessons from anthropologic and cross-cultural research. Ann Intern Med 1978;88:251–8.
64. Bokhour BG, Cohn ES, Cortes DE, et al. The role of patients' explanatory models and daily-lived experience in hypertension self-management. J Gen Intern Med 2012;27:1626–34.
65. Office of Admissions, Refugee Processing Center. Summary of Refugee Admissions. Series Editor: Department of State, Bureau of Population, Refugees, and

Migration. Available at: http://www.wrapsnet.org/Reports/AdmissionsArrivals/tabid/211/Default.aspx. Accessed November 8, 2014.

66. Bhatta MP, Shakya S, Assad L, et al. Chronic disease burden among Bhutanese refugee women aged 18-65 years resettled in Northeast Ohio, United States, 2008-2011. J Immigr Minor Health 2014. Available online at: http://link.springer.com/article/10.1007/s10903-014-0040-9.

67. Kumar GS, Varma S, Saenger MS, et al. Noninfectious disease among the Bhutanese refugee population at a United States urban clinic. J Immigr Minor Health 2014;16:922–5.

68. Yanni EA, Naoum M, Odeh N, et al. The health profile and chronic diseases comorbidities of US-bound Iraqi refugees screened by the International Organization for Migration in Jordan: 2007-2009. J Immigr Minor Health 2013;15:1–9.

69. Culhane-Pera KA, Her C, Her B. "We are out of balance here": a Hmong cultural model of diabetes. J Immigr Minor Health 2007;9:179–90.

70. Peterman JN, Wilde PE, Liang S, et al. Relationship between past food deprivation and current dietary practices and weight status among Cambodian refugee women in Lowell, MA. Am J Public Health 2010;100:1930–7.

71. Salti I, Benard E, Detournay B, et al. A population-based study of diabetes and its characteristics during the fasting month of Ramadan in 13 countries: results of the epidemiology of diabetes and Ramadan 1422/2001 (EPIDIAR) study. Diabetes Care 2004;27:2306–11.

72. Bravis V, Hui E, Salih S, et al. Ramadan Education and Awareness in Diabetes (READ) programme for Muslims with Type 2 diabetes who fast during Ramadan. Diabet Med 2010;27:327–31.

73. Al-Arouj M, Assaad-Khalil S, Buse J, et al. Recommendations for management of diabetes during Ramadan: update 2010. Diabetes Care 2010;33:1895–902.

74. Lee E, Ryan S, Birmingham B, et al. Rosuvastatin pharmacokinetics and pharmacogenetics in white and Asian subjects residing in the same environment. Clin Pharmacol Ther 2005;78:330–41.

75. Liao JK. Safety and efficacy of statins in Asians. Am J Cardiol 2007;99:410–4.

76. Office of Refugee Resettlement, history. 2014. Available at: http://www.acf.hhs.gov/programs/orr/about/history. Accessed November 14, 2014.

FURTHER READINGS

GENERAL MEDICAL CARE FOR THE REFUGEE PATIENT

Annamalai A, editor. Refugee health care: an essential medical guide. New York: Springer; 2014.

Walker P, Barnett E, editors. Immigrant medicine. Saunders-Elsevier; 2007.

HealthReach: Health Information in Many Languages. From the U.S. National Library of Medicine. Available online at: https://healthreach.nlm.nih.gov.

CROSS-CULTURE MEDICINE

Ethnomed website. Available at: http://ethnomed.org.

OVERSEAS AND DOMESTIC EVALUATION FOR US REFUGEES

CDC website. Available at: http://www.cdc.gov/immigrantrefugeehealth/.

MANAGEMENT OF LATENT TUBERCULOSIS

Curry Tuberculosis Center website. Available at: http://www.currytbcenter.ucsf.edu/.
McGill University's TST-in-3D website. Available at: http://www.tstin3d.com.

FEMALE GENITAL CUTTING

Hearst AA, Molnar AM. Female genital cutting: an evidence-based approach to clinical management for the primary care physician. Mayo Clin Proc 2013;88:618–29.

SURVIVORS OF TORTURE

Healing invisible wounds: paths to hope and recovery in a violent world by Richard Mollica. Nashville (TN): Vanderbilt University Press; 2006.
Refuge: Caring for survivors of torture. Available from Refuge Media Project. 47 Halifax Street Jamaica Plain, MA 02130. Email: refuge@refugemediaproject.org.
The Center for Victims of Torture website. Available at: http://www.cvt.org.

Primary Care of the Childhood Cancer Survivor

Anna Volerman, MD

KEYWORDS

- Childhood cancer survivor • Primary care • Treatment summary • Care plan

KEY POINTS

- As advanced therapies are developed, childhood cancer survivorship is increasing; however, these individuals face increased morbidity and mortality.
- Primary care providers play a fundamental role in the care of childhood cancer survivors and must monitor for late effects or recurrence and provide tailored preventive care.
- The individualized treatment summary and care plan provide crucial information for the long-term follow-up care of childhood cancer survivors.

CASE

A 25-year-old woman presents to your clinic to establish care. She has no acute concerns today. In reviewing her past medical history, she reports that she was diagnosed with leukemia at age 5. After receiving chemotherapy and radiation, she was told she was cured at age 10. She no longer sees an oncologist and was told to follow up regularly with a doctor. She asks if any testing is needed because of her cancer history.

INTRODUCTION

Childhood cancer affects 1 out of every 285 children younger than age 20 in the United States, with most common malignancies including leukemia, central nervous system (CNS) tumors, and lymphoma.[1] Because of advances in treatment, survival has steadily increased since the 1970s. Today more than 80% of children diagnosed with cancer are alive 5 years after diagnosis, thus considered cured.[1] With increasing survival rates, there are currently more than 375,000 survivors of childhood cancer in the United States with 70% of them age 20 or older.[1,2]

As survival rates increase, childhood cancer survivors encounter short- and long-term effects of their cancer and treatments. They face an increased risk for

Department of Medicine and Pediatrics, University of Chicago, 5841 South Maryland Avenue, MC 3051, Chicago, IL 60637, USA
E-mail address: avolerman@uchicago.edu

Med Clin N Am 99 (2015) 1059–1073
http://dx.doi.org/10.1016/j.mcna.2015.05.005
medical.theclinics.com

long-term morbidity and mortality in their adult years, compared with their siblings who serve as control subjects.[3–5] A multicenter, longitudinal cohort study of children in the United States diagnosed with cancer between 1970 and 1986 demonstrated that 75% of childhood cancer survivors develop a chronic health condition by age 40.[5] This condition is severe or life threatening in more than 40% of survivors.

Because of increased rates of morbidity and mortality from late effects, childhood cancer survivors require long-term follow-up care with a medical provider. With less than 20% of childhood cancer survivors receiving care at a cancer center or with an oncologist as adults, primary care providers play a vital role in the long-term care of childhood cancer survivors and thus need to have an understanding of survivorship care.[6]

HISTORY

In the primary care clinic, a patient's report of a history of childhood cancer should initiate the collection of specific information needed to appropriately manage the patient in the short and long term. Because of advances in cancer care for children, there is considerable variation in treatment; thus, details related to the patient's diagnosis, treatment, and complications are crucial for determining long-term follow-up care.

A treatment summary and survivorship plan should be developed by an oncologist at the end of a patient's cancer treatment. The treatment summary details the cancer diagnosis and treatment, including cancer type, location, and stage; chemotherapy names and cumulative doses; radiation types and cumulative doses; and surgical procedures. Individualized care plans also provide recommendations for the type and frequency of office visits, laboratory tests, and imaging, and surveillance areas and potential late effects. **Table 1** provides key information in the treatment summary and care plan.

Survivorship guidelines have been developed by the Children's Oncology Group, with abbreviated and comprehensive versions of care plan templates available at http://www.survivorshipguidelines.org.[7] If the patient does not have a treatment summary or survivor plan, a treatment summary or available medical records should be requested to guide decision-making about long-term care.

MANAGEMENT GOALS

The primary care provider focuses on three aspects of care for childhood cancer survivors: (1) recurrence and subsequent malignancies, (2) late effects of treatment, and (3) preventive care. There are many models of care for survivors of pediatric cancers in academic and community settings. It is important for primary care providers to understand their role in coordination with the oncologist.

The management of childhood cancer survivors is informed by longitudinal studies that have followed survivors throughout adulthood. In North America, the primary group examining outcomes for this population is the Childhood Cancer Survivor Study.[8] The study population includes an original cohort of more than 14,000 childhood cancer survivors who were diagnosed between 1970 and 1986 and treated at multiple centers in North America, along with approximately 4000 siblings as control subjects. Because of the advances made in therapy, the cohort is being expanded to include an additional 14,000 survivors diagnosed between 1987 and 1999 who are also being followed over time. Based on the data available with this cohort, more than 150 studies looking at specific late effects have been published.

Table 1
Information about cancer treatment of childhood cancer survivors

	Key Information	Additional Information
Diagnosis	Diagnosis/type of cancer Date of diagnosis Date therapy completed	Age at diagnosis Sites involved/stage/diagnostic details Laterality Hereditary/congenital history Treatment center Oncologist contact information
Relapse	Sites Treatment	Date Laterality Date therapy completed
Subsequent malignancies	Type Sites Treatment	Date Stage Date therapy completed
Treatment protocol	—	Acronym/number Title/description Date initiated and completed On-study
Chemotherapy	Drug name Cumulative dose	Route Additional information
Radiation	Site/field Total dose (Gy)	Laterality Start and stop date Initial dose, fractions, and dose per fraction Boost site and dose Type Radiation oncologist/institution
Hematopoietic cell transplant	Type Chronic graft-versus-host disease	Source Infusion date Conditioning regimen Graft-versus-host disease prophylaxis/treatment Treating physician/institution
Surgery	Date Procedure	Site Laterality Surgeon/institution
Other therapeutic modalities	Radioiodine therapy (I-131) Systemic MIBG Bioimmunotherapy	Other modalities
Complications/late effects	Problem	Date onset Date resolved Status
Adverse drug reactions/allergies	Drug Reaction	Date Status

Adapted from Children's Oncology Group. Summary of cancer treatment. Available at: http://www.survivorshipguidelines.org/. Accessed November 1, 2014.

RECURRENCE AND SUBSEQUENT MALIGNANCIES

Although 5-year disease-free survival signifies that the cancer has been cured, recurrence may occur after this time and is referred to as late recurrence. In fact, 4.4% of childhood cancer survivors have recurrence of their primary cancer within 10 years after diagnosis and 6.2% at 20 years after diagnosis. The highest rates of late recurrence are seen in Ewing sarcoma and astrocytoma, whereas the lowest rates occur with renal cancers. Most late recurrences occur at 5 to 10 years after diagnosis (69.1%), although recurrence can rarely occur up to 30 years later.[9]

In addition to recurrence, childhood cancer survivors face an increased risk of subsequent cancers. Within 30 years following diagnosis of the childhood cancer, 20.5% of survivors were diagnosed with a second cancer, including 7.9% diagnosed with a malignant neoplasm.[10] **Table 2** provides cumulative incidence of subsequent neoplasms in childhood cancer survivors based on childhood cancer diagnosis and subsequent neoplasm. The mean age of survivors at the time of subsequent neoplasm diagnosis was 29.5 years. The median time between primary and secondary diagnosis was 17.8 years, with a range of 5 to 29 years.[10]

The most frequent subsequent neoplasms were nonmelanoma skin cancer, affecting 9.1% of all childhood cancer survivors, and breast cancer, occurring in 5% of all childhood cancer survivors and making up 23% of subsequent cancers.[10] Survivors of Hodgkin lymphoma and Ewing sarcoma were also at highest risk of a subsequent cancer, with an 18.4% and 10.1% cumulative incidence, respectively.[10] Factors associated with a higher risk of subsequent cancer included female gender, older age at primary cancer diagnosis, treatment with radiation therapy, and primary cancer of Hodgkin lymphoma. It should be noted that these risks differed based on the primary diagnosis; for example, younger age at diagnosis of the primary cancer was associated with certain subsequent cancers, such as meningioma and thyroid cancer.[10]

Table 2
Cumulative incidence of subsequent neoplasms in childhood cancer survivors based on childhood cancer diagnosis and subsequent neoplasm

Childhood Cancer Diagnosis	30-y Cumulative Incidence[a] (%)	Subsequent Neoplasm	30-y Cumulative Incidence[a] (%)
All primary cancers	20.5	All (benign and malignant)	20.5
Hodgkin lymphoma	18.4	Malignant only[b]	7.9
Ewing sarcoma	10.1	Nonmelanoma skin cancer	9.1
Soft tissue sarcoma	8.8	Breast cancer (female only)	5
Medulloblastoma	7.8	Meningioma	3.1
Osteosarcoma	6.0	Thyroid cancer	1.4
Neuroblastoma	5.9	Soft tissue sarcoma	0.9
Non-Hodgkin lymphoma	5.8	Central nervous system tumor	0.7
Leukemia	5.6	Bone cancer	0.4
Astrocytoma	4.7	Lymphoma	0.4
Kidney cancer	4	Small intestine and colorectal cancer	0.4
—	—	Head and neck cancer	0.3
—	—	Leukemia	0.3
—	—	Lung cancer	0.1

[a] Cumulative incidence for all first or subsequent neoplasms at 30 years following childhood cancer diagnosis.
[b] Excluding nonmelanoma skin cancer.
Data from Friedman DL, Whitton J, Leisenring W. Subsequent neoplasms in 5-year survivors of childhood cancer: The Childhood Cancer Survivor Study. J Natl Cancer Inst 2010;102(14):1083–95.

The risk of recurrence and subsequent malignancies varies considerably based on the cancer diagnosis, cancer site, and treatment modalities. Continued surveillance of childhood cancer survivors is crucial. Patients should monitor for symptoms that may suggest cancer and report these to a medical provider. In addition, childhood cancer survivors should have a yearly comprehensive visit that includes a history and physical. For individuals who received radiation, a dermatologic examination of irradiated fields should also be performed annually.

Routine cancer screening guidelines should be followed for all survivors. However, earlier start or increased frequency of testing may be necessary based on the type of cancer and treatment received. For example, children who received chest radiation should begin breast cancer screening with mammogram and breast MRI 8 years after radiation or age 25, whichever occurs later.[7] In addition to examinations and screening tests, survivors should be advised to adopt habits that minimize their risk of cancer, including avoiding cigarettes, using sun protection, and maintaining a healthy diet. Close surveillance may decrease recurrence and subsequent neoplasms.

LATE EFFECTS

Although cancer therapy has become more effective and survival rates are increasing, childhood cancer survivors continue to encounter late effects, defined as side effects from the cancer treatment that can occur months to years after treatment ends.

Based on a Childhood Cancer Survivor Study that followed survivors and their siblings for a mean of 17.5 years from cancer diagnosis, childhood cancer survivors are significantly more likely to have any chronic disease (relative risk, 3.3; 95% confidence interval, 3–3.5) and two or more chronic diseases (relative risk, 4.9; 95% confidence interval, 4.4–5.5) when compared with their siblings.[6] Childhood cancer survivors were 8.2 times as likely to have a severe or life-threatening chronic health condition, such as myocardial infarction, heart failure, premature gonadal failure, subsequent neoplasm, or severe cognitive dysfunction. Survivors of bone tumors, CNS tumors, and Hodgkin lymphoma faced the highest risk of having a severe or life-threatening chronic disease, and multiple conditions.[6]

Thirty years after the cancer diagnosis, 73.5% of childhood cancer survivors reported at least one chronic health condition.[6] In addition, the incidence of chronic diseases increased with time from cancer diagnosis and did not plateau. Late effects can occur anywhere in the body and can include physical, cognitive, and psychosocial problems, in addition to subsequent malignancies.

Physical

The late effects related to physical health vary considerably based on individual factors (eg, age, gender, and genetic factors) and treatment factors (eg, the timing, intensity, and duration of therapy). **Table 3** provides late effects in adult survivors of childhood cancer according to organ system.

The Children's Oncology Group's Long-Term Follow-Up Guidelines[7] detail late effects according to treatment modality (chemotherapy, radiation, surgery), therapeutic agents (medication, radiation site and dose, surgical procedure), and organ system. For each therapy, late effects and risk factors are described. **Table 4** provides late effects based on chemotherapy agent and radiation site. In addition, recommendations for evaluation, including history, physical, and screening, and health counseling and other considerations are provided. Using an individualized treatment summary, a primary care physician can enact a survivor care plan that is based on with guidelines.

Table 3
Late effects in adult survivors of childhood cancer, according to organ system

Organ System	Late Effects
Cardiac	Atherosclerotic heart disease
	Myocardial infarction
	Valvular disease
	Cardiomyopathy
	Congestive heart failure
	Arrhythmia
	Pericarditis or pericardial fibrosis
	Carotid or subclavian artery disease
	Thrombosis/vascular disease
Pulmonary	Obstructive lung disease
	Restrictive lung disease
	Chronic bronchitis
	Bronchiectasis
	Bronchiolitis obliterans
	Interstitial pneumonitis
	Pulmonary fibrosis
Gastrointestinal/hepatic	Esophageal stricture
	Bowel obstruction or stricture
	Fecal incontinence
	Chronic enterocolitis
	Fistula
	Malabsorption
	Nutritional deficiency
	Cholelithiasis
	Cholecystitis
	Hepatic dysfunction
	Hepatic fibrosis
	Chronic hepatitis
	Cirrhosis
Renal/urinary	Hypertension
	Hydronephrosis
	Single kidney
	Renal insufficiency
	Renal glomerular hyperfiltration
	Renal tubular acidosis
	Renal Fanconi syndrome
	Hypophosphatemic rickets
	Renal calculi
	Bladder fibrosis
	Hemorrhagic cystitis
	Dysfunction voiding
	Urinary incontinence
	Vesicoureteral reflux
	Chronic urinary tract infection
	Urinary tract obstruction/stricture

(continued on next page)

Table 3 (*continued*)	
Organ System	**Late Effects**
Endocrine/metabolic	Hypothyroidism
	Hyperthyroidism
	Thyroid nodule
	Gonadal dysfunction or failure
	Adrenal insufficiency
	Hyperprolactinemia
	Short stature
	Growth hormone deficiency
	Metabolic syndrome
	Obesity or overweight
	Failure to thrive
	Impaired glucose tolerance
	Diabetes mellitus
	Dyslipidemia
Reproductive	Female:
	Primary ovarian failure
	Premature menopause
	Pregnancy/delivery complications
	Infertility
	Dyspareunia
	Ovarian cysts
	Vaginal stenosis or fibrosis
	Uterine vascular insufficiency
	Breast tissue hypoplasia
	Psychosexual dysfunction
	Male:
	Azoospermia/oligospermia
	Infertility
	Hypogonadism
	Erectile dysfunction
	Anejaculation
	Retrograde ejaculation
	Hydrocele
Musculoskeletal	Amputation
	Phantom pain
	Prosthesis malfunction or difficulty
	Avascular necrosis
	Contractures
	Fibrosis
	Hypoplasia
	Reduced growth
	Limb length discrepancy
	Osteopenia or osteoporosis
	Fracture
	Kyphosis
	Scoliosis
	Craniofacial abnormalities
Dermatologic	Dysplastic nevi
	Skin pigmentation alterations
	Vitiligo
	Skin fibrosis
	Scleroderma
	Alopecia
	Nail dysplasia
	Telangiectasias

(*continued on next page*)

Table 3 (continued)	
Organ System	**Late Effects**
Immune	Asplenia
	Hypogammaglobulinemia
	IgA deficiency
	Chronic graft-versus-host disease
	Chronic hepatitis B
	Chronic hepatitis C
	Human immunodeficiency virus
Neurologic	Seizures
	Stroke
	Moyamoya
	Cavernomas
	Occlusive cerebral vasculopathy
	Leukoencephalopathy
	Movement disorder
	Ataxia
	Motor deficit
	Paralysis
	Neurogenic bladder or bowel
	Peripheral neuropathy
Ocular	Cataract
	Enophthalmos
	Glaucoma
	Keratitis
	Xeroophthalmia
	Lacrimal duct atrophy
	Retinopathy
	Maculopathy
	Visual impairment
	Ocular nerve palsy
	Gaze paresis
	Nystagmus
	Papilledema or papillopathy
	Optic atrophy
	Optic chiasm neuropathy
Auditory	Eustachian tube dysfunction
	Hearing loss
	Otosclerosis
	Tympanosclerosis
	Tinnitus
	Vertigo
Dental	Enamel dysplasia
	Root thinning/shortening
	Agenesis of tooth/root
	Microdontia
	Periodontal disease
	Tooth decay
	Malocclusion
	Xerostomia
	Osteoradionecrosis
	Temporomandibular joint dysfunction

Adapted from Children's Oncology Group. Long-term follow-up guidelines for survivors of childhood, adolescent, and young adult cancers. Available at: http://www.survivorshipguidelines.org/. Accessed November 1, 2014.

Cognitive

In addition to physical effects, childhood cancer survivors experience neurocognitive impairment at higher rates compared with siblings, as a result of their prior treatments. Late effects may manifest as decreased overall intellectual ability and impaired

---

Table 4
Late effects based on chemotherapy agent and radiation site

Chemotherapy	Late Effects

Alkylating agents
  Busulfan
  Carmustine (BCNU)
  Chlorambucil
   Cyclophosphamide
  Ifosfamide
  Lomustine (CCNU)
   Mechlorethamine
  Melphalan
  Procarbazine
  Thiotepa
  Cisplation
  Carboplatin
	Gonadal dysfunction
	Acute myeloid leukemia, myelodysplasia
	Pulmonary fibrosis (busulfan, BCNU, CCNU)
	Cataracts (busulfan)
	Urinary tract toxicity (cyclophosphamides/ifosfamide)
	Bladder malignancy (cyclophosphamide)
	Renal toxicity (ifosfamide, platinum)
	Ototoxicity (platinum)
	Peripheral sensory neuropathy (platinum)
	Dysplipidemia (platinum)

Anthracyclines
  Daunorubicin
  Doxorubicin
  Epirubicin
  Idarubicin
  Mitoxantrone
	Acute myeloid leukemia
	Cardiac toxicity

Antimetabolites
  Cytarabine
  Mercaptopurine (6MP)
   Thioguanine (6TG)
  Methotrexate
	Neurocognitive deficits
	Clinical leukoencephalopathy
	Hepatic dysfunction
	Veno-occlusive disease
	Reduced bone mineral density
	Renal toxicity

Antitumor antibiotics Bleomycin	Pulmonary toxicity

Corticosteroids
  Dexamethasone
  Prednisone
	Reduced bone mineral density
	Osteonecrosis
	Cataracts

Topoisomerase II inhibitors
  Etoposide
  Teniposide
	Acute myeloid leukemia

Vinca alkaloids
  Vinblastine
  Vincristine
	Peripheral sensory or motor neuropathy
	Raynaud phenomenon

Radiation Site	**Late Effects**
All sites	Secondary benign or malignant neoplasm Bone malignancies Dysplastic nevi, skin cancer Dermatologic changes

(continued on next page)

Table 4
(continued)

Radiation Site	Late Effects
Cranial/head	Brain tumor Neurocognitive deficits Clinical leukoencephalopathy Cerebrovascular complications Craniofacial abnormalities Chronic sinusitis Overweight or obesity Metabolic syndrome Growth hormone deficiency Precocious puberty Hyperprolactinemia Central hypothyroidism Gonadotropin deficiency Central adrenal insufficiency Cataracts Ocular toxicity Ototoxicity Xerostomia, salivary gland dysfunction Dental abnormalities Osteoradionecrosis Thyroid abnormalities, nodules, cancer Carotid artery disease
Neck	Xerostomia Salivary gland dysfunction Dental abnormalities Osteoradionecrosis Thyroid abnormalities Thyroid nodules, cancer Carotid/subclavian artery disease Musculoskeletal growth problems Radiation-induced fracture
Mantle	Xerostomia, salivary gland dysfunction Dental abnormalities Osteoradionecrosis Thyroid abnormalities, nodules, cancer Carotid/subclavian artery disease Breast cancer, breast tissue hypoplasia Pulmonary toxicity Esophageal stricture Musculoskeletal growth problems Scoliosis, kyphosis Radiation-induced fracture
Chest	Thyroid abnormalities, nodules, cancer Carotid/subclavian artery disease Breast cancer, breast tissue hypoplasia Pulmonary toxicity Cardiac toxicity Musculoskeletal growth problems Scoliosis, kyphosis Radiation-induced fracture

(continued on next page)

Table 4 (*continued*)	
Radiation Site	**Late Effects**
Abdomen/pelvis	Cardiac toxicity Functional asplenia Hepatic fibrosis, cirrhosis Cholelithiasis Bowel obstruction Chronic enterocolitis, fistula, strictures Colorectal cancer Renal or urinary tract toxicity Hemorrhagic cystitis, bladder malignancy Uterine vascular insufficiency Gonadal dysfunction Vaginal fibrosis/stenosis Musculoskeletal growth problems Scoliosis, kyphosis Radiation-induced fracture
Spine (based on location in spine)	Thyroid abnormalities, nodules, cancer Carotid/subclavian artery disease Cardiac toxicity Bowel obstruction Esophageal stricture Chronic enterocolitis, fistula, strictures Colorectal cancer Uterine vascular insufficiency Gonadal dysfunction Musculoskeletal growth problems Radiation-induced fracture

Adapted from Children's Oncology Group. Long-term follow-up guidelines for survivors of childhood, adolescent, and young adult cancers. Available at: http://www.survivorshipguidelines.org/. Accessed November 1, 2014.

functioning in specific domains, such as attention, executive function, memory, and visual and motor processing.[11,12]

In survivors of CNS tumors, neurosurgery and/or cranial radiation have been demonstrated to cause a decline in neurocognitive functioning. Overall intellectual ability is affected, with a decline in intelligence quotient scores by 20 to 40 points in survivors of brain tumors.[11,13] Secondary effects of treatment, such as hearing loss, visual impairment, and stroke, are significantly associated with greater impairment.[11]

Survivors of non-CNS tumors also experience neurocognitive impairment, with one study demonstrating 13% to 21% of these survivors affected.[12] Cranial radiation and chemotherapy (systemic and intrathecal) are associated with cognitive impairment. The chemotherapy agents most commonly associated with neurotoxic effects include methotrexate and corticosteroids.[12]

Risk factors for greater cognitive impairment include female gender, younger age at cancer diagnosis, and higher doses of radiation. Younger children have developing brains, which may be more vulnerable to the neurotoxic effects. Higher doses of cranial radiation are associated with larger intelligence quotient declines, thought to be secondary to white matter changes.[11–13]

Deficits in intellectual ability and specific cognitive domains can impact survivors' quality of life and overall functioning in society. Primary care doctors caring for childhood cancer survivors should identify each patient's neurocognitive deficits and ensure appropriate resources and supports are in place to overcome these deficits.

Psychosocial

The diagnosis of childhood cancer and its associated treatment may affect social and emotional development, leading to a long-term impact on employment, social relationships, and psychological status.

Childhood cancer survivors are three times more likely to be unemployed as adults in the United States compared with healthy control subjects.[14] Factors associated with unemployment include brain tumors, high doses of cranial radiation, younger age at cancer diagnosis, female gender, and chronic medical conditions.[15] Among survivors who are employed, they are more likely to have lower-skill occupations and to receive a lower income, even after adjustment for educational level.[16] Unemployment and lower income may impact independent living, thus affecting survivors' quality of life.

In addition to unemployment, childhood cancer survivors experienced higher levels of impaired social functioning. In one Dutch study, young adult (age 18–30) survivors of cancer indicated they have fewer friends and are less likely to spend time with friends. In addition, they were older at the time of their first dating and sexual relationships and were less likely to engage in risky behaviors.[17] These findings may have lifelong implications, because studies show that childhood cancer survivors are less likely to marry than their peers. Once married, divorce rates were similar among survivors and peers. Individuals with a history of CNS tumors and cranial radiation have a lower rate of marriage, based on studies in United States and Britain.[18,19]

Social functioning and employment status impact psychological status. When examining rates of depression, anxiety, and somatization, childhood cancer survivors report more psychological distress than their siblings; however, both groups have fewer symptoms than the general population. Factors associated with worse psychological health are similar to the national population and include female gender, lower educational level, unemployment, lower income, unmarried or no long-term relationship, major health conditions, and worse health status.[20,21]

Although childhood cancer survivors have overall low levels of psychosocial distress and high level of life satisfaction, it is important to monitor for depression, anxiety, somatization, and other psychosocial disability to provide the support necessary to minimize impairment and maximize functioning in society.[21]

PREVENTIVE CARE

The primary care provider is responsible for providing general health care maintenance for childhood cancer survivors to minimize the chance of late effects. Childhood cancer survivors should undergo routine cancer screening based on their age and risk factors. Additional screening may be necessary based on their cancer treatment. For example, children who received radiation should have dermatologic examinations annually, because of high rates of nonmelanoma skin cancer. Children who had chest radiation as part of their treatment face an increased risk of breast cancer, with nearly 20% of this population developing breast cancer by age 45.[22] As a result, they should have annual breast cancer screening with mammography and breast MRI starting 8 years after radiation or at age 25, whichever is later. In addition, childhood cancer survivors who received abdominal or pelvic radiation are at 11 times higher risk of colorectal cancer.[23] Based on the cumulative dose of radiation received, they may require a colonoscopy starting 10 years after radiation or age 35, whichever is later.

Box 1
General counseling for the childhood cancer survivor

Avoid excessive sun or ultraviolet light exposure and use sun protection

Avoid tobacco or achieve smoking cessation

Maintain a healthy weight and lifestyle, including nutrition and physical fitness

Use safe sexual practices and contraception

Wear a seat belt properly and consistently

Be aware of risk of fractures

Report symptoms that may indicate late effects or recurrence (patient specific)

Adopt necessary practices based on late effects, for example limited sports participation for survivors with one kidney or need for endocarditis prophylaxis in certain valvular disease cases

Adapted from Children's Oncology Group. Long-term follow-up guidelines for survivors of childhood, adolescent, and young adult cancers. Available at: http://www.survivorshipguidelines.org/. Accessed November 1, 2014.

In addition to surveillance, the primary care provider should counsel survivors about practices that may increase the chance of developing late effects. **Box 1** provides specific counseling to provide to childhood cancer survivors. Counseling and prevention are instrumental to diminish the risks of late effects.

SUMMARY

Childhood cancer survivors are at high-risk for long-term morbidity and mortality as a result of their cancer diagnosis and treatment. Primary care providers play a key role in their long-term care, which includes monitoring for recurrence and secondary malignancies, evaluating for and treating late effects, and providing preventive care and counseling. Providers can use the recommendations for long-term follow-up care for childhood cancer survivors developed by The Children's Oncology Group, along with input from the patient's oncologist. The "Long-Term Follow-up Guidelines for Survivors of Childhood, Adolescent, and Young Adult Cancers" is publicly accessible at http://www.survivorshipguidelines.org, including patient education materials in the form of "Health Links." By providing ongoing surveillance and follow-up care, primary care providers can help childhood cancer survivors lead long and fulfilling lives.

CASE REVISITED

It is important to obtain and treatment summary and survivor care plan to guide follow-up care in this patient, based on the long-term follow-up guidelines. A comprehensive history and physical should be performed annually by the primary care physician, including a psychosocial assessment. If she received radiation, a yearly dermatologic examination should be performed. The primary care provider should counsel the patient to avoid smoking, eat healthy and exercise regularly, use sun protection, and avoid cigarettes and other substances. Additional surveillance and testing is guided by the specific treatment the patient received.

ACKNOWLEDGMENT

The author thanks Tara Henderson, MD, MPH, for her input on the article.

REFERENCES

1. American Cancer Society. Cancer facts & figures 2014. Atlanta (GA): American Cancer Society; 2014.
2. Howlader N, Noone AM, Krapcho M, et al, editors. SEER cancer statistics review, 1975-2011. National Cancer Institute. Available at: http://seer.cancer.gov/csr/1975_2011. Accessed November 1, 2014.
3. Armstrong GT, Liu Q, Yasui Y, et al. Late mortality among 5-year survivors of childhood cancer: a summary from the Childhood Cancer Survivor Study. J Clin Oncol 2009;27:2328–38.
4. Mertens AC, Yasui Y, Neglia JP, et al. Late mortality experience in five-year survivors of childhood and adolescent cancer: the Childhood Cancer Survivor Study. J Clin Oncol 2001;19:3163–72.
5. Oeffinger KC, Mertens AC, Sklar CA, et al, for the Childhood Cancer Survivor Study. Chronic health conditions in adult survivors of childhood cancer. N Engl J Med 2006;355:1572–82.
6. Oeffinger KC, Mertens AC, Hudson MM, et al. Health care of young adult survivors of childhood cancer: a report from the Childhood Cancer Survivor Study. Ann Fam Med 2004;2:61–70.
7. Children's Oncology Group. Long-term follow-up guidelines for survivors of childhood, adolescent, and young adult cancers. Available at: http://www.survivorshipguidelines.org/. Accessed November 1, 2014.
8. St. Jude Children's Research Hospital. The Childhood Cancer Survivor Study. Available at: https://ccss.stjude.org/. Accessed October 23, 2014.
9. Wasilewski-Masker K, Liu Q, Yasui Y, et al. Late recurrence in pediatric cancer: a report from the Childhood Cancer Survivor Study. J Natl Cancer Inst 2009; 101(24):1709–20.
10. Friedman DL, Whitton J, Leisenring W. Subsequent neoplasms in 5-year survivors of childhood cancer: the Childhood Cancer Survivor Study. J Natl Cancer Inst 2010;102(14):1083–95.
11. Ellenberg L, Liu Q, Gioia G, et al. Neurocognitive status in long-term survivors of childhood CNS malignancies: a report from the Childhood Cancer Survivor Study. Neuropsychology 2009;23(6):705–17.
12. Kadan-Lottick NS, Zeltzer LK, Liu Q, et al. Neurocognitive functioning in adult survivors of childhood non-central nervous system cancers. J Natl Cancer Inst 2010; 102(12):881–93.
13. Mulhern RK, Merchant TE, Gajjar A, et al. Late neurocognitive sequelae in survivors of brain tumours in childhood. Lancet Oncol 2004;5(7):399–408.
14. deBoer AG, Verbeek JH, van Dijk FJ, et al. Adult survivors of childhood cancer and unemployment: a metaanalysis. Cancer 2006;107(1):1–11.
15. Gurney JG, Krull KR, Kadan-Lottick N, et al. Social Outcomes in the Childhood Cancer Survivor Study Cohort. J Clin Oncol 2009;27(14):2390–5.
16. Kirchhoff AC, Krull KR, Ness KK, et al. Occupational outcomes of adult childhood cancer survivors: a report from the Childhood Cancer Survivor Study. Cancer 2011;117(13):3033–44.
17. Stam H, Grootenhuis MA, Last BF. The course of life of survivors of childhood cancer. Psychooncology 2005;14:227–38.
18. Janson C, Leisenrig W, Cox C, et al. Predictors of marriage and divorce in adult survivors of childhood cancers: a report from the Childhood Cancer Survivor Study. Cancer Epidemiol Biomarkers Prev 2009;18(10):2626–35.

19. Frobisher C, Lancashire ER, Winter DL, et al. Long-term population-based marriage rates among adult survivors of childhood cancer in Britain. Int J Cancer 2007;121(4):846–55.
20. Zebrack BJ, Zevon MA, Turk N, et al. Psychological distress in long-term survivors of solid tumors diagnosed in childhood: a report from the Childhood Cancer Survivor Study. Pediatr Blood Cancer 2007;49(1):47–51.
21. Zeltzer LK, Lu Q, Leisenring W, et al. Psychosocial outcomes and health-related quality of life in adult childhood cancer survivors: a report from the Childhood Cancer Survivor Study. Cancer Epidemiol Biomarkers Prev 2008;17(2):435–46.
22. Kenney LB, Yasui Y, Inskip PD. Breast cancer after childhood cancer: a report from the Childhood Cancer Survivor Study. Ann Intern Med 2004;141(8):590–7.
23. Henderson TO, Oeffinger KC, Whitton J, et al. Secondary gastrointestinal cancer in childhood cancer survivors: a cohort study. Ann Intern Med 2012;156(11):757–66.

Primary Care of the Solid Organ Transplant Recipient

Christopher J. Wong, MD*, Genevieve Pagalilauan, MD

KEYWORDS

- Primary care • Immunocompromised host • Immunosuppressive agents
- Solid organ transplantation • Liver transplantation • Heart transplantation
- Kidney transplantation • Lung transplantation

KEY POINTS

- Care of the solid organ transplant (SOT) recipient includes assessment of function of the transplanted organ, symptoms and signs of infection and rejection, and medication toxicities.
- Common metabolic complications of immunosuppressants include chronic kidney disease, hypertension, hyperlipidemia, diabetes, gout, and decreased bone density.
- Increased risk of malignancy, especially skin cancers and posttransplant lymphoproliferative disorder, is an important long-term complication of immunosuppressive medications used in SOT recipients.
- Infections in SOT recipients tend to follow a pattern depending on time since transplant; increased immunosuppression used to treat rejection effectively "resets the clock" with respect to timing of infections.
- Live vaccines are contraindicated in SOT recipients receiving immunosuppressive medications.

INTRODUCTION

Solid organ transplantation (SOT) is one of the most remarkable advances in modern medicine. Between 2009 and 2013, an average of 28,533 SOTs were performed each year in the United States.[1] The most commonly transplanted organ is the kidney, followed by the liver, heart, and lung (**Table 1**). The life expectancy of SOT recipients is increasing: the 50% survival for liver and kidney transplants now exceeds 10 years[2]; 5-year survival rates are shown in **Table 2**.[3]

With SOT, the certainty of death from a failing organ is supplanted by the promise and expectation of restored life. This transformation requires accepting the upfront risk of transplantation, facing the morbidity of a host of potential complications, and

Division of General Internal Medicine, Department of Medicine, University of Washington, 4245 Roosevelt Way Northeast, Box 354760, Seattle, WA 98105, USA
* Corresponding author.
E-mail address: cjwong@uw.edu

Med Clin N Am 99 (2015) 1075–1103
http://dx.doi.org/10.1016/j.mcna.2015.05.002
0025-7125/15/$ – see front matter © 2015 Elsevier Inc. All rights reserved.

medical.theclinics.com

Table 1
Average number of transplants per year in the United States, between 2009 and 2013

Organ	Average Number of Transplants per Year
Kidney	16,785
Liver	6333
Heart	2355
Lung	1786
Kidney-Pancreas	808
Pancreas	302
Intestine	135
Heart-Lung	30

Data from Health Resources and Services Administration, US Department of Health & Human Services. Transplants in the US by recipient age, US transplants performed: January 1, 1988–September 30, 2014. Organ Transplantation and Procurement Network. Available at: http://optn.transplant.hrsa.gov/converge/latestData/step2.asp. Accessed December 13, 2014.

then committing to sustained maintenance efforts to stay as healthy as possible. The increase in survivors of SOT beckons generalists to have continued and expanding roles in treating SOT recipients. Patients with complex medical and social problems are common in primary care, but there are nevertheless specific considerations to the care of SOT recipients that are essential to optimizing their health.

INITIAL ASSESSMENT OF THE SOLID ORGAN TRANSPLANT RECIPIENT

Case

A 54-year-old man presents for a first visit to a primary care provider, stating he has "graduated" from the liver transplant program. He is feeling well.

Table 2
Approximate 5-year survival of solid organ transplant recipients in the United States, 1997–2004

Organ	Approximate 5-y Survival, %	
	Women	Men
Kidney	86	84
Liver	73	72
Heart	69	73
Lung	47	47
Kidney-Pancreas	84	86
Pancreas	80	85
Intestine	46	49
Heart-Lung	42	36

Data from Health Resources and Services Administration, US Department of Health & Human Services. All Kaplan-Meier patient survival rates for transplants performed: 1997–2004, based on OPTN data as of December 5, 2014. Organ Procurement and Transplantation Network. Available at: http://optn.transplant.hrsa.gov/converge/latestData/step2.asp. Accessed December 13, 2014.

Recipients of SOTs typically are followed closely by the transplant team before and immediately after transplantation. Patients who have an uncomplicated postoperative course (a well-functioning graft, without opportunistic infections or rejection) will often return to the care of the primary care provider with periodic evaluations by the transplant specialist. The extent of specialty follow-up versus transition to primary care is not uniform and should be individualized; for example, a liver transplant recipient who is doing well several years after transplantation might see a primary care provider regularly but the transplant hepatologist yearly, whereas a heart transplant recipient may continue to see the transplant cardiologist frequently for life.

History-Taking Elements

The initial assessment should include identifying the patient's recommended follow-up schedule and the relevant specialty providers involved. The key facts to gather at the initial primary care visit are summarized in **Table 3**.

Basic data
The date of transplantation is an important consideration with regard to the differential diagnosis of infectious complications, as well as the risk of malignancy from cumulative immunosuppressive burden. The reason for transplantation, and the extent of organ failure and complications before transplantation, should be reviewed.

Laboratory data
The recipient and donor status for the viruses Epstein-Barr virus (EBV) and cytomegalovirus (CMV) should be documented. The highest risk for opportunistic CMV infection is in CMV-negative recipients of CMV-positive grafts. Similarly, the highest risk for EBV-related complications, such as posttransplant lymphoproliferative disorder (PTLD) is in the recipient-negative host who receives a donor-positive organ.

Status of the transplanted organ
Previous tests assessing the function of the transplanted organ should be reviewed carefully. Dysfunction of the transplanted organ may be due to rejection by the recipient's immune system, return of the underlying disease, or development of a new illness. Protocols for laboratory, radiologic, and pathologic surveillance vary by transplant center. Monitoring is frequent in the first 6 to 12 months after transplantation, and moderates over time if there are no complications. The indication for transplantation may warrant additional monitoring: although some diseases are not expected to recur in the transplanted organ (eg, chronic obstructive pulmonary disease [COPD] in a lung transplant recipient who no longer smokes), others may be expected to cause disease and merit surveillance (eg, hepatitis C in liver transplant recipients). Patients should be assessed for being up to date with their individualized monitoring protocol. General guidelines are summarized in **Table 4**.

Rejection
Previous episodes of rejection should be documented, including how they presented, how they were confirmed (eg, biopsy), and what treatment was initiated (typically an increase in immunosuppression). Rejection may be classified as cellular or antibody-mediated, in addition to other pathologic features, or as early or late with regard to time since transplantation.

Infectious complications
A thorough history of infections, both opportunistic and nonopportunistic but serious (eg, community-acquired pneumonia) should be obtained.

Table 3
History-taking elements for the solid organ transplant recipient

Topic	History	Example
1. Basic data	History of organ failure/ indication for transplant. Date of transplant?	Cirrhosis due to hepatitis C diagnosed 2004. Before transplantation developed ascites, encephalopathy, GI bleeding. Liver transplant, cadaveric, June 2009.
2. Laboratory data	Patient and donor's CMV and EBV status.	CMV: donor positive, recipient positive. EBV: donor positive, recipient negative.
3. Last state of the transplanted organ	May include symptoms, laboratory studies, imaging, and biopsy results (See **Table 4**). Assess if the original disease for which the organ was transplanted is likely to reoccur.	For a liver transplant: AST, ALT 50–70, total bilirubin 1.0, INR 1.0, albumin 4.0, creatinine 0.9, platelets 139. Last liver biopsy June 2014: mild inflammation, no evidence of rejection.
4. History of rejection?	Previous episodes of rejection. Previous treatment (eg, increased immunosuppression).	Acute rejection in 2010 diagnosed by biopsy, treated with corticosteroids.
5. Infectious complications	Opportunistic and other infections.	CMV gastritis 2011. Community-acquired pneumonia 2012.
6. Medications	Current immunosuppressive medication regimen, including how well it is tolerated, goal level(s) of immunosuppressant medications, adherence. Anti-infectious prophylaxis, if applicable.	Prednisone 5 mg once daily. Tacrolimus 1.5 mg twice daily (goal level 4–6). Taking medications.
7. Other complications	Organ-specific complications. Metabolic complications.	Diabetes since 2012 and mild CKD thought due to tacrolimus.

Abbreviations: ALT, alanine aminotransferase; AST, aspartate aminotransferase; CKD, chronic kidney disease; CMV, cytomegalovirus; EBV, Epstein-Barr virus; GI, gastrointestinal; INR, international normalized ratio.

Medications

A careful medication history should be obtained for dosages, goal levels, and adherence. In most cases, the transplant specialist monitors and adjusts the immunosuppressant levels. Drug levels, when followed, are typically drawn as trough levels just before the morning dose, and although the generalist should not be adjusting immunosuppressant medications, a working knowledge of what is the target level for a given patient is useful. The target level usually decreases over time if there is no rejection. Immunosuppressant brand names should be identified, as the formulations have different milligram dosing. Antirejection medications are discussed in more detail in a

Table 4
Typical surveillance schedules for graft function in asymptomatic solid organ transplant recipients

Transplanted Organ	Laboratory	Other Testing	Biopsy
Kidney	Urine volume, protein every 3 mo in first year, then annually. Serum creatinine frequently in the first 6 mo, then monthly for the remainder of the first year, then every 2–3 mo lifelong.[4]	BK virus may be screened or followed depending on the patient's risk and presence of disease.	Biopsies for surveillance are commonly performed, vary by transplant center, and are individualized for a given patient. A typical schedule is at 6 mo, 12 mo, and 2 y after transplantation.
Liver	Transaminases, alkaline phosphatase, bilirubin, albumin, INR, electrolytes, BUN, creatinine, CBC. Frequent in the first 6 mo, then typically every 3 mo lifelong. The frequency should be individualized by the transplant center.[5]	Varies by transplant center: Liver ultrasound with Doppler: annually.	Varies by transplant center and by indication for transplant. Typical schedule is at 6 mo, 12 mo, then yearly for hepatitis C, every 5 y for other indications.
Heart	—	Coronary angiography (to assess for cardiac allograft vasculopathy): yearly but adjusted balancing risk of disease and risk of procedure.	Varies by transplant center. Endomyocardial biopsy is frequent in first 1–2 y, then less frequently afterward.
Lung	—	Spirometry at every transplant follow-up visit; frequency of visits varies by transplant center.	The use of transbronchial biopsy varies by transplant center.
All SOT recipients	Typically receive monitoring for immunosuppressive medication side effects and drug levels every 3 mo once stable.	—	—

These are shown for reference only; the patient's transplant team individualizes the surveillance for a given patient.
Abbreviations: BUN, blood, urea, nitrogen; CBC, complete blood count; INR, international normalized ratio; SOT, solid organ transplantation.

later section (Medications: interactions and side effects). Patients should be asked about supplements and over-the-counter preparations. A patient's laboratory monitoring schedule should be obtained (typically complete blood count, comprehensive metabolic panel, and drug levels every 3 months). It should be clearly defined who is responsible for laboratory monitoring. Adherence should be assessed, as side effects and expense may be barriers to consistent use.

Other Medical History

In addition to taking the usual full medical history of unrelated conditions, illnesses related to the transplant should be reviewed.

Systemic illnesses that lead to transplantation

Some systemic illnesses may lead to organ transplantation but still cause disease after transplantation. Examples include patients with cystic fibrosis who receive bilateral lung transplantation but continue to have gastrointestinal disease; patients with systemic lupus erythematosus who require a kidney transplant due to lupus nephritis, but still continue to intermittently have active disease elsewhere. The activity and treatment of these conditions, if present, should be assessed.

Other complications common to solid organ transplant recipients

All SOT recipients are at risk for the following:

Chronic kidney disease Chronic kidney disease (CKD) is one of the most common complications of all SOTs: it occurs in 30% to 80% of liver transplant recipients with a risk of progression to end-stage renal disease (ESRD) of 5% to 8%.[5] Etiology may be multifactorial, but often at least partially caused by toxicity from the calcineurin inhibitors cyclosporine and tacrolimus. Treatment includes blood pressure control, eliminating other nephrotoxins, including nonsteroidal anti-inflammatory drugs (NSAIDs), and consideration of reduction in calcineurin inhibitor dose if possible. Consultation is usually warranted with a nephrologist familiar with the care of SOT recipients. If ESRD develops, the treatment of choice is renal transplantation.

Hypertension Hypertension is common and may be in part caused by immunosuppressive medications. Calcium channel blockers (eg, amlodipine, felodipine) may be used, but diltiazem and verapamil are avoided (see Medications: interactions and side effects, later in this article). Angiotensin-converting enzyme inhibitors and angiotensin receptor blockers may be used, but creatinine and potassium should be monitored carefully. Diuretics should be used with caution, as magnesium wasting that can occur due to calcineurin inhibitors may be worsened, and thiazide diuretics may increase hyperuricemia.

Metabolic complications Hyperlipidemia is common and may in part be caused by calcineurin inhibitors. Statin therapy should be considered for SOT recipients at increased cardiovascular risk, and is recommended for all heart transplant recipients (see Organ-specific Issues, later in this article). Drug interactions with statins are common with medications given to SOT recipients and careful selection is important. In general, high doses of simvastatin, lovastatin, and atorvastatin should be avoided because of the greatest interaction risk, especially in patients receiving cyclosporine.

Hyperuricemia from calcineurin inhibitors may cause symptomatic gout. Acute gout may be managed in the usual way; however, many SOT recipients have CKD and cannot receive NSAIDs. Chronic urate-lowering therapy, when indicated, is usually managed with allopurinol. Other medications that may increase uric acid levels should be avoided if possible. Patients taking azathioprine require dose adjustment and close monitoring if allopurinol must be used, and the transplant specialist should be consulted.

Diabetes may be caused by calcineurin inhibitors and corticosteroids, and is usually screened for in the SOT recipient (see Preventive health in SOT recipients, later in this article).

Review of Systems

Review of systems should assess for symptoms of infection, specific organ dysfunction, and medication side effects.

Physical Examination

Examination should assess the transplanted organ, as well as any other primary care–related concerns.

The renal transplant is most often located in the lower pelvis and is palpable on examination. Patients may have had hemodialysis before transplantation and may still have a functioning arterio-venous fistula or other vascular access. Although pancreas transplants are sometimes performed in isolation, they are most commonly performed in combination with a renal transplant, and situated in the opposite lower quadrant of the abdomen. Pancreas transplants are increasingly performed with enteric drainage rather than bladder drainage to reduce risk of urinary tract complications and acidosis.

The liver transplant scar is typically a 3-spoked incision radiating from the epigastrium. Stigmata of chronic liver disease often resolves after transplantation. There should not be evidence of recurrence of cirrhosis in a well-functioning transplant. In the liver transplant recipient who had previous portal hypertension, splenomegaly may persist for years after transplantation despite the resolution of portal hypertension.[5]

Heart transplant recipients have a median sternotomy scar; examination may otherwise be normal in patients with well-functioning grafts. Rejection can include signs of heart failure and tachycardia.

Lung transplants may be single or bilateral. Single lung transplant recipients may still have disease in the native lung, and can cause ensuing complications (eg, pneumonia, pneumothorax in a patient with COPD). Graft dysfunction, usually caused by chronic rejection (bronchiolitis obliterans syndrome) may be subtle and not heard on auscultation, but may also present with rales and rhonchi.

For all patients, look for signs of complications of medications: hypertension, fever, steroid complications (striae, skin thinning, compression fractures).

FOLLOW-UP VISITS
Routine Follow-up

The frequency of follow-up with a primary care provider, if not determined by the patient's other medical conditions, should be at least yearly, but closer routine follow-up should be considered. Patients will receive more frequent laboratory monitoring depending on the transplant center's protocols and individualized for the patient, and follow-up visits with the transplant specialist depending on the patient's type of transplant, indication for transplant, risk factors, and complications.

Visits for Medical Conditions or Symptoms

At visits for acute concerns or other medical conditions, the primary care provider will need to assess whether the problem is potentially related to the patient's transplantation. If the visit is not primarily to assess the transplant, the minimum assessment of the transplanted organ is to recheck medication dosage and adherence and whether the patient is due for any surveillance studies. A review of systems should be geared toward the transplanted organ's function and for other complications.

Common primary care symptoms require an expanded differential diagnosis in SOT recipients, and earlier workup for complications is often warranted. In general, patients many years from transplantation with a well-functioning graft will typically be at less risk for most opportunistic infections, but at greater risk for malignancy from cumulative years of immunosuppression.

Organ-specific Issues

In addition to the previously discussed general considerations for all SOT recipients, organ-specific complications include the following:

Kidney transplantation

Renal transplant recipients may develop posttransplant erythrocytosis, which remits in some patients, and in uncommon cases, may be severe and symptomatic. BK polyoma virus nephropathy may contribute to graft failure, is monitored in many transplant protocols, and is distinguished from rejection by biopsy. In contrast to rejection, the transplant nephrologist may manage BK virus nephropathy by a reduction in immunosuppression. Renal transplant graft rejection, although it can occasionally present with pain and tenderness of the transplanted kidney, is usually manifested as an increase in serum creatinine, thus necessitating surveillance laboratory monitoring. Unlike other organ transplants, should graft failure occur, patients have the option of starting renal replacement therapy with dialysis; such therapy will depend on candidacy for repeat transplantation, overall health, quality of life, and patient preferences.

Pancreas transplantation

Pancreas transplants are often performed in combination with a kidney transplant; the blood supply is anastomosed to the iliac artery system, and the exocrine ducts are drained to either the bladder or small bowel. Rejection may manifest as a decrease in pancreatic endocrine function, increase in urine amylase (if bladder drained), or an increase in serum amylase.

Liver transplantation

In addition to rejection, assessment of recurrent disease is very important in liver transplant recipients, as the most common causes of liver transplantation can both recur. Hepatitis C commonly reoccurs in the transplanted liver, and usually requires more frequent liver biopsies: yearly instead of every 5 years. Alcohol use also may reoccur and should be screened at every visit. Liver transplant rejection causes elevated transaminases, bilirubin, and alkaline phosphatase. Severe cases may present with right upper quadrant pain and symptoms of liver failure.

Heart transplantation

Cardiovascular disease in the transplanted heart may arise from the donor heart, de novo due to traditional cardiovascular risk factors, or from cardiac allograft vasculopathy. Statin therapy is recommended for *all* heart transplant recipients regardless of lipid levels.[6] Cardiac allograft vasculopathy is a form of coronary artery disease and a major source of morbidity in heart transplant recipients. It often presents as diffuse coronary vessel stenosis, and can progress to ischemia, heart failure, and arrhythmia. Because of denervation, patients usually do not present with classic anginal symptoms. Cardiac allograft vasculopathy is monitored by yearly coronary angiography. Patients with severe CKD, as from calcineurin inhibitors, are at increased risk from coronary angiography; if they have had previous negative evaluations, then surveillance may either be discontinued or replaced by stress echocardiogram in select patients at the discretion of their cardiologist.[6]

In heart transplant recipients, rejection may manifest as symptoms of heart failure. Cardiac function is assessed by the patient's history and examination, and surveillance for rejection relies on biopsy. Endomyocardial biopsy remains the gold standard to assess for rejection and is performed frequently in the first year after transplantation. After the first year, biopsies may continue depending on the patient's risk and if there has been previous rejection.[6] Other modalities to assess for rejection include gene expression profiling, which is sometimes used as one component of the evaluation. Echocardiograms are frequently performed for other reasons, but are not recommended purely to assess for rejection.[6] Biopsy schedules tend to be more frequent in heart transplant patients compared with liver and kidney transplant recipients.

Lung transplantation

As with care of the heart transplant recipient, there are no blood tests for lung function. Monitoring for lung function is usually accomplished by spirometry: more frequently in the first 2 years, and at every follow-up visit with the transplant specialist, with some patients additionally performing home spirometry. Bronchiolitis obliterans, a form of chronic graft rejection, is the most common cause of graft failure. Rejection in lung transplant recipients may present with dyspnea, cough, and hypoxia. The frequency of surveillance biopsy via bronchoscopy varies by transplant center, but when performed by protocol, is typically more common in the first 2 years, then afterward as needed.

When to Consult with Transplant Team/Specialist

There should be a low threshold to consult with the transplant specialist. Infections, hospitalization, anticipated surgery, systemic symptoms, symptoms or signs of graft problems, altered mental status, any condition that interferes with the ability to take or absorb transplant medications, should all prompt consultation with the transplant team.

PREVENTIVE HEALTH IN SOLID ORGAN TRANSPLANT RECIPIENTS

Case

A 62-year-old woman with idiopathic pulmonary fibrosis status post lung transplant 6 years ago returns for a preventive health visit.

SOT recipients should continue to receive preventive health measures to reduce risky behaviors, identify diseases at an earlier stage, and lower risk of acquiring new illnesses. Because of their immunosuppressed status and other risks, however, preventive health measures require modification compared with an otherwise healthy patient (**Tables 5** and **6**).

Immunizations

General considerations

- Live vaccines are contraindicated in the SOT recipient. Any anticipated live vaccines should be administered before transplantation.[8]
- During periods of increased immunosuppression (eg, treatment of a rejection episode) vaccinations should generally be held with the exception of inactivated influenza vaccination during an outbreak.[8]
- In general, routine vaccinations should start 2 to 6 months after transplantation and not in the immediate posttransplant period when immunosuppression is expected to be at its highest levels.[8]

Table 5
Preventive health measures in a solid organ transplant recipient

Measure	Frequency/Indication	Notes
Metabolic complications		
Blood pressure	Every visit.	—
Lipid panel	Every 6–12 mo.	Increased risk in patients receiving calcineurin inhibitors.
Diabetes screening (fasting blood sugar or A1c)	Every 6–12 mo.	Increased risk in patients receiving calcineurin inhibitors and glucocorticoids.
Cancer screening		
Breast cancer Colorectal cancer Lung cancer Prostate cancer	No change in frequency—follow standard guidelines.	—
Cervical cancer	No change in frequency, or yearly.	Increased risk—some investigators advocate yearly screening.
Skin cancer	Annual skin examinations.	With a dermatologist or experienced primary care provider.
Bone density		
Dual-energy X-ray absorptiometry	1 y after transplantation, then every 2–3 y if not osteopenic.	Adjust frequency based on risk factors and previous results. Some guidelines recommend checking in the first 3 mo after transplantation.
Substance use		
Smoking	At each visit.	—
Alcohol	At each visit.	Especially in liver transplant recipients who had alcoholic cirrhosis.
Recreational drugs	At each visit.	—
Contraception		
Assessment	Women of child-bearing age with a male partner: provide for first 1–2 y after transplant, and then as needed.	All options available. Use combined oral contraceptives with caution if heart disease or liver disease.
Mental health		
Depression screening	Screen periodically.	Exact frequency uncertain.

- Household contacts of SOT recipients may receive vaccinations based on Centers for Disease Control and Prevention guidelines, including the live vaccines measles-mumps-rubella, varicella, zoster, and rotavirus, provided they meet indications. However, oral polio vaccine should not be given to household contacts, and SOT recipients should not handle diapers of infants vaccinated with rotavirus for 4 weeks after vaccination. Immunocompetent persons who develop skin lesions after either the varicella or herpes zoster vaccine should avoid contact with SOT recipients.[8]

Recommendations for specific vaccines are shown in **Table 6**.

Table 6
Preventive health measures in a solid organ transplant recipient: immunizations

Vaccinations[7]	Recommendation	Notes
Note: *all live virus vaccines contraindicated*	Contraindicated	Varicella: Varicella immune status is checked before transplantation and patients who are not immune to varicella zoster should be immunized before transplantation if they are not immunosuppressed for other reasons and it is at least 4 wk before transplantation.[8] After transplantation, varicella vaccine (VAR), a live virus, is contraindicated due to high levels of immunosuppression. Herpes zoster: Reactivation of varicella zoster (herpes zoster, or shingles) is common in the SOT population: approximate incidence 9%, high rates in the first year after transplantation, approximately 40% chance of post herpetic neuralgia.[9] The shingles vaccine, also a live virus, is contraindicated when receiving immunosuppression after solid organ transplantation, and therefore should be given before transplantation if the patient meets standard indications (age 60 or older and if it can be given at least 4 wk before transplantation; can consider age 50–59).[8] Other common live vaccines: The measles mumps rubella (MMR), live attenuated intranasal influenza vaccine, and the live oral typhoid vaccine (often given to travelers) are also contraindicated after transplantation.
Influenza	Yearly (inactivated vaccine)	Live attenuated intranasal influenza vaccinations are contraindicated.
Pneumococcal[10]	Pneumococcal polysaccharide vaccine (PPSV23) Conjugated pneumococcal vaccine (PCV13)	If no prior vaccination: PCV13 single dose if not received previously, followed by PPSV23 at least 8 wk later, and then PPSV23 5 y later, and then, if applicable, PPSV23 after age 65 and at least 5 y after last dose. If prior PPSV23: Give PCV13 at least 1 y after last PPSV23. If subsequent PPSV23 required, then give at least 8 wk after PCV13 (and 5 y after last PPSV23).
Human papilloma virus (HPV)	—	3 doses through age 26 y.
Td/Tdap	—	One-time booster of pertussis (currently given as Tdap, a tetanus, diphtheria, and acellular pertussis vaccine) in adulthood. Tetanus booster (Td) every 10 y.

Cancer Screening

Cancer screening for SOT recipients should be modified to be more frequent in some cases because of increased risk of malignancy due to immunosuppression, or less frequent if life expectancy is diminished due to poor graft function, medical comorbidities, or other complications.

Most patients receive cancer screening according to standard indications before transplantation. In some cases, an increase in posttransplant cancer risk arises from the same risk factor that caused disease in the transplanted organ. For example, liver transplant patients who were transplanted because of alcoholic liver disease have an increased risk of oropharyngeal and upper gastrointestinal tract cancers,[11,12] most likely because of the previous alcohol exposure, and those with inflammatory bowel disease have an increased risk of colorectal cancer.[13]

SOT recipients are at particularly increased risk for PTLD and nonmelanoma skin cancers. The incidence of other solid tumors is variable; a recent review showed an increased incidence of a large variety of both infection-related and infection-unrelated cancers.[14] There may be variability in risk depending on the organ transplanted and the population studied; in one study of heart transplant patients, solid tumor incidence was similar to that of nontransplant patients.[15]

Despite the increased incidence of cancer, studies have not been conducted in SOT recipients that would define whether patients have better outcomes with screening. Recommendations are generally therefore based on expert opinion. As with any screening, the risks of harms, the patient's overall health, and the individual's values and preferences, must be considered along with the potential benefit of screening.

Colorectal, breast, prostate, and lung cancer screening

Recommendations for SOT recipients are unchanged from those of the general population. Lung cancer after transplantation has been shown to be increased in all SOT recipients, although greatest in lung transplant recipients.[14] One study found a decreased incidence of breast cancer and prostate cancer in SOT recipients,[14] but this observation may have been attributable to pretransplant screening.

Cervical cancer screening

General guidelines for cervical cancer screening, such as those from the US Preventive Services Task Force (USPSTF), specifically do not address the immunosuppressed population.[16] Immunosuppression increases the risk of HPV-associated cancers. In patients with human immunodeficiency virus (HIV), guidelines recommend cervical cancer screening twice in the first year after diagnosis of HIV, and then annually.[17] For SOT recipients, however, there has been conflicting evidence and divergent recommendations. Although there is a clear increase in risk of cervical cancer in renal transplant recipients, another study did not identify an increased risk in SOT recipients in general.[14,18] Annual cervical cancer screening was recommended for renal transplant recipients by previous guidelines (2000),[19] but updated guidelines recommend screening as per the general population (2010), although acknowledging an increased risk.[20] Other authors and guidelines continue to recommend yearly screening.[18] Given the lack of controlled studies in patients with SOT, it is reasonable to offer cervical cancer screening at least according to standard guidelines for patients who would benefit based on their overall health, and, on an individual basis, more frequent screening may be considered.

Skin cancer screening

The USPSTF concluded there was insufficient evidence to recommend for or against skin cancer screening in the general population.[21] Nonmelanoma skin cancers, however, are among the most common of all malignancies in SOT recipients.[14] Risk factors include age, fair skin, sun exposure, geographic location, and previous nonmelanoma skin cancers.[22] General recommendations for SOT recipients include sun protection with clothing and sunscreen, and annual skin examinations with an experienced primary care provider or dermatologist.[6] Patients should be encouraged to bring any suspicious skin lesions to attention.

Bone Density Screening

Current guidelines for nontransplant recipients are for screening women age 65 and older, and younger women with an equivalent risk.[23] SOT recipients are at increased risk of bone loss and fractures due to corticosteroid exposure. It is recommended to assess bone mineral density for both male and female SOT recipients at 1 year after transplantation, and then yearly if osteopenic, and every 2 to 3 years if not osteopenic.[5,6] Renal transplant guidelines recommend checking bone mineral density in the first 3 months after transplantation if the patient is receiving corticosteroids or has other risk factors, provided the glomerular filtration rate is greater than 30 mL/min per 1.73 m^2.[24] Rechecking sooner than 2 to 3 years if a patient has received high-dose glucocorticoids to treat rejection is reasonable. Prevention includes lowering of the glucocorticoid dose, but the rate at which steroid therapy may be decreased or discontinued depends on the transplant center's practice, the type of organ transplanted, and any history of rejection. Patients may present to primary care with symptoms of an osteoporotic fracture, and recognition of the increased risk is critical to make the diagnosis.

Substance Use

Smoking is a relative contraindication to SOT; nevertheless patients may start smoking after transplantation and should be screened. Metabolic complications are common in the SOT recipient, and smoking adds to this already increased cardiovascular risk, as well as increasing the risk of malignancy. Alcohol use is assessed carefully before transplantation and recurrent use is a cause of graft failure in liver transplant patients. Marijuana use has been reported to have severe adverse effects in bone marrow transplant recipients. For SOT recipients, however, there are limited data regarding adverse effects, but invasive aspergillosis has been reported.[25] Despite increasing legalization by states of recreational and medical marijuana, because of potential for infection and other possible adverse health effects, its use should be generally discouraged in SOT recipients.

Exposures

Recipients of SOTs should avoid exposures to infections that may be overwhelming because of their immunosuppressed state. Foodborne exposures to avoid include unpasteurized dairy products, uncooked or undercooked meats, and unfiltered water.[5] Exposures to high-risk animals, such as rodents, reptiles, and birds, should be avoided because of the risk of bacterial infection.[5] SOT recipients should avoid exposure to others who have active infections. SOT recipients who are seronegative for varicella and who are exposed to varicella or herpes zoster are candidates for postexposure prophylaxis[26] and should receive consultation with an infectious disease specialist experienced with transplant recipients.

Pregnancy

With improving care and reduced complications, pregnancy in a patient with an SOT is now feasible, with the most clinical experience occurring in renal transplant recipients, and more recent successes in heart and lung transplantation.[27] Pregnancy poses additional risks in SOT recipients, including prematurity and preeclampsia.[28,29] Most recommendations include consultation with a high-risk pregnancy center well before conception and close coordination with the transplant team, ensuring immunosuppression is at a low level, with no infectious complications. If present, metabolic complications should be well controlled. Some guidelines recommend postponing conception for at least 1 year after transplantation, with other organizations recommending postponing conception for up to 2 years.[5,30] Mycophenolate, azathioprine, and sirolimus are avoided because of teratogenicity.

Contraception should be provided to all SOT recipients who are women of childbearing age with a male partner in the first 1 to 2 years after transplantation, and then afterward if pregnancy is not desired. Although all options for contraception are theoretically available, combined oral contraceptives via any delivery route should be used with caution because of drug interactions, and should be avoided in patients with cardiovascular or liver disease, such as heart transplant patients with cardiac allograft vasculopathy, or liver transplant recipients with recurrent liver disease.[30] Intrauterine devices are considered reasonably safe and effective options for SOT recipients.[30]

Mental Health

Depressive disorders are widely prevalent in the SOT recipient, both before and after transplantation.[31] Depression has been associated with increased mortality in SOT recipients, but not in all types of organ transplants, and if this association represents a true causal relationship, the mechanism is not known.[31] The development of psychiatric illness after transplantation may represent a recurrence of a previous disorder or a newly acquired syndrome. Depression, anxiety disorders, posttraumatic stress disorder, and other conditions should be treated to improve quality of life, adherence to other medications, and treatment of comorbidities. Screening for depression is recommended by the USPSTF[32] and it is reasonable to apply this guideline to SOT recipients, even without data to support outcomes in this population.

Screening for Metabolic and Other Conditions

Medication side effects produce a number of metabolic abnormalities. These are often screened with periodic laboratory testing by the transplant team. The primary care provider is likely to be involved in screening and treatment of these other conditions. Blood pressure should be checked at every clinic visit and at least yearly. Lipid panels are checked annually, with some protocols checking more frequently in the first year. Although gout is common, uric acid screening is not typically performed. Diabetes testing with either a fasting glucose or hemoglobin A1c should be performed at least annually.

MEDICATIONS: INTERACTIONS AND SIDE EFFECTS

> **Case**
>
> A 45-year-old woman with an orthotopic heart transplant for idiopathic dilated cardiomyopathy presents for follow-up. She has been diagnosed with *Helicobacter pylori* infection, and also would like to start medication therapy for depression.

After confirmation that treatment for *H pylori* is indicated, a regimen not containing clarithromycin is chosen due to clarithromycin's increasing calcineurin inhibitor levels. For her depression, she is started on mirtazapine and continued on cognitive behavioral therapy.

Medication History

Knowledge of transplant medications is essential in the care of SOT recipients to be familiar with side effects and drug interactions. Complications are shown in **Table 7**.

Calcineurin inhibitors

The widespread use of calcineurin inhibitors cyclosporine and tacrolimus (FK506) has allowed increased graft survival by reducing rejection. These drugs reduce T-cell lymphocyte proliferation by inhibiting calcineurin. Unfortunately, CKD is a dose-limiting side effect and ultimately remains a major source of morbidity in the SOT recipient. Laboratory monitoring is conducted every 3 months in a stable patient, although protocols vary. Cyclosporine and tacrolimus are both capsules and are usually dosed twice daily. Trough levels are drawn immediately before the next scheduled dose. Goal levels are typically decreased according to time since transplantation. Target levels may be increased if there are episodes of rejection, or decreased because of infections or cancer. Side effects of calcineurin inhibitors are common and must be recognized by the generalist. In addition to renal toxicity, both medications can cause tremors. Metabolic effects include magnesium wasting, hypertension, hyperkalemia, hyperuricemia, and hyperglycemia. Rare side effects include thrombotic microangiopathy with either drug, and gingival hyperplasia with cyclosporine.

Medication refills must be handled carefully and are usually performed by the transplant specialist: calcineurin inhibitor dosing is not the same across brand-name formulations, and formulations should not be switched without consultation with a transplant pharmacist. Common names are listed in **Table 8**. Statin drugs, antifungals, macrolide antibiotics, and diltiazem are commonly used medications that interact with calcineurin inhibitors.

Mycophenolate

Mycophenolate is a purine synthesis inhibitor that inhibits B and T lymphocytes. Mycophenolate is often combined with calcineurin inhibitors to allow lower doses of calcineurin inhibitors, and therefore reduce risk of renal disease. Like cyclosporine, the dosing of mycophenolate is not consistent between different formulations, and

Table 7 Long-term risks of immunosuppressive medications	
Complication	**Examples**
Metabolic	Diabetes (prednisone and calcineurin inhibitors) Hypertension (prednisone) Hyperlipidemia (calcineurin inhibitors) Gout (cyclosporine) Magnesium wasting
Malignancy	Posttransplant lymphoproliferative disorder Skin cancer Risk of multiple other cancers increased
Infection	Multiple: see "Infectious complications in solid organ transplant recipients" in the text
Renal disease	Calcineurin inhibitor toxicity

Table 8
Immunosuppression medications used in solid organ transplant recipients

Drug	Brand/Generic	Dosing	Levels	Side Effects	Common Drug Interactions	Notes
Calcineurin inhibitors						
Cyclosporine	Generic Neoral Gengraf Sandimmune 25-mg, 50-mg, 100-mg capsules	Twice daily	Trough levels followed regularly. Target levels lowered over time in uncomplicated cases.	Renal toxicity Tremor Hypertension Diabetes Hyperkalemia Hyperuricemia Gingival hyperplasia Infection Malignancy	Statins, Antifungals, Diltiazem	Formulations not equivalent. Sandimmune no longer routinely used.
Tacrolimus	Generic Prograf 0.5-mg, 1-mg, 2-mg capsules	Twice daily	Trough levels followed regularly. Target levels lowered over time in uncomplicated cases.	Renal toxicity Tremor Hypertension Diabetes Hyperkalemia Hyperuricemia Infection Malignancy	Statins, Antifungals, Diltiazem	—

Antimetabolites

Mycophenolate	CellCept 250 mg, 500 mg, Myfortic 180 mg, 360 mg	Twice daily	Levels not usually followed.	Cytopenias, Diarrhea, Infection, Malignancy	—	Formulations not equivalent; 720 mg of Myfortic is approximately equivalent to 1000 mg of CellCept.
Azathioprine	50-mg, 75-mg, 100-mg tablets	Once daily	Some protocols follow 6-thioguanine levels.	Cytopenias	Allopurinol, Trimethoprim/Sulfa	Less frequently used. Complete blood count, liver panel followed frequently. Thiopurine methyl-transferase (TPMT) checked before starting.

Mammalian target of rapamycin inhibitors

Sirolimus Everolimus	Sirolimus 0.5-mg, 1-mg, 2-mg tablets. Everolimus: different formulations	Once daily	Trough levels usually followed.	Cytopenias, Hyperlipidemia, Diarrhea, Impaired wound healing	—	Used only in certain protocols. Sirolimus also known as Rapamune. Everolimus has multiple formulations, not equivalent dosing.

Glucocorticoids

Prednisone	Multiple strengths	Once daily	Not followed.	Infection, Hyperglycemia, Low bone density, Hypertension, Weight gain	—	Doses reduced over time; some protocols allow discontinuation.

knowledge of the brand-name medications (Myfortic, CellCept) is important: 720 mg of Myfortic is approximately equivalent to 1000 mg of CellCept. Unlike calcineurin inhibitors, drug levels can be checked but are not routinely followed. Similarly to calcineurin inhibitors, mycophenolate increases the risk of infection and malignancy (although the lymphoma risk may be higher with calcineurin inhibitors). In contrast, it does not commonly have renal toxicity or neurologic side effects, although it frequently has gastrointestinal side effects (diarrhea and an inflammatory bowel disease–like illness) and myelosuppression. Mycophenolate is class "D" for pregnancy.

Prednisone

There are different weaning protocols for corticosteroids depending on patient risk, complications from corticosteroids, and transplant center preferences. In some cases, patients are able to be tapered off of corticosteroids within the first year. Side effects of glucocorticoids are well known and increase with dose and duration.

Azathioprine

Azathioprine, also an antimetabolite, is used less frequently in modern practice compared with mycophenolate. Its side effects include cytopenias and liver toxicity, and complete blood count (CBC) and liver enzymes are checked every 3 months in stable patients. Azathioprine has fewer gastrointestinal side effects compared with mycophenolate. The most important drug interaction is allopurinol, and most likely febuxostat as well, both of which generally should be avoided in patients taking azathioprine. Additionally, concurrent use of trimethoprim-sulfa increases the risk of leukopenia.

Mammalian target of rapamycin inhibitors

Sirolimus, a macrolide antibiotic, and its metabolite everolimus are lymphocyte inhibitors. They are used in certain transplant center protocols, more commonly in renal transplants and heart transplants, and usually not as initial therapy, although protocols vary. Some examples include patients in whom calcineurin inhibitor toxicity, such as CKD or PTLD is to be minimized, and in liver transplant patients transplanted for hepatocellular carcinoma (HCC).[5] Side effects include cytopenias and hyperlipidemia, and there are concerns for impaired wound healing. Drug interactions are similar to tacrolimus.

Drug interactions

Drug interactions should be checked before prescribing any new medication to an SOT recipient. The most common serious drug interactions in primary care are with anti-infectives, cardiovascular medications, and psychiatric medications. The oral antifungal azole class of medications and macrolide antibiotics increase calcineurin inhibitor concentrations. Azithromycin may interact less compared with clarithromycin.[33] Amiodarone and non-dihydropyridine calcium channel blockers (diltiazem, verapamil) may increase drug levels of calcineurin inhibitors. Even the dihydropyridine calcium channel blockers may interact with cyclosporine and should be used with caution. Additionally, cyclosporine may increase levels of statin drugs. Selective serotonin reuptake inhibitors (SSRIs) may have variable increase on calcineurin inhibitor levels. Citalopram has fewer interactions with the cytochrome p450 system than other SSRIs, but it also may increase the QT interval in combination with tacrolimus; although sertraline and fluoxetine and paroxetine inhibit the cytochrome system, its clinical effect in SOT recipients is less certain. Mirtazapine may be considered safe, whereas monoamine oxidase inhibitors should be avoided. The use of St John's Wort is contraindicated, as its efficacy is uncertain and it causes enzyme induction that may reduce immunosuppressant levels.

Common drug interactions are shown in **Table 9**.

Table 9
Common drug interactions between medications encountered in primary care and immunosuppressant medications used in solid organ transplant recipients

Category	Interaction	
Anti-infectives	Antifungals: oral azoles	Avoid: Increases levels of cyclosporine, tacrolimus, mTOR inhibitors. If must be given consult with transplant specialist for dose adjustment and monitoring.
	Antibacterials: macrolides	Avoid clarithromycin: increases levels of cyclosporine, tacrolimus and may increase QT interval. Also avoid oral erythromycin. Azithromycin is less of a risk with calcineurin inhibitors; consult with transplant specialist if used with mTOR inhibitors.
	Antibacterials: trimethoprim-sulfa	May increase risk of hyperkalemia and renal toxicity in combination with calcineurin inhibitors; if must be used, monitor renal function and potassium. May increase risk of cytopenias in combination with azathioprine.
Cardiovascular	Statins	Cyclosporine may increase levels of any statin drug; if both drugs are required, start at a low dose of statin and monitor for side effects. Pravastatin may have fewer interactions. Tacrolimus is considered to have fewer interactions with statins compared with cyclosporine.
	Amiodarone	May increase drug levels of tacrolimus, cyclosporine, and mTOR inhibitors. Avoid unless necessary.
	Calcium channel blockers	Avoid diltiazem and verapamil; increase levels of cyclosporine and tacrolimus, mTOR inhibitors. Dihydropyridine calcium channel blockers are preferred, although they may still interact with cyclosporine.
Psychiatric	Antidepressants: SSRIs	May have variable increase on calcineurin inhibitor levels Citalopram has fewer interactions with the cytochrome p450 system than other SSRIs, but it also may increase the QT interval in combination with tacrolimus. Although sertraline and fluoxetine and paroxetine inhibit the cytochrome system, its clinical effect in SOT recipients is less certain.
	MAO inhibitors	Should be avoided.
Supplements	—	St John's Wort contraindicated.

Abbreviations: MAO, monoamine oxidase; mTOR, mammalian target of rapamycin; SOT, sold organ transplantation; SSRI, selective serotonin reuptake inhibitor.

INFECTIOUS COMPLICATIONS IN SOLID ORGAN TRANSPLANT RECIPIENTS

Case

A 40-year-old woman who has received a kidney transplant because of lupus nephritis presents with watery, nonbloody diarrhea for 4 weeks. Her transplant was 3 years before presentation, complicated by BK virus positivity. Her creatinine is normal and her last biopsy showed no rejection. She takes tacrolimus, mycophenolate mofetil, prednisone, and rapamycin.

Comprehensive stool studies were obtained, including enteric pathogens, *Clostridium difficile*, *Giardia*, norovirus polymerase chain reaction (PCR), fecal ova, and parasite for *Cryptosporidium*, *Isospora*, *Cyclospora*, microsporidia, and fecal leukocytes. Laboratory studies included CBC with differential, serum CMV PCR, C-reactive protein, erythrocyte sedimentation rate, and a comprehensive metabolic panel. When her symptoms persisted despite an unrevealing workup, a colonoscopy was conducted with biopsies showing CMV. She was treated with ganciclovir.

SOT recipients are at increased risk for infections due to their immunosuppressant drugs. Transplant medications inhibit T-cell and B-cell function, and cause infectious complications analogous to those of a patient with HIV. Time course is essential to knowing what infections a patient is at risk for experiencing (**Box 1**). Episodes of rejection that lead to increased immunosuppression "reset" the clock with regard to typical infections after transplantation.[34] The standard of care at most transplant centers is for the transplant center to follow patients in the early posttransplant period; this lasts from the day of transplantation to 3 months after transplantation. At 3 months, barring complications, patients are often referred back to their primary care provider.

Early: Immediate Posttransplant to 1 Month

Most primary care providers will not be responsible for the assessment and treatment of infectious complications of the early posttransplant period. Nosocomial infections, infections from the donor (graft), and infections due to colonization of the recipient cause the bulk of infections in this period.[35]

Nosocomial infections

Common nosocomial infections include resistant organisms, such as methicillin-resistant *Staphylococcus aureus*, high-level aminoglycoside resistant enterococcus, including vancomycin-resistant *Enterococcus*, methicillin-resistant coagulase-negative

---

Box 1
General approach to working up infections in solid organ transplant recipients

- At the 3-month posttransplant mark when patients are transferred back to their primary care providers, they are at the highest degree of immunosuppression and most at risk for opportunistic infections.

- Episodes of rejection that require intensification of antirejection medications "reset the clock" for risk of infection.

- Infectious symptoms may be blunted or absent in patients with solid organ transplantation because of the anti-inflammatory effect of medications. Prolonged symptoms, even if milder (eg, cough, diarrhea, new malaise), should trigger an aggressive workup.

- More aggressive workup is often necessary, as serologic testing can be negative. Direct tissue sampling (via endoscopy, bronchoscopy, or biopsy), and advanced imaging are often warranted if a diagnosis is not immediately apparent.

Staphylococcus, and extended-spectrum beta-lactamase (ESBL)-resistant gram-negative rods.[36,37] Other early infections include albicans and nonalbicans candida; hospital-based infections, such as *C difficile*; and infectious complications from the surgical sites, central lines, drains, and urinary catheters; ventilator use; and aspiration.

Donor-derived infections
Donor-derived infections are mostly viral in this time period, and include West Nile virus, herpes simplex virus (HSV), lymphocytic choriomeningitis virus, and rabies.

Common recipient colonizers
Common recipient colonizers that cause active infections after transplantation include *Pseudomonas aeruginosa* and *Aspergillus*.[34] Most transplant recipients receive antibiotic prophylaxis for 6 to 12 months. Use of prophylactic trimethoprim/sulfa (TMP/Sulfa) against *Pneumocystis jiroveci pneumonia* (PJP) also is effective prophylaxis against toxoplasmosis, diarrheal illnesses due to *Isospora* and *Cyclospora*, and some *Nocardia* and *Listeria* species. Valganciclovir and acyclovir help with prophylaxis against cytomegalovirus (CMV), but also are effective against HSV, EBV, and varicella zoster virus.

Mid: 1 to 6 Months After Transplantation

The immunosuppressive effects of antirejection medications are maximally manifest 1 to 6 months after transplantation. Patients are apt to develop opportunistic infections and reactivation of latent infections from either the donor or the recipient. It is also at the 3-month mark that many patients will transfer back to their primary care provider for their comprehensive care.

Viral infection
Antiviral prophylaxis against CMV using valganciclovir or intravenous (IV) ganciclovir is typically provided to patients in the first 3 months after transplantation if either the donor or recipient is CMV positive. Duration may be extended for higher-risk patients, including CMV-negative recipients whose donor organ is CMV positive. Hepatitis B may cause reinfection in patients with hepatitis B cirrhosis who receive a liver transplant. Reinfection rates have dropped markedly with the use of hepatitis B immune globulin and lamivudine or entecavir. Patients may also receive hepatitis B–positive donor organs; for liver transplant recipients, chemoprophylaxis is used, as antibodies (hepatitis B surface antibody) from previous hepatitis B vaccination are not adequately protective when receiving a liver from a recipient who is hepatitis B core antibody positive.

In nonliver solid organ transplants, 2 options are possible: surveillance for the development of hepatitis B DNA with every 3-month to 6-month serology paired with early treatment (before the development of symptoms or transaminitis) or empiric treatment.[38]

For patients who receive antiviral prophylaxis directed against CMV and hepatitis B, other viral infections, such as BK polyoma virus, hepatitis C virus, adenovirus, and influenza, are likely.[34]

Bacterial infections
In the setting of TMP/Sulfa prophylaxis for PJP, many bacterial opportunistic infections are addressed. TMP/Sulfa also may offer some protection, although certainly not ideal, against common bacterial infections seen in primary care, including urinary tract infections (UTIs), cellulitis, and sinusitis. Although it is not first line for community-acquired pneumonia (CAP), it is biologically active against *Streptococcus pneumoniae*, and *Staphylococcus aureus*. Hence, although patients with SOT remain on

TMP/Sulfa, primary care providers should be vigilant for the development of other pneumonias (atypical), reactivation of tuberculosis, and the development of *C difficile* infection.

Fungal infections

Invasive fungal infections more commonly occur within the first 3 months after transplantation. In one series of liver transplant recipients, the most common fungal infections were due to *Candida* and *Aspergillus*, and usually followed a course of broad-spectrum antibiotics.[39] In this same series, *Candida* found only in the urine or bronchial alveolar lavage samples always represented colonization. Chemoprophylaxis with fluconazole is recommended for high-risk patients, and pragmatic use of antibiotics as well as early definitive diagnosis are other strategies that have reduced the incidence and morbidity related to invasive fungal infections in patients with SOT. Complicating matters for providers are the major drug interactions that occur with the use of azole antifungal therapy and immunosuppressive medications. Azoles are potent inhibitors of cytochrome P450 and risk toxic levels of cyclosporine, tacrolimus, and sirolimus.[40]

Endemic mycoses, such as coccidioidomycosis, blastomycosis, and histoplasmosis, are typically indolent regional infections in immunocompetent patients, but coccidioidomycosis can cause infection rates of 6.9% in patients with SOT in endemic areas (blastomycosis and histoplasmosis are rare, causing <1% of infections). The portal for infection is through the respiratory tract. Coccidioidomycosis is prevalent in the desert southwest of the United States, specifically in the San Joaquin Valley, but has been reported in other regions in the western states. In patients with SOT in endemic regions, the rate of infection is as high as 6.9%, mostly due to reactivation from either the donor or recipient. Donor-derived infections occur within the first month and are severe. Recipient-derived reactivation infections occur within the first year. Symptoms include fevers, chills, pleurisy, cough, and shortness of breath; severe pneumonias and disseminated multiorgan infection and failure can occur.[39]

Late: More than 6 Months After Transplantation

Community-acquired infections are the predominant types of infections in this time period, but they may have more severe manifestations in patients with SOT compared with nonimmunosuppressed hosts. In SOT recipients, the degree of immunosuppression is reduced over time, and some patients discontinue their antiproliferative agent. CAP, UTIs, and diarrhea are common in both the SOT and general population. However, unique to SOT recipients is the increased risk in this period for later viral infections, including CMV, HSV, hepatitis B and C viruses, and less common viruses such as JC and BK virus.[34]

Providers also must recognize that patients who require escalation of immunosuppression medications due to episodes of rejection are at increased risk for opportunistic, nosocomial, and community-acquired infections; the immunosuppression timeline has reset and the patient may be at risk for infections from the early to mid posttransplant period.

COMMON INFECTIOUS SYNDROMES (CAP, UTI, DIARRHEA)
Community-acquired Pneumonia

CAP is a common cause of morbidity and mortality in the SOT population. In the late posttransplant period, more than half of pneumonias are CAP, followed closely by health care–associated pneumonia, with a much smaller percentage being hospital-acquired pneumonia.[41,42] Bacterial infections are most common with a combination of typical community infections (*Haemophilus influenzae, S pneumoniae*) and multidrug-resistant bacterial species (*P aeruginosa*, ESBL-producing Enterobacteriaceae, *Stenotrophomonas maltophilia*) being common pathogens. Fungal infections, including *Aspergillus fumigatus,* were the second most common, followed by viral causes of CAP.[40,41] Most episodes of pneumonia occur more than 6 months after transplantation, although more than 30% were in the 1-month to 6-month period and 10% in the early posttransplant period. Risk factors for pneumonia included male gender, older age, tobacco use, acute and chronic graft rejection, and comorbid chronic conditions, such as hypertension, coronary artery disease, and diabetes.[40]

Diagnostic considerations
The diagnostic workup in patients with SOT with symptoms concerning for a lower respiratory infection, such as fever, cough, and dyspnea, include blood tests, such as a CBC, chemistry panel, blood cultures, and also sputum culture and a chest radiograph. If the chest radiograph shows pulmonary infiltrates, primary care providers should consider a computed tomography (CT) scan of the chest and bronchoscopy after consultation with a pulmonologist. Use of advanced imaging and invasive procedures, such as bronchoscopy, have been shown to distinguish between infectious and noninfectious processes in immunosuppressed patients.[43,44] Tools that determine the severity of CAP and the need for admission (eg, CURB-65, Pneumonia Severity Index) should be used in patients with SOT.[45]

Therapeutic considerations
Providers should not delay initiation of antibiotics in patients with SOT suspected of pneumonia. Empiric therapy for CAP includes fluoroquinolones, macrolides, or ESBLs plus a macrolide. Guidelines recommend tailoring of the antibiotic choices to reflect the pattern of antibiotic resistance in the community.[42] The use of clarithromycin should be avoided, as it is a potent inhibitor of the metabolism of some immunosuppressive agents used in SOT populations. Its use even for short-term treatment of infections can lead to toxic levels of these medications. Azithromycin, however, remains a reasonable treatment option.

Urinary tract infections UTIs occur in all SOT recipients, but are most common in kidney transplant patients. UTIs in nonrenal transplant patients tend to occur in the first month after transplantation, but occur most frequently between 3 and 6 months after renal transplantation, and up to 16% of UTIs occur after 6 months.[46,47] Not only are UTIs more common in renal transplant recipients, but they also are more severe; UTI-related bacteremia is seen in 39% of renal transplant recipients, and less than 3% for other types of SOT.[46] The major predictors for bacterial UTI and pyelonephritis in this population are female gender and increased immunosuppression. For candiduria, risk factors are female gender, intensive care unit care, and neurogenic bladder. Risk factors for UTIs occurring more than 6 months after transplantation are prednisone use of more than 20 mg per day, serum creatinine more than 2 mg/dL, and increased immunosuppression.[46]

Diagnostic considerations
The diagnostic criteria from the Infectious Disease Society of America (IDSA) are the same for the general population as they are for patients with SOT, but notably all patients with SOT with symptomatic UTI symptoms should be considered "complicated." The Canadian Guidelines Committee recommends an individually tailored approach in patients with complicated UTIs.[48] The usual symptoms for UTI in the

general population are replicated in most patients with SOT: dysuria, frequency, urgency, and suprapubic pain, although atypical presentation of fever, malaise, or septic symptoms are not uncommon. Clinicians should palpate the renal allograft and costovertebral angles; tenderness in either location is suggestive of an upper tract infection. All patients should have a urinalysis and urine culture, and consideration for CBC, chemistry panel, and blood cultures, especially if there is suspicion for an upper tract infection.[45] Renal ultrasound or abdominal CT scan should be considered if obstruction or abscess is suspected.[46]

Therapeutic considerations
Escherichia coli, Enterococcus, and *Pseudomonas* are the most common major pathogens in renal transplant UTIs, but other causative organisms include *Staphylococcus, Klebsiella, Enterobacter, Proteus*, and *Candida*.[45] The practice of screening and treating asymptomatic renal transplant patients is common at many transplant centers, although this is controversial and not supported by evidence. When asymptomatic bacteruria is found, expert opinion is for consideration of treatment after repeat urinalysis with a straight catheterization evidences bacteria greater than 10^3 colonies in the first 3 months after renal transplantation. However, treatment of asymptomatic bacteruria should be avoided in patients more than 3 months after transplantation.[46] For patients with UTIs and mild symptoms, empiric therapy is with ciprofloxacin ± amoxicillin for 5 to 7 days. For UTIs with moderate symptoms, empiric 14-day therapy is ciprofloxacin, amoxicillin/sulbactam, or ceftriaxone, with narrowing to appropriate therapy based on culture results. For UTIs with severe symptoms, empiric therapy is piperacillin-tazobactam or cefepime ± a carbapenem ± vancomycin depending on the risk for multidrug-resistant organisms in the community/hospital.[46]

Diarrhea Diarrhea commonly occurs with variable presentations and causes in the SOT population, and is more serious than similar infections in the general population. Infectious causes may be viral, bacterial, and parasitic, whereas noninfectious causes include medication side effects, posttransplant lymphoproliferative disease, and rarely graft-versus-host disease.[49,50]

Diagnostic considerations
IDSA guidelines address the approach to infectious diarrhea for clinicians. Immunosuppression, as seen in SOT, is only considered in the management of diarrhea that persists for more than 7 days.[51] However, patients with SOT are more susceptible to acute diarrhea of any cause, and bouts of infectious diarrhea can be more severe. Providers must aggressively workup diarrhea with typical red flags (fever, associated hematochezia, high volume or frequency, severe abdominal pain, recent antibiotic exposure, or hospitalization), but also be aggressive in the assessment of milder diarrhea that persists for more than 7 days in patients with SOT. Noninvasive diagnostic studies are well described in other resources and are appropriate to pursue in patients with SOT, but intensification to abdominal CT and endoscopy with biopsy is rapidly necessary in more ill patients or for those whose noninvasive workup is unrevealing.[49] Early consultation with infectious disease and gastroenterology specialists is appropriate.

Therapeutic considerations
Patients with SOT may benefit from empiric fluoroquinolone therapy in acute diarrhea when there is a low suspicion for *C difficile* and enterohemorrhagic *E coli*.

- *C difficile*–associated diarrhea (CDAD) typically occurs early after transplantation as a nosocomial infection, but is an important cause of community-acquired diarrhea, graft loss, and mortality in patients with SOT. Providers should order tests for *C difficile* early in the evaluation of patients with SOT with acute diarrhea, pursue invasive testing if noninvasive testing is negative but suspicion exists, and consider hospitalization to expedite the workup in more acutely ill patients.[52]

- Cryptosporidia, a water-borne parasite, should be considered in patients with SOT with a recent travel history, and exposure to water parks.
- Norovirus causes a biphasic illness in patients with SOT. The acute illness is characterized by usual symptoms of profuse, watery diarrhea, which may be accompanied by fever, nausea, vomiting, and abdominal pain. This phase can be longer and more severe than in immunocompetent patients, and causes up to 18% of hospital admissions for diarrhea in patients with SOT. The chronic phase is characterized by cycles of normal stool with intermittent bouts of loose stool. During this time, viral shedding can continue to occur. Diagnosis is via PCR of infected fluids and treatment is supportive, although some evidence suggests holding or reducing immunosuppression for a time may shorten the illness.[53]
- CMV is most problematic in CMV-negative transplant recipients, especially those with lung, small bowel, and pancreas transplants (liver and kidney are lowest risk). CMV infection can affect multiple organs; in the gastrointestinal tract, colitis is most common, with symptoms of abdominal pain, diarrhea, and fever. Severe cases cause bleeding and ulceration. Serum PCR should be obtained but can be falsely negative in 15% of cases, hence endoscopy with characteristic findings, biopsy, and histologic findings of "owl's eye inclusions" or pathognomonic staining may be required. Treatment is with the antivirals IV ganciclovir or oral valganciclovir depending on severity of illness.[52]

RISK OF MALIGNANCY IN SOLID ORGAN TRANSPLANT RECIPIENTS: POSTTRANSPLANT LYMPHOPROLIFERATIVE DISORDER AND OTHER CANCERS

Case

A 56-year-old man presents with 1 month of nonproductive cough 8 months after liver transplantation for cirrhosis due to nonalcoholic steatohepatitis. He had a single episode of rejection resulting in the addition of mycophenolate to his previous regimen of tacrolimus. He is EBV negative and received an EBV-positive graft. Both he and the donor were CMV positive. He has traveled to Ohio and is a nonsmoker. A chest radiograph is obtained, which reveals multiple pulmonary masses. Biopsy is obtained and is positive for B-cell lymphoma. Patient is treated with chemotherapy and lowering of his immunosuppression.

Posttransplant lymphoproliferative disorder (PTLD) is critically important for providers to be familiar with, as it is one of the most common posttransplant malignancies, may present clinically to nontransplant providers, and there is currently no screening for it.

PTLD is a disease of immune suppression and is thought to be due to proliferation of EBV. The highest risk is in EBV-seronegative recipients who receive a seropositive donor organ.[54] Patients present with lymphadenopathy or B symptoms due to lymphoma, and, compared with non-SOT recipients, more commonly present with extranodal involvement of specific organs, including liver, lungs, gastrointestinal tract, kidneys, and central nervous system.[55] Additionally, there are myeloma and T-cell forms of PTLD.

In this case of a patient presenting with pulmonary masses after transplantation, the potential etiologies include infectious causes (eg, *Aspergillus*, *Cryptococcus*, histoplasmosis) and malignancy, both primary, metastatic, and PTLD. PTLD may present early in the first year after transplantation, and then tends to arise again later, and earlier presentations may be more likely to be recipient EBV negative.[56] Nevertheless, late presentations also are common, and these patients develop disease at a time when they may be no longer followed predominantly by transplant physicians. The high incidence, often late presentation, and extranodal organ involvement requires a high level of suspicion for and recognition of symptoms or signs of PTLD.

Approaches to treatment of PTLD include lowering of immunosuppression, chemotherapy, and antiviral therapy. Radiation or surgery is sometimes required for local control.

In addition to PTLD, SOT recipients are at substantially increased risk for other malignancies, including skin cancers, such as squamous cell carcinoma and basal cell carcinoma, Kaposi sarcoma, cancers of the transplanted organ, and others. Despite the increased risk of multiple different cancers, other than skin cancer surveillance, there are neither conclusive data nor consensus recommendations regarding whether screening for other malignancies is effective in this population. Thus, with late presentations and no screening, it is essential that primary care providers have a high index of suspicion for emergence of malignancy in SOT recipients.

SUMMARY

Care of the SOT recipient is complex, and continued partnership with the transplant specialist is essential to manage and treat complications and maintain health. The increased longevity of SOT recipients will lead to their being an evolving part of primary care practice, with ever more opportunities for care, education, and research of this rewarding patient population.

REFERENCES

1. Health Resources and Services Administration, U.S. Department of Health & Human Services. Organ Transplantation and Procurement Network. Transplants in the U.S. by recipient age, U.S. transplants performed 1988-September 30, 2014. Available at: http://optn.transplant.hrsa.gov/converge/latestData/step2.asp. Accessed December 13, 2014.
2. Lodhi SA, Lamb KE, Meier-Kriesche HU. Solid organ allograft survival improvement in the United States: the long-term does not mirror the dramatic short-term success. Am J Transplant 2011;11:1226–35.
3. Health Resources and Services Administration, U.S. Department of Health & Human Services. Organ Procurement and Transplantation Network. All Kaplan-Meier patient survival rates for transplants performed: 1997–2004, based on OPTN data as of December 5, 2014. Available at: http://optn.transplant.hrsa.gov/converge/latestData/step2.asp. Accessed December 13, 2014.
4. Kidney Disease: Improving Global Outcomes (KDIGO) Transplant Work Group. KDIGO clinical practice guideline for the care of kidney transplant recipients. Am J Transplant 2009;9(Suppl 3):S1–155.
5. Lucey MR, Terrault N, Ojo L, et al. Long-term management of the successful adult liver transplant: 2012 practice guideline by the American Association for the Study of Liver Diseases and the American Society of Transplantation. Liver Transpl 2013;19(1):3–26.
6. Costanzo MR, Dipchand A, Starling R, et al. The International Society of Heart and Lung Transplantation Guidelines for the care of heart transplant recipients. J Heart Lung Transplant 2010;29(8):914–56.

7. Centers for Disease Control and Prevention. Vaccines that might be indicated for adults based on medical and other indications. Effective September 19, 2014. Available at: www.cdc.gov/vaccines/schedules/hcp/imz/adult-conditions.html. Accessed March 11, 2014.

8. Rubin LG, Levin MJ, Ljungman P, et al, Infectious Diseases Society of America. 2013 IDSA clinical practice guideline for vaccination of the immunocompromised host. Clin Infect Dis 2014;58(3):e44–100.

9. Gourishankar S, McDermid JC, Jhangri GS, et al. Herpes zoster infection following solid organ transplantation: incidence, risk factors and outcomes in the current immunosuppressive era. Am J Transplant 2004;4(1):108–15.

10. Centers for Disease Control and Prevention (CDC). Use of 13-valent pneumococcal conjugate vaccine and 23-valent pneumococcal polysaccharide vaccine for adults with immunocompromising conditions: recommendations of the Advisory Committee on Immunization Practices (ACIP). MMWR Morb Mortal Wkly Rep 2012;61(40):816–9.

11. Baccarani U, Adani GL, Montanaro D, et al. De novo malignancies after kidney and liver transplantations: experience on 582 consecutive cases. Transplant Proc 2006;38(4):1135–7.

12. Jain A, DiMartini A, Kashyap R, et al. Long-term follow-up after liver transplantation for alcoholic liver disease under tacrolimus. Transplantation 2000;70(9): 1335–42.

13. Silva MA, Jambulingam PS, Mirza DF. Colorectal cancer after orthotopic liver transplantation. Crit Rev Oncol Hematol 2005;56(1):147–53.

14. Engels EA, Pfeiffer RM, Fraumeni JF Jr, et al. Spectrum of cancer risk among US solid organ transplant recipients. JAMA 2011;306(17):1891–901.

15. Kellerman L, Neugut A, Burke B, et al. Comparison of the incidence of de novo solid malignancies after heart transplantation to that in the general population. Am J Cardiol 2009;103(4):562–6.

16. Moyer VA, U.S. Preventive Services Task Force. Screening for cervical cancer: U.S. Preventive Services Task Force recommendation statement. Ann Intern Med 2012;156(12):880–91.

17. ACOG Committee on Practice Bulletins–Gynecology. ACOG Practice Bulletin No. 117: gynecologic care for women with human immunodeficiency virus. Obstet Gynecol 2010;116(6):1492–509.

18. Nguyen ML, Flowers L. Cervical cancer screening in immunocompromised women. Obstet Gynecol Clin North Am 2013;40(2):339–57.

19. EBPG Expert Group on Renal Transplantation. European best practice guidelines for renal transplantation. Section IV: long-term management of the transplant recipient. IV.6.3. Cancer risk after renal transplantation. Solid organ cancers: prevention and treatment. Nephrol Dial Transplant 2002;17(Suppl 4): 32, 34–6.

20. Kasiske BL, Zeier MG, Chapman JR, et al. KDIGO clinical practice guideline for the care of kidney transplant recipients: a summary. Kidney Int 2010;77(4): 299–311.

21. U.S. Preventive Services Task Force. Screening for Skin cancer Clinical summary of U.S. Preventive Services Task Force Recommendation. 2009. Available at: http://www.uspreventiveservicestaskforce.org/uspstf/uspsskca.htm. Accessed June 12, 2014.

22. Tessari G, Girolomoni G. Nonmelanoma skin cancer in solid organ transplant recipients: update on epidemiology, risk factors, and management. Dermatol Surg 2012;38(10):1622–30.

23. U.S. Preventive Services Task Force. Screening for osteoporosis: U.S. Preventive Services Task Force Recommendation Statement. Ann Intern Med 2011;154: 356–64.

24. Kidney Disease: Improving Global Outcomes (KDIGO) CKD-MBD Work Group. KDIGO clinical practice guideline for the diagnosis, evaluation, prevention, and treatment of chronic kidney disease-mineral and bone disorder (CKD-MBD). Kidney Int Suppl 2009;113:S1–130.

25. Marks WH, Florence L, Lieberman J, et al. Successfully treated invasive pulmonary aspergillosis associated with smoking marijuana in a renal transplant recipient. Transplantation 1996;61(12):1771–4.

26. Pergam SA, Limaye AP, AST Infectious Diseases Community of Practice. Varicella zoster virus in solid organ transplantation. Am J Transplant 2013;13(Suppl 4): 138–46.

27. Vos R, Ruttens D, Verleden SE, et al. Pregnancy after heart and lung transplantation. Best Pract Res Clin Obstet Gynaecol 2014;28(8):1146–62.

28. Deshpande NA, James NT, Kucirka LM, et al. Pregnancy outcomes of liver transplant recipients: a systematic review and meta-analysis. Liver Transpl 2012;18(6): 621–9.

29. Deshpande NA, James NT, Kucirka LM, et al. Pregnancy outcomes in kidney transplant recipients: a systematic review and meta-analysis. Am J Transplant 2011;11(11):2388–404.

30. Deshpande NA, Coscia LA, Gomez-Lobo V, et al. Pregnancy after solid organ transplantation: a guide for obstetric management. Rev Obstet Gynecol 2013; 6(3–4):116–25.

31. Corbett C, Armstrong MJ, Parker R, et al. Mental health disorders and solid-organ transplant recipients. Transplantation 2013;96(7):593–600.

32. U.S. Preventive Services Task Force. Screening for depression in adults: U.S. Preventive Services Task Force recommendation statement. Ann Intern Med 2009;151(11):784–92.

33. Paterson DL, Singh N. Interactions between tacrolimus and antimicrobial agents. Clin Infect Dis 1997;25(6):1430–40.

34. Pagalilauan GL. Limaye AP infections in transplant patients. Med Clin North Am 2013;97(4):581–600.

35. Fishman JA. Introduction: infection in solid organ transplant recipients. Am J Transplant 2009;9(Suppl 4):S3–6.

36. Kawecki D, Chmura A, Pacholczyk M, et al. Bacterial infections in the early period after liver transplantation: etiological agents and their susceptibility. Med Sci Monit 2009;15(12):CR628–37.

37. Kawecki D, Wszola M, Kwiatkowski A, et al. Bacterial and fungal infections in the early post-transplant period after kidney transplantation: etiological agents and their susceptibility. Transplant Proc 2014;46(8):2733–7.

38. John S, Andersson KL, Kotton CN, et al. Prophylaxis of hepatitis B infection in solid organ transplant recipients. Therap Adv Gastroenterol 2013;6(4):309–19.

39. Sganga G, Bianco G, Frongillo F, et al. Fungal infections after liver transplantation: incidence and outcome. Transplant Proc 2014;46(7):2314–8.

40. Miller R, Assi M. Endemic fungal infections in solid organ transplantation. Am J Transplant 2013;13(Suppl 4):250–61.

41. Dizdar OS, Ersoy A, Akalin H. Pneumonia after kidney transplant: incidence, risk factors, and mortality. Exp Clin Transplant 2014;12(3):205–11.

42. Giannella M, Munoz P, Alarcon JM, et al. Pneumonia in solid organ transplant recipients: a prospective multicenter study. Transpl Infect Dis 2014;16(2):232–41.

43. Ramirez P, Valencia M, Torres A. Bronchoalveolar lavage to diagnose respiratory infections. Semin Respir Crit Care Med 2007;28(5):525–33.
44. Waite S, Jeudy J, White CS. Acute lung infections in normal and immunocompromised hosts. Radiol Clin North Am 2006;44(2):295–315, ix.
45. Mandell LA, Wunderink RG, Anzueto A, et al. Infectious Diseases Society of America/American Thoracic Society consensus guidelines on the management of community-acquired pneumonia in adults. Clin Infect Dis 2007;44(Suppl 2):S27–72.
46. Vidal E, Torre-Cisneros J, Blanes M, et al. Bacterial urinary tract infection after solid organ transplantation in the RESITRA cohort. Transpl Infect Dis 2012; 14(6):595–603.
47. Parasuraman R, Julian K. Urinary tract infections in solid organ transplantation. Am J Transplant 2013;13(Suppl 4):327–36.
48. Nicolle LE. Complicated urinary tract infection in adults. Can J Infect Dis Med Microbiol 2005;16(6):349–60.
49. Krones E, Hogenauer C. Diarrhea in the immunocompromised patient. Gastroenterol Clin North Am 2012;41(3):677–701.
50. Rice JP, Spier BJ, Cornett DD, et al. Utility of colonoscopy in the evaluation of diarrhea in solid organ transplant recipients. Transplantation 2009;88(3):374–9.
51. Guerrant RL, Van Gilder T, Steiner TS, et al. Practice guidelines for the management of infectious diarrhea. Clin Infect Dis 2001;32(3):331–51.
52. Boutros M, Al-Shaibi M, Chan G, et al. *Clostridium difficile* colitis: increasing incidence, risk factors, and outcomes in solid organ transplant recipients. Transplantation 2012;93(10):1051–7.
53. Lee LY, Ison MG. Diarrhea caused by viruses in transplant recipients. Transpl Infect Dis 2014;16(3):347–58.
54. Sampaio MS, Cho YW, Shah T, et al. Impact of Epstein-Barr virus donor and recipient serostatus on the incidence of post-transplant lymphoproliferative disorder in kidney transplant recipients. Nephrol Dial Transplant 2012;27(7):2971–9.
55. Penn I. Post-transplant malignancy: the role of immunosuppression. Drug Saf 2000;23(2):101–13.
56. Morton M, Coupes B, Roberts SA, et al. Epidemiology of posttransplantation lymphoproliferative disorder in adult renal transplant recipients. Transplantation 2013;95(3):470–8.

Primary Care of the Human Immunodeficiency Virus Patient

Fred R. Buckhold III, MD

KEYWORDS

- HIV infection • Chronic disease management • Primary care
- Antiretroviral therapy • Preventive care

KEY POINTS

- Human immunodeficiency virus (HIV) is a treatable disease that requires expert care in treatment of the virus.
- Patients with HIV have higher levels of comorbidity than non–HIV infected patients who require management.
- Prevention and early detection of disease is vital in HIV patients, as they tend to have higher rates of infections and cancer.
- Primary care physicians play a vital role in improving access and quality for HIV-infected patients.

INTRODUCTION

The evolution of the approach to the patient with human immunodeficiency virus (HIV) has transitioned in the era of highly effective treatment of the virus. In the early part of the HIV/AIDS epidemic, treatment goals were focused on managing the many opportunistic infections and malignancies that commonly occurred when the HIV patient developed AIDS. The approach to treating HIV-infected persons has changed, as most patients diagnosed with HIV are currently receiving long-term antiretroviral therapy (ART). Given the marked success of ART in suppressing levels of HIV, a diagnosis of HIV can now be considered a chronic illness. This article discusses aspects of care relevant to a primary care physician, with an emphasis on long-term consequences of HIV infection and treatment with ART. Attention to comorbid disease is also discussed.

Internal Medicine Residency Training Program, Division of General Internal Medicine, Department of Medicine, Saint Louis University School of Medicine, 1402 South Grand Boulevard, FDT 14th Floor, Saint Louis, MO 63104, USA
E-mail address: buckhold@slu.edu

Med Clin N Am 99 (2015) 1105–1122
http://dx.doi.org/10.1016/j.mcna.2015.05.010
0025-7125/15/$ – see front matter © 2015 Elsevier Inc. All rights reserved.

medical.theclinics.com

MANAGEMENT GOALS
Detection and Screening

The Centers for Disease Control and Prevention (CDC) estimated that in 2012 910,541 persons living in the United States were infected with HIV. Approximately 50,000 new HIV diagnoses are made every year, and it is estimated that 180,900 persons living in the United States have HIV but have yet to be diagnosed.[1] As of 2012, the number of people classified as having AIDS was 27,928.[2] Transmission of the virus still disproportionately affects younger patients, minorities, and men who have sex with men (**Table 1**). However, with the continued success of ART in improving mortality, the number of patients who have HIV in the middle to later years in life continues to increase (**Fig. 1**).

The US Preventive Services Task Force and CDC recommend screening all adults aged 15 to 65 for HIV infection.[3,4] Testing can be done annually or even more frequently in high-risk patients. The most current CDC guidelines also recommend an "opt-out" strategy of testing all patients who interact with the United States health care system to facilitate acceptance in screening and improve HIV detection.[4] However, health care providers must be aware of the state laws regarding HIV screening, which supersede CDC guidelines.[5] A compendium of state laws regarding HIV screening is available at: http://nccc.ucsf.edu/clinical-resources/hiv-aids-resources/state-hiv-testing-laws/.

Until recently, screening was performed using an HIV enzyme-linked immunoassay with confirmation with a Western blot, providing excellent sensitivity and specificity except when patients are in the "window" between acute infection and antibody seroconversion.[3] Recently, the CDC updated their recommended screening test to a combined antigen/antibody screen that can detect an acute infection even in the absence of HIV antibodies.[6] Acute primary HIV infection, or acute retroviral syndrome (ARS), is usually a febrile illness with a variety of nonspecific symptoms. Clinical suspicion for ARS should be high when individuals present with an illness and a diagnosis of infectious mononucleosis is entertained.[5] During ARS, viral loads of HIV are very high, and the risk for transmission is high because of elevated levels of virus and the likelihood that the infected person is unaware of the diagnosis. Detecting HIV early can lead to reduced rates of transmission when treatment begins early.[7]

Goals of Antiretroviral Therapy

The goals of starting HIV-infected patients on ART are to[8]:

- Improve the survival and quality of life

Table 1
Estimated diagnoses of HIV infection, by age, race/ethnicity, and transmission route for 2013

Age (y)	Estimated Number of Diagnoses	Race/Ethnicity	Estimated Number of Diagnoses	Route of Transmission	Estimated Number of Diagnoses
Age 20 to 34	22,327	Black/African American	21,853	Male-to-male sexual contact	31,023
Age 35 to 49	14,905	White	13,105	Heterosexual contact	4021
Age 50 or greater	8793	Hispanic/Latino	10,888	Injection drug use	2051
		Multiple Races	1039	Male-to-male and injection drug use	1284

Data from Centers for Disease Control and Prevention. HIV Surveillance Report, vol. 25. 2013. Available at: http://www.cdc.gov/hiv/library/reports/surveillance/. Published February 2015. Accessed June 22, 2015.

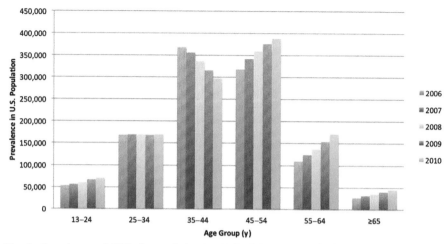

Fig. 1. Prevalence of HIV diagnosis in the United States stratified by age group on an annual basis, 2006 to 2010. (*Adapted from* Centers for Disease Control and Prevention. Monitoring selected national HIV prevention and care objectives by using HIV surveillance data—United States and 6 dependent areas, 2011. HIV Surveillance Supplemental Report 2013;18(5).)

- Reduce the complications of HIV infection
- Improve immunologic function
- Suppress the viral load to undetectable levels for a prolonged duration
- Prevent transmission

Multiple expert panels recommend treatment for all patients infected with HIV regardless of CD4 count or viral load, as early as possible in the diagnosis or when AIDS-defining illness is present.[8–10] This recommendation accounts for the fact that reduced viral counts limit the perinatal and sexual transmission of the virus and improve the complications HIV can add to morbidity (**Table 2**). Treatment with ART reduces the incidence of HIV complications and the deleterious inflammation caused by high levels of virus, but while blunting the process of inflammation it does not control it completely.[11,12] Even with treatment, chronic inflammation with or without ART contributes to non–HIV-related morbidity and mortality.[12–14] Thus, early initiation of ART reduces exposure to chronic inflammation and prevents the progressive loss of CD4 counts and the risk of opportunistic infections.

Presence of Comorbidities

Given that many infected with HIV are advancing in age, it is understandable that many chronic diseases prevalent in the United States would also affect HIV-infected patients. One center reviewed records of 1478 patients in an HIV clinic and found a high prevalence of chronic disease, including coronary artery disease, hypertension, diabetes, and chronic renal disease as the age of the patients increased (**Fig. 2**).[22] Another survey of 3 HIV clinics for veterans for patients undergoing ART found that there are much higher levels of general medical conditions than HIV-related conditions.[23] Other studies have confirmed a high prevalence of comorbid conditions as patients age.[24,25] The use of injection drugs and concomitant infection with hepatitis C increase the risk of comorbid chronic illness even further (**Box 1**).[24,25]

Table 2
Common morbidities associated with HIV infection

Opportunistic infections
  Mycobacterium tuberculosis
  Other *Mycobacterium*
  Pneumocystis pneumonia
  Cryptococcal meningitis
  Toxoplasmosis
  Candidiasis
	All are AIDS-defining illness, concomitant treatment usually with early initiation of ART

Hepatitis B (HBV) and/or hepatitis C (HCV) coinfection	Associated with more rapid progression of liver disease[15] ART should include drugs with activity active against HBV May consider treatment of HCV first before starting ART
HIV-associated nephropathy[16]	Seen with advanced HIV More common in African Americans

Malignancy
  AIDS-defining:
    Kaposi sarcoma
    Non-Hodgkin lymphoma
    Invasive cervical cancer
  Non–AIDS-defining (much higher incidence than non-HIV controls)[17,18]
    Lung
    Anal
    Oropharyngeal
    Skin and melanoma
  Hodgkin lymphoma
	Survival of any cancer depends on CD4 count[19]
	ART reduces risk of AIDS-defining malignancies

Cardiovascular disease	HIV patients are at higher risk for myocardial infarction than age-matched controls[20] Also increased with the use of some ART drugs[20] Still unclear whether HIV itself is a risk factor or if dysmetabolic effects of chronic infection or ART increases risk. Higher rates of smoking in HIV patients likely plays a role[21]
Neurologic complications[8]	With HIV infection: wide spectrum of mild cognitive or motor dysfunction to encephalopathy and dementia On ART: mild cognitive impairment Peripheral neuropathy associated with duration of untreated HIV

Many drugs used in the treatment of HIV can cause renal disease, and kidney disease is prevalent in 4.7% to 9.7% of HIV patients.[16] For HIV patients, there is significant overlap between substance abuse, depressive symptoms, and comorbid medical conditions (**Fig. 3**).[22–24]

Treatment with ART has reduced mortality and increased life expectancy over time.[26] Despite these improvements, mortality rates are still much higher than for the general population,[27] with one analysis suggesting that an HIV-infected person aged 33 has a life expectancy 11.92 years shorter than an age-matched control.[28]

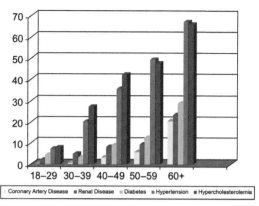

Fig. 2. Percentage of HIV-infected patients with comorbid disease, stratified by age group. (*From* Vance DE, Mugavero M, Willig J, et al. Aging with HIV: a cross-sectional study of comorbidity prevalence and clinical characteristics across decades of life. J Assoc Nurses AIDS Care 2011;22(1):23; with permission.)

Substance abuse, non–AIDS-related cancer, and cardiovascular disease account for 76% of non–HIV-related deaths in HIV patients; however, most (74.2%) AIDS patients continue to die from HIV-related causes.[29]

HIV infection is associated with higher rates of cancer[17,18,30] and cardiovascular disease,[31] suggesting that HIV infection and treatment with ART affects the long-term health of HIV patients. Although traditional risk factors such as lifestyle choices (smoking, alcohol, recreational drug use), environmental, and dietary factors are important to address, it is clear that untreated HIV leads to inflammation and endothelial dysfunction that may put patients at higher risk for cardiovascular disease. Some different ART regimens can increase the risk of cardiovascular disease slightly, particularly with the use of certain protease inhibitors (PIs).[20] Treatment with ART can have effects on body fat and insulin resistance, and can lead to an atherogenic lipid profile. However, initiation of ART does lead to improved endothelial function.[32]

Smoking is much more prevalent in HIV patients than in noninfected controls,[33] and smokers with HIV have higher rates of non–HIV-related mortality compared with either

---

Box 1
Predictors of increased mortality in HIV-infected persons

- Depression[27]
- Substance abuse, injection drug use[27,29]
- Active hepatitis B or C[27]
- Late initiation or early termination of ART[28]
- Black or Hispanic race
- Cardiovascular disease
- Cancer
- Untreated HIV
- Tobacco use

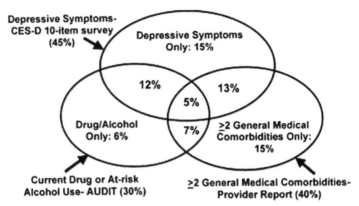

Fig. 3. Venn diagram of overlap of comorbid conditions, substance abuse, and depressive symptoms in 768 HIV-infected patients undergoing ART at 3 Veterans Association medical centers. (*From* Kilbourne AM, Justice AC, Rabeneck L, et al. General medical and psychiatric comorbidity among HIV-infected veterans in the post-HAART era. J Clin Epidemiol 2001;54(Suppl 1):S22–8; with permission.)

nonsmokers with HIV or non-HIV patients who smoke.[34,35] Rates of cancer and cardiovascular disease are also higher in smokers with HIV than in nonsmokers with HIV.[34]

Approach to the Patient

Although many practice guidelines recommend that persons infected with HIV be managed by experts familiar with the treatment of HIV using ART,[36,37] it is possible that primary care providers will diagnose most newly infected HIV patients. Furthermore, given the chronic nature of HIV infection, patients will still need the expertise of a primary care provider in providing preventive care and managing comorbid acute and chronic diseases.

In evaluating the patient with HIV, full attention must be given to a complete history and physical examination. Patients should be queried about past opportunistic infections, malignancies, and other comorbid illness. In addition to surgical history, the medical history must include previous exposure to other sexually transmitted diseases, previous cervical or anal cytology, varicella exposure, and previous tuberculosis testing. Immunization status, travel history, and medications and allergies should be obtained. Patients should be screened for mental illness and intimate partner violence; a detailed sexual history, and the use of tobacco, alcohol, or other recreational drugs should be elicited. A review of systems should include questions directed at the possibility of opportunistic infections, malignancy, and symptoms of chronic diseases such as obstructive airway disease, diabetes, and cardiovascular disease. The examination should be detailed, including a thorough examination of the skin, genitalia, and anus, and for lipodystrophy, lipoatrophy, or wasting.[37]

Baseline Evaluation

Recognizing the importance of a thorough history and examination in initially evaluating the HIV-infected patient, subsequent laboratory testing is required to help determine treatment of the virus, screening for opportunistic infections, and evaluation of the presence of comorbid disease. Recommended initial laboratory evaluations are listed in **Tables 3** and **4**.[8,37]

PHARMACOLOGIC STRATEGIES
Antiretroviral Therapy

Table 5 describes the recommended regimens for ART. The goal of ART for an HIV-infected patient is to maintain a sustained, suppressed HIV viral load, with resultant improvements in a depressed CD4 count (if present) and improved morbidity and mortality. Current regimens are often once daily, and consist of 2 nucleoside analog reverse transcriptase inhibitors (NRTIs) combined with either a PI, a nonnucleoside reverse transcriptase inhibitor (NNRTI), or an integrase strand transfer inhibitor (INSTI). As ART is a lifelong treatment, choices of therapy should provide maximum adherence and minimal toxicity.[8,10] A list of common interactions and side effects for certain ART drugs is listed in **Box 2**, and **Table 6** provides a list of follow-up tests for monitoring while on ART, including intervals of laboratory monitoring.

Prevention of Opportunistic Infections

Effective treatment with ART will lower viral levels of HIV to undetectable levels, and subsequently CD4 counts will either recover or maintain a normal level. However, when CD4 counts are low, opportunistic infections need to be prevented using antimicrobials targeted at common organisms.[38] A guide to prophylactic treatment is given in **Table 7**.

Treatment of Comorbid Chronic Conditions

Cardiovascular disease
As mentioned previously, cardiovascular disease is a common comorbidity for the HIV patient. On the whole, treatment of HIV with ART does improve the overall risk of myocardial infarction. Patients with HIV still have higher rates of cardiovascular disease than the non-HIV patient, although it is unclear whether this is due to the effects of chronic infection and treatment or whether the HIV-infected patient is comparable epidemiologically with non-HIV patients in making inferences about the risk of cardiovascular disease.[39,40]

Table 3	
Initial HIV laboratory monitoring for HIV-infected patients on entry into care or at ART initiation	
Laboratory or Screening Measure	**Rationale or Comment**
HIV Serology	Confirm diagnosis (if not done) or undetectable viral load
CD4 count and percentage	Assess need for opportunistic infection prophylaxis
Plasma HIV RNA (viral load)	
HIV resistance testing	Genotype preferred if not on therapy
Coreceptor tropism assay	If use of CCR5 antagonist considered
HLA B*5701	If abacavir is considered for treatment

Data from World Health Organization. March 2014 supplement to the 2013 consolidated guidelines on the use of antiretroviral drugs for treating and preventing HIV infection: recommendations for a public health approach. Available at: http://apps.who.int/iris/bitstream/10665/104264/1/9789241506830_eng.pdf?ua=1. Accessed May 11, 2015; and Vance DE, Mugavero M, Willig J, et al. Aging with HIV: a cross-sectional study of comorbidity prevalence and clinical characteristics across decades of life. J Assoc Nurses AIDS Care 2011;22(1):17–25.

Table 4
Initial screening for coinfection and comorbidities in HIV-infected patients

Selected Test	Comments
Complete blood cell count with differential	
Liver function testing with total protein and albumin	
Electrolyte panel (basic metabolic panel) including fasting glucose	
Fasting lipid panel	
Hemoglobin A$_{1c}$	Can be screen or confirmation of suspected diabetes
Urinalysis	
Anti-CMV IgG	CMV screen
NAAT (preferred) or culture for gonorrhea/chlamydia	Sites tested should be based on route of sexual exposure (rectal, nasopharyngeal, cervical, urethral)
RPR	Screen for syphilis
Antitoxoplasma IgG	Latent *Toxoplasma gondii* infection
Tuberculin skin test or IGRA (preferred if BCG vaccinated)	Screen latent/active TB
HBsAg, HBsAb, anti-HBc, HCV antibody, HAV antibody (total or IgG)	Hepatitis screen; order RNA level of HBV or HCV if positive HBsAg or HCV antibody, respectively
Antivaricella IgG	If no known varicella exposure or immunization
Glucose-6-phosphate dehydrogenase	Appropriate to screen in ethnically appropriate groups
Trichomoniasis screen	For women

Abbreviations: BCG, bacillus Calmette-Guérin; CMV, cytomegalovirus; HAV, hepatitis A virus; HBc, hepatitis B core; HBsAb, hepatitis B surface antibody; HBsAg, hepatitis B surface antigen; HCV, hepatitis C virus; IgG, immunoglobulin G; IGRA, interferon-γ release assay; NAAT, nucleic acid amplification testing; RPR, rapid plasma reagin; TB, tuberculosis.

Data from World Health Organization. March 2014 supplement to the 2013 consolidated guidelines on the use of antiretroviral drugs for treating and preventing HIV infection: recommendations for a public health approach. Available at: http://apps.who.int/iris/bitstream/10665/104264/1/9789241506830_eng.pdf?ua=1. Accessed May 11, 2015.

Earlier regimens of ART had high rates of adverse effects that included dyslipidemia, metabolic syndrome, and lipodystrophy, which are less frequent with newer ART regimens. Patients who have been on ART for a long time (whereby they would have taken older ART regimens) should be monitored for such changes. Patients should be screened for risk factors for cardiovascular disease and treated according to guidelines (**Table 8**). It is important to bear in mind that many ART regimens (particularly those using PIs) have interactions with statins, as described in **Table 9**.

Bone mineral density is often affected by the presence of HIV, concomitant hepatitis C infection, and treatment with ART. If osteoporosis is present, treatment with a bisphosphonate or alternative agent is reasonable.[49] Vitamin D supplementation at 800 to 1000 IU with 1000 mg of calcium daily may also help with bone health.[49,50]

Chronic kidney disease is also common in HIV-infected patients, occurring in 4.7% to 9.7%. Disease can occur in the setting of advanced HIV infection or as a result of

Table 5
Recommended regimens of ART

Regimen Type	Drug Combination	Comments
INSTI plus 2 NRTIs	Dolutegravir plus tenofovir/emtricitabine Dolutegravir plus abacavir/lamivudine Elvitegravir/cobicistat/tenofovir/emtricitabine Raltegravir plus tenofovir/emtricitabine	INSTIs will be chelated with divalent cations given at same time (calcium, magnesium, etc) May have less effect on lipids Better to use if getting concomitant chemotherapy
NNRTI plus 2 NRTIs	Efavirenz/tenofovir/emtricitabine Efavirenz plus abacavir/lamivudine Rilpivirine/tenofovir/emtricitabine	Efavirenz best taken on empty stomach and at night Rilpivirine should not be taken with PPI
Ritonavir-boosted PI plus 2 NRTIs	Atazanavir/ritonavir plus tenofovir/emtricitabine Atazanavir/ritonavir plus abacavir/lamivudine Darunavir/ritonavir plus tenofovir/emtricitabine	Do not take these combinations with food Avoid PPI or H2 blockers

Abbreviations: INSTI, integrase strand transfer inhibitor; NNRTI, nonnucleoside reverse transcriptase inhibitor; NRTI, nucleoside analogue reverse transcriptase inhibitor; PI, protease inhibitor; PPI, proton-pump inhibitor.

Data from Panel on Antiretroviral Guidelines for Adults and Adolescents. Guidelines for the use of antiretroviral agents in HIV-1-infected adults and adolescents. Department of Health and Human Services. Available at: http://www.aidsinfo.nih.gov/ContentFiles/AdultandAdolescentGL.pdf. Accessed May 11, 2015; and Günthard HF, Aberg JA, Eron JJ, et al. Antiretroviral treatment of adult HIV infection: 2014 recommendations of the International Antiviral Society—USA panel. JAMA 2014;312(4):410–25.

Box 2
Common adverse effects of ART drugs

- Hypersensitivity: usually in HLA B*5701–positive patients
- Hepatotoxicity: usually with PIs and NNRTIs with coexisting viral hepatitis
- Lactic acidosis: rare, with use of NRTIs
- Lipodystrophy
- Alteration of lipid levels, especially certain protease inhibitors
- Nephrotoxicity: common with tenofovir, more common with concomitant use of PI or with existing kidney disease
- Kidney stones: can occur with atazanavir/ritonavir, perhaps darunavir. Idinivir historically (no longer routinely given)
- Neuropathy: uncommon; seen with didanosine (was also common with DDC and D4t)
- Pancreatitis: mostly reported with didanosine, or as a complication of hyperlipidemia from PIs
- Rash: potentially Stevens-Johnson syndrome
- Diarrhea: typically with PIs
- Central nervous system effects, especially with efivarenz

Data from Gallant JE. What does the generalist need to know about HIV infection? Adv Chronic Kidney Dis 2010;17(1):5–18.

Table 6
Recommend subsequent laboratory monitoring for HIV-infected patients while on ART

Laboratory Test	Frequency	Comments
CD4 count	Every 3–6 mo	If viral load suppressed >2 y, can do yearly
HIV viral load	2–8 wk after initiation, then every 3 mo	Can prolong to 6 mo on adherent patients with viral loads suppressed >2 y
Resistance testing	Treatment failure	—
Basic chemistry	2–8 wk after initiation, then every 3–6 mo	—
ALT, AST, total bilirubin	2–8 wk after initiation, then every 3–6 mo	—
CBC with differential	2–8 wk after initiation, then every 3–6 mo	—
Fasting lipid profile	Consider 4–8 wk after starting ART, if abnormal recheck 6 mo. Otherwise every year	—
Fasting glucose or hemoglobin A_{1c}	Every year, unless abnormal then 6 mo	—
Urinalysis	Every year	—

Tests should always be ordered at other times if clinically indicated.
Abbreviations: ALT, alanine aminotransferase; AST, aspartate aminotransferase; CBC, complete blood count.

treatment of ART. Many drugs used in ART affect renal physiology, and a nephrologist should be consulted for a 25% change in glomerular filtration rate (GFR), hematuria, and albuminuria, or if a GFR is less than 60 mL/min/1.73 m^2 and does not improve after removing nephrotoxic drugs.[16] Kidney stones have been associated with the use of

Table 7
Prophylaxis to prevent first occurrence of opportunistic infections in HIV/AIDS patients

Infection	Indication	Recommended Treatment	When to Discontinue
Pneumocystis pneumonia	CD4 count <200 or oropharyngeal candidiasis	TMP-SMX 1 double-strength daily	CD4 count >200 for 3 mo
Toxoplasmosis	Toxoplasma IgG-positive patients with CD4 count <100	TMP-SMX 1 double-strength daily	CD4 count >200 for 3 mo
Mycobacterium tuberculosis	Positive screen for latent TB, or close contact with TB-infected person	Isoniazid 300 mg with pyridoxine 25 mg daily for 9 mo	After treatment
Mycobacterium avium complex	CD4 count <50	Azithromycin 1200 mg weekly	After treatment course (usually 12 mo, if needed) and CD4 count >100 for 3 mo

Data from Masur H, Brooks JT, Benson CA, et al. Prevention and treatment of opportunistic infections in HIV-infected adults and adolescents: Updated Guidelines from the Centers for Disease Control and Prevention, National Institutes of Health, and HIV Medicine Association of the Infectious Diseases Society of America. Clin Infect Dis 2014;58(9):1308–11.

Table 8 Screening and treatment of cardiovascular risk factors		
Cardiovascular Risk Factor	Screening Guidance	Treatment Goals
Blood pressure	Adults ≥18[41] *Annually in all HIV patients*[37]	• Age >60: treat for BP >150/90 mm Hg, with a goal for <150/90 mm Hg • Treat when BP >140/90, with a goal of BP <140/90 (includes diabetics and those with CKD) • Black population: treat initially with a thiazide diuretic (or CCB) • Nonblack population: treat with thiazide diuretic, CCB, ACEI, or ARB • An ACEI or ARB should be given to CKD patients[42]
Cholesterol	*Men:* Age ≥35, 20–35 if other risk factors present *Women:* Age ≥45, 20–45 if other risk factors present[43] *Yearly screening if on ART*[37]	Moderate dose statin for ASCVD risk >7.5%, diabetes with ASCVD risk <7.5% High-dose statin for known ASCVD, LDL >190, or diabetes with ASCVD risk >7.5%[44] (see **Table 10**)
Diabetes	Asymptomatic adults with sustained BP >135/80 mm Hg[45] *Every 6–12 mo*[37]	Treat according to ADA guidelines for a goal hemoglobin A_{1c} of 7.0% or 8.0% depending on comorbidities[37,46]
Smoking	Every visit	Counsel and assist with cessation. Nicotine replacement is effective[47] Varenicline might be more effective than nicotine replacement and may be used with concurrent ART[48]

Abbreviations: ACEI, angiotensin-converting enzyme inhibitor; ADA, American Diabetes Association; ARB, angiotensin receptor blocker; ASCVD, atherosclerotic cardiovascular disease; BP, blood pressure; CCB, calcium-channel blocker; CKD, chronic kidney disease; LDL, low-density lipoprotein.

the PI atazanavir boosted with ritonavir.[51] The reason for this is unclear, although high levels of atazanavir are excreted in the urine and exist in high concentrations in the calculi of affected patients. Of note, darunavir also reached high concentrations in the urine but is less clearly linked to nephrolithiasis.[52]

NONPHARMACOLOGIC STRATEGIES
Screening and Preventive Care

Given the longevity afforded the HIV-infected patient who undergoes treatment, it remains imperative for a primary care physician to screen for preventable illness or detect severe illness early according to established guidelines. Measures to screen for are listed in **Box 3**.

Vaccinations are also vital in the prevention of common infections of the HIV-infected patient. Current CDC vaccine guidance is listed in **Table 10**.

Strategies to reduce high-risk behavior, namely unprotected sexual intercourse and injection drug use, in HIV patients may not only improve the health of patients but also reduce the transmission of HIV. Although best approaches are not well defined, providers should inquire about whether patients engage in high-risk behavior, and at a minimum should counsel and educate on ways to reduce or avoid HIV

Table 9
Recommended statins by potency for HIV-infected patients on ART (all doses daily unless noted)

Statin Dosing	Use of PIs	Use of NNRTIs
Medium intensity		
Atorvastatin 10–20 mg	Use lowest dose	May need higher dose
Rosuvastatin 5–10 mg	Lopinavir/ritonavir and tipranavir/ritonavir increase potency	Acceptable
Pravastatin 40–80 mg	Acceptable, but darunavir may increase potency	May need higher dose with efavirenz
Lovastatin 40 mg	Contraindicated	Acceptable
Fluvastatin 40 mg BID	Not recommended with nelfinavir	May need lower dose with etravirine
Simvastatin 20–40 mg	Contraindicated	May need higher dose
High intensity		
Atorvastatin 40–80 mg	Use lowest dose	May need higher dose
Rosuvastatin 20–40 mg	Lopinavir/ritonavir and tipranavir/ritonavir increase potency	Acceptable

Data from Stone NJ, Robinson JG, Lichtenstein AH, et al. 2013 ACC/AHA guideline on the treatment of blood cholesterol to reduce atherosclerotic cardiovascular risk in adults: a report of the American College of Cardiology/American Heart Association Task Force on Practice Guidelines. Circulation 2014;129(25 Suppl 2):S1–45; and Aberg JA, Gallant JE, Ghanem KG, et al. Primary care guidelines for the management of persons infected with HIV: 2013 update by the HIV Medicine Association of the Infectious Diseases Society of America. Clin Infect Dis 2014;58(1):e1–34.

transmission.[37,53] Referrals to providers that provide counseling on drug use reduction or treatment for comorbid psychiatric illness should be made if possible if the patient is able to undergo treatment. Ideally, care could be provided in a well-integrated facility that has such resources present and available.[36]

EVALUATION, ADJUSTMENT, AND RECURRENCE

The current therapy for HIV can result in long-term viral suppression and maintenance of normal immune function, resulting in a near-normal quality of life and prolonged life expectancy.[26] However, success in treatment requires adherence to ART regimens and quality care. On a population level, success has proved elusive: only 28% of the United States population has had sustained viral suppression,[54] and 59% of HIV-infected patients routinely receive health care.[55] This situation has led an international panel to make a series of recommendations to improve entry of HIV-infected persons into health care environments and to provide supportive educational, behavioral health, and improved service delivery to improve adherence in ART regimens.[56] Selected recommendations are listed in **Box 4**.

In general, decisions to initiate and monitor ART therapy are usually done by experts familiar with ART who have clinical care models that are able to monitor adherence and effects of therapy.[5,36] It is feasible that primary care providers might be providing more comprehensive HIV care in the future. At present, patients with HIV need primary care and chronic comorbid disease management in a coordinated relationship between a primary care physician, an HIV expert, and the patient, to maintain ongoing care and adherence.[37,56]

Box 3
Screening and preventive care for the HIV-infected patient

- Screen for selected sexually transmitted diseases based on clinical suspicion and exposure
- Men and women should be screened for gonorrhea and chlamydia annually (including syphilis, anal human papillomavirus (HPV), and *Trichomonas* if at risk)
- Men and women infected with HPV should have an anal Papanicolaou (Pap) test, including men who have sex with men, women who have had receptive anal intercourse, women with abnormal cervical Pap tests, and persons with genital warts
  - Biopsy should be performed if abnormal; duration/interval of screening unclear
- Women should have a cervical Pap screen every 6 mo in the first year of diagnosis, then annually
  - Abnormal testing should be referred to gynecologist for colposcopy
- Hepatitis C testing annually
- Colorectal cancer screening at age 50
- Annual mammography for women aged 50 or older
- Bone density screen: baseline examination at age 50 and then at 65 if no other risk factors present (start age 60 if risk factors present)
- Screen for abdominal aortic aneurysm for men aged 65–75 who have smoked
- Annual low-dose computed tomography of the lungs for lung cancer screening for patients aged 55–80 years with a 30 pack-year smoking history who currently smoke or have quit within the last 15 years
- Annual depression screening

Data from Aberg JA, Gallant JE, Ghanem KG, et al. Primary care guidelines for the management of persons infected with HIV: 2013 update by the HIV Medicine Association of the Infectious Diseases Society of America. Clin Infect Dis 2014;58(1):e1–34; and US Preventive Services Task Force. Published recommendations. Available at: http://www.uspreventiveservicestaskforce.org/BrowseRec/Index/browse-recommendations. Accessed May 11, 2014.

Table 10
Recommend vaccines (if not previously completed) for HIV-infected patients

Tetanus, diphtheria, pertussis (Td/Tdap)	One dose of Tdap booster, then Td every 10 y
Varicella[a]	Two doses 4–8 wk apart
Human papillomavirus	Three doses up to age 26: second 4–8 wk after first, third 24 wk after first
Measles, mumps, rubella[a]	If not already given
Pneumococcal 13-valent (PCV13) or polysaccharide (PPSV23)	If naïve, should receive PCV13 then PPSV23 4–8 wk later If previously received one, provide the other, preferably 8 wk after first
Meningococcal	Only if other risk factors present
Hepatitis A	For men who have sex with men, can consider in all patients
Hepatitis B	Three doses at 0, 1, and 6 mo

[a] Contraindication if CD4 count <200.
Data from Kroger AT, Atkinson WL, Marcuse EK, et al. General recommendations on immunization: recommendations of the Advisory Committee on Immunization Practices (ACIP). MMWR Recomm Rep 2006;55(Rr–15):1–48; and Advisory Committee on Immunization Practices. Recommended adult immunization schedule: United States, 2013. Ann Intern Med 2013;158(3):191–9.

Box 4
Selected recommendations for improving access of care for HIV treatment adherence

- Systematic monitoring of successful entry in HIV care
- Self-reported adherence should be obtained routinely
- Once-daily regimens of ART are recommended, when safe and possible
- Education and counseling with adherence related tools and one-on-one education
- Nurse or community counselor based care has similar outcomes to doctor or clinic based care in underresourced settings
- Offering buprenorphine or methadone to opioid-dependent patients is recommended
- Screening, management, and treatment of depression and other mental illnesses in combination with adherence counseling

Data from Thompson MA, Mugavero MJ, Amico KR, et al. Guidelines for improving entry into and retention in care and antiretroviral adherence for persons with HIV: evidence-based recommendations from an International Association of Physicians in AIDS care panel. Ann Intern Med 2012;156(11):817–33.

Aside from improving entry of HIV-infected patients into health care settings and treating patients with ART, it is important to monitor and assess metrics of quality care as a means of improvement of clinical care. Some measures have been created and endorsed by the National Quality Foundation, and are undergoing testing as a feasible means of monitoring improvement in the HIV clinical setting (**Box 5**).[57] The future goal of HIV care, therefore, is to continue to develop efforts to promote the diagnosis of HIV, prevention of transmission, improved access to quality clinical environments with effective primary care, improvement in the quality of care provided.

Box 5
Selected HIV quality measures endorsed by the National Quality Forum

1. Retention in care
2. CD4 count
3. Gonorrhea/chlamydia screening
4. Syphilis screening
5. Injection drug use screening
6. High-risk sex screening
7. Tuberculosis screening
8. Hepatitis B screening
9. Hepatitis C screening
10. Hepatitis B vaccination
11. Pneumocystis pneumonia prophylaxis
12. Maximal viral control achieved

Data from Horberg MA, Aberg JA, Cheever LW, et al. Development of national and multi-agency HIV care quality measures. Clin Infect Dis 2010;51(6):732–8.

SUMMARY AND FUTURE CONSIDERATIONS

Although marked advances in the care of the HIV-infected patient have been made, it remains underdiagnosed and undertreated. Those who do receive care have the opportunity for long-term survival, but tend to have higher rates of mental health needs and chronic disease. Although many benefit from expert care in ART administration and adjustment, the other needs of the HIV-infected patient are best suited for the skill set of primary care providers. It is likely that such providers will continue to have a key role in the care of these complex patients for the foreseeable future.

REFERENCES

1. Centers for Disease Control and Prevention. Monitoring selected national HIV prevention and care objectives by using HIV surveillance data—United States and 6 U.S. dependent areas, 2011. HIV Surveillance Supplemental Report 2013;18(No. 5). Available online at: http://www.cdc.gov/hiv/library/reports/surveillance/. Accessed June 22, 2015.
2. Centers for Disease Control and Prevention. HIV Surveillance report, 2013; Available online at: http://www.cdc.gov/hiv/library/reports/surveillance/. Accessed June 22, 2015.
3. Moyer VA. Screening for HIV: U.S. Preventive Services Task Force Recommendation Statement. Ann Intern Med 2013;159(1):51–60.
4. Branson BM, Handsfield HH, Lampe MA, et al. Revised recommendations for HIV testing of adults, adolescents, and pregnant women in health-care settings. MMWR Recomm Rep 2006;55(Rr–14):1–17 [quiz: CE1–4].
5. Gallant JE. What does the generalist need to know about HIV infection? Adv Chronic Kidney Dis 2010;17(1):5–18.
6. Centers for Disease Control and Prevention, Association of Public Health Laboratories. Laboratory testing for the diagnosis of HIV infection: Updated Recommendations. Available online at: http://stacks.cdc.gov/view/cdc/23447. Accessed June 22, 2015.
7. Cohen MS, Chen YQ, McCauley M, et al. Prevention of HIV-1 infection with early antiretroviral therapy. N Engl J Med 2011;365(6):493–505.
8. Panel on Antiretroviral Guidelines for Adults and Adolescents. Guidelines for the use of antiretroviral agents in HIV-1-infected adults and adolescents. Department of Health and Human Services. Available online at: http://www.aidsinfo.nih.gov/ContentFiles/AdultandAdolescentGL.pdf. Accessed June 22, 2015.
9. WHO. March 2014 supplement to the 2013 consolidated guidelines on the use of antiretroviral drugs for treating and preventing HIV infection: recommendations for a public health approach. Geneva (EU): WHO; 2014.
10. Günthard HF, Aberg JA, Eron JJ, et al. Antiretroviral treatment of adult HIV infection: 2014 recommendations of the international antiviral society—USA panel. JAMA 2014;312(4):410–25.
11. Hunt PW, Martin JN, Sinclair E, et al. T cell activation is associated with lower CD4+ T cell gains in human immunodeficiency virus-infected patients with sustained viral suppression during antiretroviral therapy. J Infect Dis 2003;187(10):1534–43.
12. Neuhaus J, Jacobs DR Jr, Baker JV, et al. Markers of inflammation, coagulation, and renal function are elevated in adults with HIV infection. J Infect Dis 2010;201(12):1788–95.

13. Borges AH, Silverberg MJ, Wentworth D, et al. Predicting risk of cancer during HIV infection: the role of inflammatory and coagulation biomarkers. AIDS 2013; 27(9):1433–41.

14. Duprez DA, Neuhaus J, Kuller LH, et al. Inflammation, coagulation and cardiovascular disease in HIV-infected individuals. PLoS One 2012;7(9):e44454.

15. Kalayjian RC, Franceschini N, Gupta SK, et al. Suppression of HIV-1 replication by antiretroviral therapy improves renal function in persons with low CD4 cell counts and chronic kidney disease. AIDS 2008;22(4):481–7.

16. Lucas GM, Ross MJ, Stock PG, et al. Clinical practice guideline for the management of chronic kidney disease in patients infected with HIV: 2014 update by the HIV Medicine Association of the Infectious Diseases Society of America. Clin Infect Dis 2014;59(9):e96–138.

17. Bedimo RJ, McGinnis KA, Dunlap M, et al. Incidence of non-AIDS-defining malignancies in HIV-infected versus noninfected patients in the HAART era: impact of immunosuppression. J Acquir Immune Defic Syndr 2009;52(2):203–8.

18. Silverberg MJ, Chao C, Leyden WA, et al. HIV infection, immunodeficiency, viral replication, and the risk of cancer. Cancer Epidemiol Biomarkers Prev 2011; 20(12):2551–9.

19. Monforte A, Abrams D, Pradier C, et al. HIV-induced immunodeficiency and mortality from AIDS-defining and non-AIDS-defining malignancies. AIDS 2008; 22(16):2143–53.

20. Friis-Moller N, Reiss P, Sabin CA, et al. Class of antiretroviral drugs and the risk of myocardial infarction. N Engl J Med 2007;356(17):1723–35.

21. Triant VA. Epidemiology of coronary heart disease in HIV patients. Rev Cardiovasc Med 2014;15(Suppl 1):S1–8.

22. Vance DE, Mugavero M, Willig J, et al. Aging with HIV: a cross-sectional study of comorbidity prevalence and clinical characteristics across decades of life. J Assoc Nurses AIDS Care 2011;22(1):17–25.

23. Kilbourne AM, Justice AC, Rabeneck L, et al. General medical and psychiatric comorbidity among HIV-infected veterans in the post-HAART era. J Clin Epidemiol 2001;54(Suppl 1):S22–8.

24. Weiss JJ, Osorio G, Ryan E, et al. Prevalence and patient awareness of medical comorbidities in an urban AIDS clinic. AIDS Patient Care STDS 2010;24(1):39–48.

25. Goulet JL, Fultz SL, McGinnis KA, et al. Relative prevalence of comorbidities and treatment contraindications in HIV-mono-infected and HIV/HCV-co-infected veterans. AIDS 2005;19(Suppl 3):S99–105.

26. Samji H, Cescon A, Hogg RS, et al. Closing the gap: increases in life expectancy among treated HIV-positive individuals in the United States and Canada. PLoS One 2013;8(12):e81355.

27. French AL, Gawel SH, Hershow R, et al. Trends in mortality and causes of death among women with HIV in the United States: a 10-year study. J Acquir Immune Defic Syndr 2009;51(4):399–406.

28. Losina E, Schackman BR, Sadownik SN, et al. Racial and sex disparities in life expectancy losses among HIV-infected persons in the United States: impact of risk behavior, late initiation, and early discontinuation of antiretroviral therapy. Clin Infect Dis 2009;49(10):1570–8.

29. Sackoff JE, Hanna DB, Pfeiffer MR, et al. Causes of death among persons with AIDS in the era of highly active antiretroviral therapy: New York City. Ann Intern Med 2006;145(6):397–406.

30. Riedel DJ, Mwangi EI, Fantry LE, et al. High cancer-related mortality in an urban, predominantly African-American, HIV-infected population. AIDS 2013;27(7):1109–17.

31. Triant VA, Lee H, Hadigan C, et al. Increased acute myocardial infarction rates and cardiovascular risk factors among patients with human immunodeficiency virus disease. J Clin Endocrinol Metab 2007;92(7):2506–12.

32. Torriani FJ, Komarow L, Parker RA, et al. Endothelial function in human immunodeficiency virus-infected antiretroviral-naive subjects before and after starting potent antiretroviral therapy: The ACTG (AIDS Clinical Trials Group) Study 5152s. J Am Coll Cardiol 2008;52(7):569–76.

33. Kaplan RC, Kingsley LA, Sharrett AR, et al. Ten-year predicted coronary heart disease risk in HIV-infected men and women. Clin Infect Dis 2007;45(8):1074–81.

34. Helleberg M, Afzal S, Kronborg G, et al. Mortality attributable to smoking among HIV-1-infected individuals: a nationwide, population-based cohort study. Clin Infect Dis 2013;56(5):727–34.

35. Cockerham L, Scherzer R, Zolopa A, et al. Association of HIV infection, demographic and cardiovascular risk factors with all-cause mortality in the recent HAART era. J Acquir Immune Defic Syndr 2010;53(1):102–6.

36. Gallant JE, Adimora AA, Carmichael JK, et al. Essential components of effective HIV care: a policy paper of the HIV Medicine Association of the Infectious Diseases Society of America and the Ryan White Medical Providers Coalition. Clin Infect Dis 2011;53(11):1043–50.

37. Aberg JA, Gallant JE, Ghanem KG, et al. Primary care guidelines for the management of persons infected with HIV: 2013 update by the HIV Medicine Association of the Infectious Diseases Society of America. Clin Infect Dis 2014;58(1): e1–34.

38. Masur H, Brooks JT, Benson CA, et al. Prevention and treatment of opportunistic infections in HIV-infected adults and adolescents: updated guidelines from the Centers for Disease Control and Prevention, National Institutes of Health, and HIV Medicine Association of the Infectious Diseases Society of America. Clin Infect Dis 2014;58(9):1308–11.

39. Stein JH. Cardiovascular risk and dyslipidemia management in HIV-infected patients. Top Antivir Med 2012;20(4):129–33 [quiz: 123–4].

40. Triant VA. HIV infection and coronary heart disease: an intersection of epidemics. J Infect Dis 2012;205(Suppl 3):S355–61.

41. Screening for High Blood Pressure. U.S. preventive services task force recommendation. Ann Intern Med 2007;147(11):I43.

42. James PA, Oparil S, Carter BL, et al. 2014 evidence-based guideline for the management of high blood pressure in adults: Report from the panel members appointed to the eighth joint national committee (JNC 8). JAMA 2014;311(5): 507–20.

43. Helfand M, Carson S. Screening for Lipid Disorders in Adults: Selective Update of 2001 US Preventive Services Task Force Review [Internet]. Rockville (MD): Agency for Healthcare Research and Quality (US); 2008. (Evidence Syntheses, No. 49).

44. Stone NJ, Robinson JG, Lichtenstein AH, et al. 2013 ACC/AHA guideline on the treatment of blood cholesterol to reduce atherosclerotic cardiovascular risk in adults: a report of the American College of Cardiology/American Heart Association Task Force on Practice Guidelines. Circulation 2014;129(25 Suppl 2):S1–45.

45. U.S. Preventive Services Task Force. Screening for type 2 diabetes mellitus in adults: U.S. Preventive Services Task Force recommendation statement. Ann Intern Med 2008;148(11):846–54.

46. American Diabetes Association. Standards of medical care in diabetes—2013. Diabetes Care 2013;36(Suppl 1):S11–66.

47. Cioe PA. Smoking cessation interventions in HIV-infected adults in North America: a literature review. J Addict Behav Ther Rehabil 2013;2(3):1000112.
48. Ferketich AK, Diaz P, Browning KK, et al. Safety of varenicline among smokers enrolled in the lung HIV study. Nicotine Tob Res 2013;15(1):247–54.
49. Cosman F, de Beur SJ, LeBoff MS, et al. Clinician's Guide to Prevention and Treatment of Osteoporosis. Osteoporosis International 2014;25(10):2359–81.
50. Yin M. Vitamin D, bone, and HIV infection. Top Antivir Med 2012;20(5):168–72.
51. Hamada Y, Nishijima T, Watanabe K, et al. High incidence of renal stones among HIV-infected patients on ritonavir-boosted atazanavir than in those receiving other protease inhibitor-containing antiretroviral therapy. Clin Infect Dis 2012;55(9): 1262–9.
52. de Lastours V, Ferrari Rafael De Silva E, Daudon M, et al. High levels of atazanavir and darunavir in urine and crystalluria in asymptomatic patients. J Antimicrob Chemother 2013;68(8):1850–6.
53. Centers for Disease Control and Prevention (CDC), Health Resources and Services Administration, National Institutes of Health. Incorporating HIV prevention into the medical care of persons living with HIV. Recommendations of CDC, the Health Resources and Services Administration, the National Institutes of Health, and the HIV Medicine Association of the Infectious Diseases Society of America. MMWR Recomm Rep 2003;52(Rr–12):1–24.
54. Vital signs. HIV prevention through care and treatment—United States. MMWR Morb Mortal Wkly Rep 2011;60(47):1618–23.
55. Marks G, Gardner LI, Craw J, et al. Entry and retention in medical care among HIV-diagnosed persons: a meta-analysis. AIDS 2010;24(17):2665–78.
56. Thompson MA, Mugavero MJ, Amico KR, et al. Guidelines for improving entry into and retention in care and antiretroviral adherence for persons with HIV: evidence-based recommendations from an international association of physicians in AIDS care panel. Ann Intern Med 2012;156(11):817–33.
57. Horberg MA, Aberg JA, Cheever LW, et al. Development of national and multi-agency HIV care quality measures. Clin Infect Dis 2010;51(6):732–8.

The Management of Sarcoidosis
A Primary Care Approach

Justin Shinn, MD[a],*, Douglas S. Paauw, MD, MACP[b]

KEYWORDS

- Sarcoidosis • Treatment • Management • Corticosteroids • Primary care
- Bilateral hilar adenopathy • Löfgren syndrome

KEY POINTS

- Sarcoidosis is an idiopathic, granulomatous inflammatory disorder, which can affect any organ system.
- Hypercalcemia and hypercalciuria in patients with sarcoid is usually caused by an increased 1,25-hydroxyvitamin D level.
- Syncope and palpitations must be aggressively evaluated in patients with sarcoid, because they may be a sign of cardiac involvement.
- Steroids are the mainstay of treatment, but they should be tapered to their lowest effective dose.
- Steroid-sparing adjuvant therapy for sarcoidosis is available, depending on the organ system involved, most commonly methotrexate, azathioprine, and occasionally biological agents.
- Death from sarcoidosis most commonly originates from involvement of the pulmonary, cardiac, and nervous system.

INTRODUCTION

Sarcoidosis is an idiopathic granulomatous disease that can affect any organ system. Commonly, diagnosis requires histologic examination with evidence of noncaseating granulomas. The clinical picture is often complex and, combined with the rarity of the disease, can make diagnosis difficult for any health care provider. Despite these challenges, it is possible to successfully manage patients with sarcoidosis in a primary care setting.

Disclosure statement: D.S. Paauw, Editor for *Medical Clinics of North America*.
[a] Department of Internal Medicine, University of Washington School of Medicine, 1959 NE Pacific Street, Seattle, WA 98115, USA; [b] Division of General Internal Medicine, Department of Medicine, University of Washington School of Medicine, 1959 NE Pacific Street, Seattle, WA 98195, USA
* Corresponding author.
E-mail address: shinnj@uw.edu

Med Clin N Am 99 (2015) 1123–1148
http://dx.doi.org/10.1016/j.mcna.2015.05.008
0025-7125/15/$ – see front matter © 2015 Elsevier Inc. All rights reserved.

medical.theclinics.com

NATURAL HISTORY OF SARCOIDOSIS

In counseling patients with sarcoidosis, it is important to understand the disease manifestation as well as its possible progression. Certain factors, organ involvement, and demographic information may give insight into the possibility of good clinical outcome. Most patients experience spontaneous remission within months to years after onset, with no long-term sequelae.

Table 1 shows risk factors for sarcoidosis. In the United States, African Americans are at increased risk of suffering from sarcoidosis at 2.4% lifetime risk and also have increased severity of disease.[1] Whites are less commonly affected, at 0.85% lifetime risk, typically have more limited disease severity, and are more likely to experience disease remission.[1] The classic presentation of sarcoidosis of asymptomatic bilateral hilar adenopathy, present in 75% of those with sarcoidosis, is also more likely to undergo spontaneous regression (70%–80% within 1 year), whereas pulmonary fibrosis, certain cutaneous manifestations, and neurologic problems are more likely to be associated with increased chronicity of disease.[1,2] Cardiac involvement and pulmonary fibrosis are the most common causes of mortality in sarcoidosis. In counseling patients, this information can be used to offer hope or to begin to prepare the patient for a more insidious or severe clinical course. **Box 1** lists indicators of good prognostic versus more worrisome clinical findings.

Sarcoidosis is a disease with an unknown cause and nonspecific treatment options. Corticosteroids are the treatment of choice, but limited data have shown that treatment does not affect disease progression but may only manage symptoms and prevent irreversible changes.

INITIAL EVALUATION

A 27-year-old African American woman presented to her primary care provider with exertional dyspnea. By report, her mother had lung problems and eventually died of sudden death. Initial examination showed no other complaints, but a chest radiograph showed bilateral hilar adenopathy. A complete blood count (CBC), electrolytes and calcium, aspartate aminotransferase, alanine transaminase, and bilirubin tests and urinalysis are obtained. An electrocardiogram (EKG), echocardiogram, and tuberculin skin test are also ordered. The laboratory values and other tests are all normal except with a mild increase of liver function test (LFT) results. Not surprisingly, the tuberculin skin test is also within normal limits.

This is a classic description of a patient with sarcoidosis, more often occurring in African Americans and females. Eighty percent of cases occur in individuals 20 to 40 years old.[1] The tuberculin skin test helps rule out other granulomatous diseases; however, 60% of patients with sarcoidosis also experience skin anergy, which

Table 1 Risk factors for sarcoidosis	
Risk Factors	**Comments**
Ethnicity/nationality	More common in African American, Scandinavian, Irish, German, and West Indian individuals. Rare in Japanese, Spanish, and Portuguese individuals
Genetic	Idiopathic complex, non-Mendelian
Age	80% of sarcoidosis occurs in individuals aged 20–40 y
Women	Marginal risk factor

> **Box 1**
> **Indicators of good prognostic versus more worrisome clinical findings**
>
> *Indicators of good clinical outcome*
>
> Löfgren syndrome
>
> White
>
> Young age
>
> Bilateral hilar adenopathy
>
> *Indicators of poor clinical outcome*
>
> African American
>
> Extrathoracic disease
>
> Cutaneous manifestations, not including erythema nodosum
>
> Neurologic and cardiac involvement
>
> Older age
>
> Parenchymal lung involvement

decreases the effectiveness of delayed-type hypersensitivity reactions.[3] Quantiferon testing can be used as an effective alternative for tuberculosis (TB) skin testing, although it may have a slightly higher indeterminate response in those with sarcoidosis and on immunosuppressive therapy.[4]

Sarcoidosis primarily affects the respiratory system but can present with extrapulmonary manifestations, sometimes as the initial problem. The lung is affected in greater than 90% of patients with sarcoidosis, with pulmonary involvement often asymptomatic, showing up as bilateral hilar adenopathy.[5] A history should be detailed and include a full systemic complement of questions, including an evaluation of risk factors and signs and symptoms of other granulomatous diseases. Other forms of granulomatous diseases are listed in **Box 2** and common extrapulmonary manifestations listed in **Table 2**. Irwin and Carrao[5] summarized the diagnosis of sarcoidosis as requiring 3 criteria: (1) A suitable clinical presentation or consistent imaging, (2) tissue demonstration of noncaseating granulomas, and (3) an exhaustive effort to rule out other potential possibilities.

> **Box 2**
> **Other granuloma forming diseases**
>
> *Granulomatous diseases*
>
> TB
>
> Atypical mycobacteria
>
> Fungal infections, particularly coccidiomycosis
>
> *Vasculitis*
>
> Pneumoconiosis
>
> Foreign body reaction
>
> Lymphoma
>
> Hypersensitivity pneumonitis

Table 2
Common extrapulmonary manifestations of sarcoidosis

Extrapulmonary Sarcoidosis	Findings
Constitutional	Low-grade fever, malaise, weight loss
Eyes	Anterior uveitis
	Posterior uveitis
	Optic neuritis
Skin	Erythema nodosum
	Lupus pernio
	Violaceous plaques
	Maculopapular lesions
	Koebner phenomenon
Cardiac	Arrhythmias
	Heart block
	Congestive heart failure
Neurologic	Unilateral or bilateral seventh cranial nerve palsy
	Cranial or peripheral neuropathy
	Small-fiber neuropathy
	Cerebellar ataxia
	Meningitis
	Hydrocephalus
	Psychiatric disease
	Cranial neuropathy
Kidney	Nephrolithiasis
	Hypercalcemia/hypercalciuria
Liver	Increased LFT test results
	Hepatomegaly, pruritus, cholestasis
	Nausea, vomiting
Spleen	Splenomegaly
Peripheral lymph nodes	Asymptomatic adenopathy
Sinuses	Epistaxis
	Sinusitis, nasal obstruction
Larynx	Hoarseness
Joints	Arthritis
	Destructive joint inflammation
Bone marrow	Reduction in cell lines
Breasts/testes	Testicular enlargement and masses, breast masses

For initial studies, there is not a standardized algorithm. The clinical picture and a high index of suspicion in context with a complement of laboratory and radiographic studies helps support the possible diagnosis. Initial laboratory tests should include CBC with differential, electrolytes including calcium, LFTs, urinalysis, and an EKG. Any EKG abnormalities should be pursued, because they can be a clue to the possibility of cardiac involvement, which can lead to life-threatening arrhythmias. A chest radiograph is not as sensitive in detecting soft tissue and intraparenchymal lung disease as computed tomography (CT); however, CT has not been shown to increase diagnostic capabilities or to affect prognosis. A chest radiograph, along with a pulmonary function test (PFT), should be obtained as part of an initial evaluation. A suggested initial battery of diagnostic studies is included in **Table 3**. Careful eye and skin examinations are important, because these are the most common extrapulmonary sites.

Table 3
Suggested initial battery of diagnostic studies

Laboratory and Radiographic Testing	
CBC	Bone marrow involvement, leukopenia (especially lymphopenia)
Serum chemistry	Hypercalcemia Hyperkalemia or hypokalemia Creatinine and blood urea nitrogen for kidney involvement
1,25-dihydroxyvitamin D	May be increased, even if 25-hydroxyvitamin D is normal
Liver enzymes	Increased alkaline phosphatase level is the most common LFT abnormality Transaminitis Cholestasis
Urinalysis/24 h urine calcium	Hypercalciuria
EKG	Heart block Arrhythmias
Chest radiograph	Bilateral hilar adenopathy Reticulonodular opacities Pulmonary fibrosis
PFT, including spirometry and diffusing capacity	Restrictive pattern, reduced DLCO (diffusing capacity of lung for carbon monoxide)
Additional Testing	
Serum angiotensin-converting enzyme level	Nonspecific, does not correlate with disease activity
Tuberculin skin testing/interferon-γ testing	Rule out TB
Total immunoglobulin levels	Common variable immunodeficiency can present with a sarcoidlike picture
6-Min walk test	Can assist with quality of life and functional status evaluation

A tissue biopsy for histologic evaluation of noncaseating granulomas is often necessary. The location of biopsy should be performed at easily accessible sites, including suspicious skin lesions, enlarged lymph nodes and salivary glands, or if required, transbronchial or mediastinal lymph nodes. The tissue should be analyzed for granulomas as well as sent for culture. In only 3 instances (Löfgren syndrome, Heerfordt syndrome [uveoparotid fever], and asymptomatic bilateral hilar adenopathy) is a biopsy not necessary for the diagnosis of sarcoidosis. This situation is because Löfgren syndrome, Heerfordt syndrome, and bilateral hilar lymphadenopathy are specific for sarcoidosis.[2,6]

Winterbauer and colleagues[2] in a retrospective review found that 74% of patients with sarcoidosis had bilateral hilar adenopathy on chest radiograph, with 29% of patients with isolated bilateral hilar adenopathy without other findings. Peritracheal adenopathy was found in 40% of patients but always occurred with bilateral hilar adenopathy. No patient suffering from sarcoidosis had findings of parenchymal nodules, effusions, or mediastinal abnormalities on chest radiograph. In that study, all asymptomatic individuals with bilateral hilar adenopathy and negative physical examination findings had sarcoidosis. In addition, all patients with bilateral hilar adenopathy and uveitis or erythema nodosum (EN) also had sarcoidosis. The same finding of all patients who were asymptomatic with bilateral hilar adenopathy having sarcoidosis was also found in Singapore.[6]

Physical examination findings in patients with sarcoidosis are variable and often unrevealing. Special attention should be given to eye, cranial nerve, nose, neck (especially evaluating for lymphadenopathy), lung, abdominal (evaluating for hepatomegaly or splenomegaly) and skin examinations.

Sarcoidosis is asymptomatic in 30% to 60% of patients and incidental findings on chest radiograph or laboratory abnormalities, including hypercalcemia, cytopenias, or increased liver enzyme levels may be the initial findings.[3] The diagnosis of sarcoidosis can be complicated and close follow-up over several months helps elicit an accurate diagnosis. Many patients with sarcoid are asymptomatic, and whatever symptoms they present for evaluation for may not be related to or caused by sarcoidosis. Serum angiotensin-converting enzyme (ACE) level is increased in 60% of patients with acute sarcoidosis, but only 10% of those with chronic sarcoidosis.[1] This test can be used to help support a diagnosis of acute sarcoid, especially because very high levels are not typically found in other granulomatous diseases. However, a high ACE level is not pathognomonic or even specific for sarcoidosis. In addition, with chronic disease, there seems to be a regression in increased levels of ACE. It is not a marker of disease progression or an adequate tool to follow disease course. Lymphopenia is more common and more severe with active sarcoidosis, and the absence of lymphopenia can be helpful in determining whether a symptom is related to active sarcoid or not.

FOLLOW-UP

A 36-year-old man came into clinic for 6-month follow-up after being diagnosed with Löfgren syndrome. A decision at that time was for watchful waiting and symptomatic nonsteroidal antiinflammatory drugs (NSAIDs) and steroid drops for his EN and uveitis, respectively.

With acute sarcoidosis, monitoring should be initially every 3 months for the first year, especially for those on immunosuppressive therapy. In the case of the 36-year-old man, the patient presented with Löfgren syndrome, which does not usually require oral prednisone or immunosuppressive therapy and is likely to undergo spontaneous remission. In this setting, 6-month follow-up is acceptable, educating the patient to seek treatment of new symptom onset. After the first year and with stable sarcoidosis, patients can be followed every 6 months. At subsequent visits, a chest radiograph can be obtained if symptoms suggest progression of pulmonary disease, and PFTs can evaluate the functional status of the lungs. An EKG is also indicated because cardiac sarcoidosis is life threatening, requires immediate treatment and subspecialty evaluation, and can be sudden in onset. Follow-up after remission should be continued for 5 years, because sarcoidosis often recurs.

Patients with active sarcoidosis should be followed closely, at least every 3 months initially, especially those on immunosuppressive therapy. A detailed history and targeted physical examination should be taken with every visit, evaluating for systemic manifestations with possible repeat chest radiographs, PFT, and EKG. PFTs seem to be the best indicator for following disease progression over time. Repeat blood testing can identify laboratory abnormalities, such as mild anemia or transaminitis, but these are often asymptomatic and rarely require treatment. Exceptions to this situation include renal insufficiency and hypercalcemia, which may need treatment depending on severity; both respond readily to systemic steroids. If disease remits, then patients should continue to be followed semiannually and then annually with suspected sarcoidosis relapse for at least 5 years. One of the most important goals of follow-up is to reduce immunosuppression whenever possible and to monitor and try to prevent the long-term negative effects of corticosteroids and other immunosuppressive medications.

RESPIRATORY SYSTEM

A 21-year-old woman presented with new-onset wheezing, not associated with exertion, weather changes, or other triggers. A chest radiograph showed bilateral hilar adenopathy and peritracheal adenopathy. Basic metabolic panel, calcium, CBC, LFTs, EKG, and a tuberculin skin test are normal. PFTs shows an increased FEV_1 (forced expiratory volume in first second of expiration)/forced vital capacity (FVC) and decreased DLCO (diffusing capacity of lung for carbon monoxide), which suggests sarcoidosis, and biopsy showed granulomatous inflammation. The patient was counseled about her disease, natural progression, and initiated on 40 mg prednisone daily. Several weeks later, her wheezing and PFTs were markedly improved. A decision is made to decrease her steroids, beginning at 20 mg of prednisone daily, and then tapering over 6 months. She was also prescribed concurrent inhaled corticosteroids. She was scheduled for follow-up in 2 weeks and 3 months.

This case highlights the overlap between asthma and sarcoidosis. In this process, PFT can be useful to help distinguish the 2 entities. Although inhaled steroids are unproved in the literature, they are a low-risk adjuvant to help alleviate symptoms, prevent relapse, and decrease steroid dosing. In this case, the patient likely required endoscopic endobronchial needle aspiration or biopsy for tissue diagnosis, because she had no other accessible biopsy sites. A specialist who is experienced in dealing with sarcoidosis, along with imaging guidance, can facilitate intrathoracic biopsies.

The lung is involved in greater than 90% of patients with sarcoidosis.[1] Many of these patients are asymptomatic, but found only with radiographic changes. Others may present with wheezing, dyspnea, chest pain, or cough. Sharp chest pain is a common symptom in patients with active pulmonary sarcoid. Chronic cough is the most frequent respiratory symptom.[7] On auscultation, the lung examination is most often without any abnormalities, particularly in early stages of disease. Chest radiograph findings are also highly variable, ranging from asymptomatic hilar adenopathy (**Fig. 1**) to parenchymal involvement, and to fibrocystic changes. These fibrocystic parenchymal changes, found in approximately 10% to 30% of those with sarcoidosis,

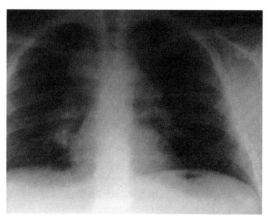

Fig. 1. Chest radiograph showing bilateral hilar adenopathy.

can be difficult to differentiate from nonfibrotic changes on chest radiograph and are irreversible.[3] They can be present at diagnosis; predispose patients to opportunistic infections, bronchiectasis and hemoptysis, diffusion abnormalities, and pulmonary hypertension; and are also one of the primary causes of mortality.

A chest radiograph is often sufficient for the workup of sarcoidosis, but chest CT is essential for atypical presentations and clinical suspicion of sarcoidosis without chest radiograph findings and can also assist with identifying pulmonary fibrosis.[7] CT findings in sarcoidosis can evaluate for more subtle parenchymal involvement and have been shown to correlate with the declines in PFTs and the severity of the inflammatory activity, unlike a chest radiograph. CT findings most typically show perilymphatic nodules predominantly in the upper and posterior portions of the lungs surrounding the lobules and fissures.

The initial diagnostic evaluation for pulmonary sarcoidosis is chest radiograph and PFT, along with a tuberculin skin test. Asymptomatic radiographic findings can be managed with watchful waiting, whereas other changes may necessitate the use of oral or inhaled corticosteroids. With active sarcoidosis, a chest radiograph should be obtained once yearly.

PFTs should be obtained initially to further evaluate lung involvement and are abnormal in 20% to 40% of patients with sarcoidosis, even in those with a normal chest radiograph.[3] PFTs correlate well with the overall disease process, particularly FVC, which is the most accurate parameter to assess sarcoidosis severity.[7] In addition, DLCO can evaluate the vitality of the respiratory membrane within the alveoli and the FEV_1/FVC ratio most often shows a restrictive pattern but can show an obstructive, restrictive, or normal pattern. The 6-minute walk test, DLCO, and FEV_1 are nonspecific and can be greatly affected by other disease and patient factors.

A challenging occurrence is a patient with both asthma and sarcoidosis, or if a patient with known asthma presents with new atypical symptoms. Asthma is more common than sarcoidosis and is always the more likely culprit. Distinguishing asthma from sarcoidosis is challenging, because both can present with wheezing and chronic cough in a young individual. Airway limitation in sarcoidosis occurs because of endobronchial granulomas, fibrosis and airway distortion, intrinsic airway narrowing and extrinsic compression from lymphadenopathy, and hyperreactivity and bronchospasm.[8] Indicators of sarcoidosis over asthma include an atypical asthmatic presentation, limited response to inhaled therapies, extrapulmonary manifestations of sarcoidosis, and a family history of sarcoidosis. A directed history should elicit atopic reactions, family history of atopy, and variation of symptoms with season and allergen exposure. The most effective means to distinguish these 2 entities is through a thorough history, but other tools can assist with the appropriate diagnosis, notably chest radiographs. PFTs in sarcoidosis can be an obstructive, restrictive, or normal pattern, depending on the area of lung involvement. A normal or increased FEV_1/FVC ratio and reduced DLCO favor sarcoidosis, whereas additional testing may be necessary with a decreased FEV_1/FVC ratio. The white blood cell differential can be a clue, because lymphopenia is common in active sarcoidosis, whereas eosinophilia is more characteristic of asthma. In some cases, a dichotomy of disease is never discovered, but the treatment of the 2 diseases is similar.

Systemic corticosteroids are the mainstay for treatment of sarcoidosis, but for minor pulmonary symptoms (especially cough), inhaled corticosteroid and bronchodilators may provide benefit, although this is unproved in the literature.[9] Budesonide 800 μg twice daily is the most extensively studied inhaled steroid in the literature, but fluticasone has also been used. They can be considered with minor disease severity, minor symptoms, or as adjuncts when tapering oral steroids.

It can be difficult to assess the appropriate timing of therapy for respiratory sarcoidosis. Oral treatment should be initiated with pulmonary symptoms, such as cough or dyspnea, or worsening pulmonary function.[1] The primary aim of therapy is to improve symptoms and pulmonary function, not the chest imaging.[5] If a patient is asymptomatic, PFTs can track lung function and it is appropriate to consider therapy with a decline in FVC of 10% or DLCO of 20%.[10] With treatment, the pulmonary manifestations and imaging characteristics of sarcoidosis begin to improve within weeks. The recommendation is to start with higher doses, typically 20 to 40 mg of prednisone daily with follow-up in 2 to 3 weeks, to control the disease processes and then begin to taper. The total length of treatment is variable but should be considered for at least 6 to 9 months with close follow-up, because recurrence is common during the time after steroid discontinuance. To mitigate the side effects of oral steroids, the goal is to taper patients completely off steroids; however, this may not be possible in patients with refractory sarcoidosis. Steroid-sparing agents are listed in **Box 4**.

After initial diagnosis, patients can be followed with symptom management, chest radiograph, and PFT. It is difficult to correlate disease progression with evolving changes on imaging, but if changes are discovered on routine chest radiograph, then PFTs can evaluate the functional status of the lungs. If a patient has persistent chest radiograph changes, they should be followed yearly indefinitely. Reactivation of latent sarcoidosis is common, but if the disease remains inactive, a patient can be monitored for at least 3 years. With burnt-out or inactive sarcoidosis, there is little clinical usefulness of repeat imaging and PFTs, but along with basic laboratory tests, these tools should be considered with any changes in baseline or new symptom onset. Much mortality in sarcoidosis is caused by end-stage fibrocystic lung disease. It is unclear whether early treatment with immunosuppressive drugs alters the natural history of these anatomic changes.

A 47-year-old woman with a long history of difficult to control sarcoidosis presented to her primary care physician's office for new-onset cough. She was diagnosed with sarcoidosis in her late 30s, with manifestations of chronic rhinosinusitis and nasal obstruction, which were controlled with oral and nasal steroids. A chest radiograph was obtained, PFTs were repeated, and after the chest radiograph showed bilateral reticulonodular patterns, chest CT showed parenchymal fibrosis and an apical mass. Serum Aspergillus antibodies were positive.

Patients with sarcoidosis that is difficult to control or of long duration are at increased risk of opportunistic infections. Chronic pulmonary aspergillosis is the most common, and with lung fibrosis, aspergillomas are also increasingly common. Invasive aspergillosis is rare. Immunosuppression, disease duration, and lung fibrosis augment the risk of opportunistic infections. It is necessary for the physician to consider these entities, particularly with new-onset or evolving neurosarcoidosis or lunglike sarcoidosis.[11] It can be difficult to treat patients diagnosed with secondary aspergillosis, because the morbidity and mortality associated with a surgical treatment is too great in those who often have a greater lung fibrotic burden. Even so, with appropriate treatment, mortality still ranges from 20% to 58%, most commonly caused by hemoptysis.[11] Referral to specialty care is important to determine definitive diagnosis and treatment, which includes tissue cultures and biopsies, surgical debridement, bronchial artery embolization, and the proper antifungal treatment.

A common problem associated with the chronic, systemic, and idiopathic nature of sarcoidosis is a patient with known sarcoidosis presenting with new complaints. Identifying relapse or progression of sarcoidosis versus other diseases can be difficult and greatly affect quality of life for the patient. Jamilloux and colleagues[11] describe sarcoidosis as a paradoxic immune response, comprising both a granulomatous proinflammatory condition of local tissue combined with a systematic anergic state. This situation potentially predisposes to opportunistic infections, of which these same investigators use the analogy of a condition similar to common variable immunodeficiency. In addition, patients suffering from sarcoidosis are frequently on immunosuppressive therapy, be it steroids, methotrexate, other immunosuppressive agents, or tumor necrosis factor α (TNF-α) inhibitors, which also may predispose them to infections.

Many opportunistic infections show increased incidence in sarcoidosis, but whether the risk is associated with the disease itself, immunodepression, or another trigger is unknown. A strategy for identifying this situation is an acute or subacute change in the clinical manifestation of a patient with sarcoidosis. Often, a patient is diagnosed with granulomatous inflammation years before the onset of opportunistic infections. At this point, it is hoped that the chronic disease has either spontaneously remitted or stabilized to expected signs and symptoms. If a patient's health status changes, opportunistic infections, shown in **Box 3**, should be a part of the differential diagnosis.

Pulmonary fibrosis, bronchiectasis, and immunosuppression lead to increased risk of infections, notably aspergillosis and aspergillomas. The most common pulmonary complaint is hemoptysis, but weight loss, fatigue, cough, and breathlessness can complicate the clinical scenario. Chronic pulmonary aspergillosis is estimated to complicate approximately 2% of all cases of sarcoidosis, and long-term corticosteroid therapy is an identified risk factor.[11] Serum IgG *Aspergillus* antibodies are an available laboratory test that can assist with diagnosis. In a recurring theme, if a patient presents with new-onset symptoms, sarcoidosis again becomes a diagnosis of exclusion, with evaluation including a chest radiograph, possibly PFT, and appropriate cultures.

In a patient with pulmonary sarcoidosis with worsening or new-onset dyspnea, wheezing, chest pain, or cough or those with worsening radiographic findings, a broad differential diagnosis needs to be considered, because sarcoidosis becomes a diagnosis of exclusion once again. Worsening dyspnea can be from pulmonary hypertension, other granulomatous diseases, inflammation, opportunistic infections, or infectious organisms found in otherwise healthy individuals. An additional consideration is whether a patient with new-onset or worsening dyspnea is being treated with methotrexate, which rarely causes methotrexate-induced pneumonitis. This risk is increased in those with renal disease.[12] Likewise, wheezing and cough can be from asthma, opportunistic infections, or the patient's underlying sarcoidosis. Asymptomatic worsening radiographic findings can be caused by sarcoid-induced fibrocystic changes, worsening intraparenchymal disease, or new-onset lung disease. A repeat chest radiograph can be helpful to rule out obvious disease or pneumonia and a CT scan may be indicated in these cases to evaluate for parenchymal fibrosis. Identification of such can give the clinician insight into withholding oral steroids, because fibrosis is irreversible and may subject patients to unnecessary steroid therapy.

Box 3
Opportunistic infections

Cryptococcus

Progressive multifocal leukoencephalopathy (JK virus)

Chronic pulmonary aspergillosis

Nocardia

Herpes zoster

CARDIAC INVOLVEMENT

A 48-year-old African American woman with a long history of cutaneous and pulmonary sarcoidosis presented with new-onset syncope. She had had brief periods of lightheadedness for several months, but this was her first time losing consciousness and falling. Initial laboratory tests were unremarkable from baseline and a syncopal workup was also negative. An EKG showed new-onset prolonged PR interval and bradycardia into the 60s. Transthoracic echocardiogram and brain natriuretic peptide levels were otherwise unremarkable.

This is a case of chronic, nonremitting sarcoidosis, which is more likely with cutaneous manifestations and in African Americans. On initial assessment, baseline sarcoid characteristics should be evaluated, including chest radiograph findings, EKG, and laboratory values, particularly hypercalcemia. The differential includes any process that can cause syncope as well as new-onset cardiac sarcoidosis. A diligent search for other manifestations should be pursued. In a patient with known sarcoidosis, cardiac disease should be suspected, and this patient should be worked up for cardiac sarcoid and begun on oral prednisone.

Sarcoid-induced cardiac disease can be life threatening, although it symptomatically occurs in only 5% of the population with sarcoid.[3,13] The disease process may result in granulomatous deposition within the myocardial muscle or conduction system, leading to atrial or ventricular arrhythmias, atrioventricular block, heart failure, or sudden death. Birnie and colleagues[13] recommended an approach for the diagnosis of cardiac sarcoidosis, which is summarized in **Table 4**.

The symptoms of syncope, lightheadedness, and palpitations in patients with sarcoid should be aggressively evaluated. An EKG should be obtained as the first step in evaluation. Holter monitoring is appropriate. An echocardiogram should also be obtained to evaluate heart function. If the echocardiogram shows abnormalities, then cardiac MRI or PET can prove useful (see **Table 4** for consensus recommendations).

Chest pain is common in patients with sarcoid and is usually caused by pulmonary disease. Patients with sarcoid who have received long-term corticosteroid therapy are at increased risk for coronary artery disease, which should be considered as a cause of chest pain. If there is suspicion for cardiac sarcoidosis, and no easily accessible or high-yield sites with low morbidity are available, an endomyocardial biopsy can be considered. Most experts do not recommend cardiac biopsy, because it is invasive, possesses a large sampling error because granulomas are commonly missed by biopsy site selection, and other laboratory and diagnostic abnormalities can adequately assist with proper diagnosis. Endomyocardial biopsy may show noncaseating granulomas in less than 25% of cases, although this may be augmented by electrophysiologic or image-guided biopsy procedures.[13] Mehta and colleagues[14] found that palpitations, Holter monitoring abnormalities, and echocardiography findings are the most predictive of cardiac sarcoidosis.

Cardiac sarcoidosis, like symptomatic lung disease and ocular sarcoidosis, should be treated early and aggressively to prevent irreversible changes in the conduction system and myocardium. The recommended starting dose is 40 to 60 mg of prednisone daily for 1 to 3 months, with periodic attempts to taper. Evidence suggests that conduction abnormalities are potentially reversible in patients who receive immunosuppressive therapy. In conjunction with oral steroids, antiarrhythmic agents can also be administered in patients with sarcoid-induced ventricular arrhythmias.[13] The data for this approach are limited, but life-threatening arrhythmias and sudden death do occur in patients with no previous symptoms. If cardiac involvement is discovered,

Table 4	
Approach for the diagnosis of cardiac sarcoidosis	
Cardiac Sarcoidosis Diagnosis	1. Pathologic diagnosis with endomyocardial biopsy showing noncaseating granulomas and with rule-out of other granulomatous disease, or
50%–90% probability of cardiac sarcoidosis with either of the following 2 scenarios	1. Clinical diagnosis with histologic evidence of extracardiac noncaseating granulomas, and 2. Either cardiomyopathy that responds to immunosuppressives, reduced left ventricular function <40%, spontaneous or induced ventricular tachyarrhythmias, Mobitz type 2 or third-degree heart block, suspicious fluorodeoxyglucose-PET uptake, positive gadolinium-enhanced cardiovascular magnetic resonance, and 3. Exclusion of other granulomatous inflammatory conditions
Suspected cardiac sarcoidosis, in the setting of extracardiac sarcoidosis	History and physical, particularly evaluating syncope and palpitations 12-lead EKG Echocardiogram If abnormalities are detected on initial screening, perform cardiac MRI or fluorodeoxyglucose-PET If no abnormalities are present on initial screening, cardiac MRI and PET scanning are not indicated
Screening indications for cardiac sarcoidosis, in the setting of suspicious cardiac presentations	If patient is <60 y old and presents with Mobitz type 2 or third-degree heart block, advanced cardiac imaging should be obtained If image screening tests are abnormal, then endomyocardial or extracardiac biopsy may be indicated to assist with diagnosis

the patient can be initially hospitalized for a thorough workup or referred to a cardiologist with experience treating patients with cardiac sarcoidosis and followed closely in the primary care office.

Monitoring cardiac sarcoidosis is challenging, because clinical indicators are essentially nonexistent. Patients presenting with arrhythmia in the setting of systemic sarcoidosis can be initiated on prednisone therapy and referred for electrophysiologic evaluation and further consideration of an implantable cardioverter defibrillator (ICD). Electrophysiologic studies should be considered to define area of conduction blockade and further assist with disease management, and ablation or ICD placement can help navigate the high-risk arrhythmias. The high-risk indicators for ICD placement include sustained ventricular tachycardia, left or right heart dysfunction, or complete heart block. Other considerations include nonresponse to immunosuppressive therapy; signs and symptoms, such as syncope; inducible ventricular tachycardia on electrophysiology; or a large intracardiac granulomatous burden based on advanced imaging. It should be noted that the American Heart Association recommends that all patients with cardiac sarcoidosis have ICD placement, but this recommendation may be impractical for all patients. Each patient should be selected based on their own presentation, symptoms, and response to therapy, with a low threshold for implantation.

NEUROLOGIC INVOLVEMENT

Neurosarcoidosis is estimated to occur in approximately 5% of those suffering with sarcoidosis and can be highly variable clinically.[15–17] Neurosarcoidosis is an isolated presentation of sarcoidosis in 1% of individuals with sarcoid, but neurosarcoidosis should be suspected with any changing neurologic concern in those already with existing sarcoidosis.[15,16] There are no identified risk factors or triggers for those who might develop or be at risk of neurologic involvement from sarcoid, although women may have a slightly higher incidence.[17] Neurosarcoidosis is a rare manifestation of an obscure disease, and it can be challenging to diagnose and manage, especially when refractory to traditional steroid treatment.

Neurologic involvement from sarcoidosis most typically affects the basal meninges but can result in focal or diffuse intracranial parenchymal plaques, spinal cord lesions, and peripheral nerve involvement.[15–17] Approximately 40% of patients with neurosarcoidosis have involvement of the basal meninges, which clinically manifests as cranial neuropathy or less commonly hydrocephalus, whereas peripheral neurosarcoidosis most commonly manifests as a small-fiber neuropathy (SFN), resulting in peripheral pain, paresthesia, or autonomic dysfunction.[1,15,16]

With intracranial neurosarcoidosis, seventh nerve palsy is the most common manifestation and cranial neuropathy, and it is usually self-limiting. Unilateral involvement of the affected cranial nerve is more likely, but neurosarcoidosis should be particularly suspected in bilateral cranial nerve VII palsy. Sarcoidosis can affect any cranial nerve, bilaterally, unilaterally, in isolation, or with other symptoms. Involvement of other cranial nerves, with presentations such as anosmia, sensorineural hearing loss, dizziness, and optic neuropathy, has been reported in the literature. Secondarily to involvement of the basal meninges, neurosarcoidosis can cause hydrocephalus as well. Hypothalamic-pituitary axis disorders (involved in 18% of patients with neurosarcoidosis) can manifest as hyperthermia, diabetes insipidus, or other endocrine manifestations, such as galactorrhea or amenorrhea. Additional central involvement includes parenchymal brain disease, possibly manifesting as seizures, cerebellar symptoms, cognitive decline, or encephalopathy. Intracranial vascular involvement has also been reported.

Spinal cord neurosarcoidosis carries a poor prognosis and typically occurs in those of older age or with long-standing sarcoid.[17] Spinal cord sarcoid can manifest as myelopathy, radiculopathy, and weakness or paresthesia of the extremities. The cervicothoracic spinal cord is more commonly affected than the caudal spinal cord, and typically more than 3 spinal cord segments.[15–17] If spinal cord neurosarcoidosis is suspected, an MRI can be obtained, which most typically shows intramedullary lesions, leptomeningeal enhancement, or fusiform enlargement.

Peripheral neurosarcoidosis can affect the perineurium and epineurium of nerves, most commonly manifesting as large-fiber or small-fiber neuropathy (SFN). Patients can present with loss of proprioception and vibratory sensation, burning pain, paresthesia, restless legs syndrome, and dry skin and decreased perspiration. Secondarily to autonomic dysfunction, sudden death has also been reported. For suspected peripheral neurosarcoidosis, electroneurography or skin biopsy is the most useful diagnostic test, depending on whether the disease is of large-fiber or SFN, respectively. In contrast to spinal cord neurosarcoidosis, peripheral involvement seems to have a better overall prognosis. Neurological symptoms are shown in **Table 5**.

Patients with neurosarcoidosis should be followed by a physician with expertise in the area, because neurologic involvement and progression can be devastating. It is important to partner with a neurologist to determine appropriate testing, possible biopsy, and the consideration of other diseases in a patient with new, chronic, or recurrent sarcoidosis. It can be particularly challenging to diagnosis new-onset central nervous system (CNS) sarcoidosis, particularly if isolated. Initial evaluation should encompass a similar workup as if diagnosing nonisolated CNS sarcoidosis, including laboratory tests, chest radiograph, and EKG. In patients presenting with neurosarcoidosis, a chest radiograph may not be so sensitive for diagnosis of sarcoidosis, and high-resolution chest CT may be appropriate if no thoracic findings are discovered on chest radiograph.[15] A diagnosis is appropriate if a patient has peripheral evidence of noncaseating granulomas with exclusion of other granulomatous inflammatory disorders, along with signs of an inflammatory nervous system response and either consistent imaging (gallium MRI, fluorodeoxyglucose [FDG]-PET, or high-resolution CT) or increased CD4:CD8 ratio.[15]

In a patient with suspected intracranial neurosarcoidosis, it is sometimes difficult to determine when to obtain a cranial MRI or FDG-PET scan or brain biopsy, because there is no standardized or consensus guidelines. MRI is the most sensitive, but

Table 5
Symptoms of neurosarcoidosis

Symptoms of Neurosarcoidosis		
Central	Miscellaneous	Headache, fatigue, fever, seizures, euphoria/depression, behavioral disturbances, cognitive decline
	Cranial neuropathies	Cranial nerve II (blurred vision, abnormal coloring, visual field defects, papilledema)
		Cranial nerve VII (most common, with unilateral > bilateral)
		Cranial nerve VIII (sensorineural hearing loss, dizziness/vertigo)
		Cranial nerve IX and X (dysphagia, vocal cord dysfunction)
	Meningeal inflammation	Hydrocephalus with communicating > noncommunicating
		Aseptic meningitis
	Hypothalamus-pituitary	Endocrine abnormalities, such as galactorrhea and amenorrhea
		Diabetes insipidus
		Hyperthermia
	Spinal cord	Myopathies/radiculopathy
		Weakness or paresthesia of extremities
Peripheral	—	Large-fiber neuropathy (loss of proprioception and vibration)
		SFN (pain and temperature disturbance, autonomic dysfunction)
Muscle	—	Muscle pain
		Muscle atrophy

Data from Hebel R, Dubaniewicz-Wybieralska M, Dubaniewicz A. Overview of neurosarcoidosis: recent advances. J Neurol 2015;262(2):258–67.

less specific. The findings in cranial MRI vary greatly, but most typically involve either the basal meninges or the hypophyseal-pituitary system.[15] The most common finding is nonenhancing white matter lesions, which have been correlated with vascular changes. Rarely, sarcoidosis can resemble neoplastic disease, but certain findings can help distinguish the cause. These findings include (1) leptomeningeal enhancement and (2) lack of central necrosis. With leptomeningeal involvement, gadolinium imaging shows diffuse or nodular enhancement on postcontrast T1-weighted MRI.[16] Other imaging findings on gadolinium enhancement imaging include multiple or solitary masses; enhancement, thickening, or cysts of the hypothalamus-pituitary region; communicating or noncommunicating hydrocephalus; osseous involvement; hyperintense lacrimal glands; and cervicothoracic intramedullary spinal cord involvement. FDG-PET is more specific for neurosarcoidosis and can show increased uptake even with a negative brain MRI scan. The usefulness of this finding is still unknown, but FDG-PET can be used to guide biopsy of any involved site, even extracranial, in unproved and suspected systemic sarcoidosis. Cranial or meningeal biopsy is the gold standard but is invasive. Other biopsy sites should be sought first before obtaining nervous tissue.

Initial treatment of neurosarcoidosis is 1 mg/kg of oral prednisone daily, tapering over many months. In more acute cases of neurosarcoidosis, 3 to 5 days of pulse therapy with 1 g intravenous methylprednisolone may be warranted, before transitioning to oral steroids.[15] The initial dose of prednisone for patients with cranial nerve involvement alone is lower, starting with 0.5 mg/kg daily. The addition of steroid-sparing agents, such as methotrexate, azathioprine, hydroxychloroquine/chloroquine, and mycophenolate mofetil, can be considered as an adjuvant to decrease steroid reliance. This treatment should be an option if unable to taper steroid therapy to less than 10 mg/d of prednisone or its equivalent within 3 to 6 months.[17] Methotrexate is first-line therapy according to expert opinion. As a patient is weaned from steroid therapy, the provider needs to maintain a vigilant effort with close follow-up, because recurrent symptoms are more common during this period. If a patient is unable to taper systemic steroids, first an immunosuppressant should be used. If this is also ineffective, anti-TNF-α therapy, such as infliximab or adalimumab, can be added to the treatment regimen to increase the likelihood that a patient can taper their steroid dose without recurring symptoms.[15] Anti-TNF-α therapy should be initiated only with a strong diagnosis of sarcoidosis, because this treatment has been associated with reactivation of latent TB, lymphoma, and multiple sclerosis.

SFN deserves special consideration, because it is difficult to diagnosis and treat and also may not respond to steroid therapy. As discussed earlier, it commonly presents as peripheral pain, paresthesia, or autonomic dysfunction. Symptom management is the most important guideline to treatment. The treatment options include neuropathic pain suppressants, anticonvulsants, antidepressants, topical anesthetics, and narcotic pain medications. In addition, intravenous immunoglobulins and ARA 290 therapy have shown some benefit, with a low risk of adverse effects.[18] TNF-α inhibitors may be necessary to treat this difficult condition, as is consistent with recalcitrant sarcoidosis.

RENAL INVOLVEMENT

A 32-year-old woman who had spontaneous remission of cutaneous and pulmonary sarcoidosis 8 months previously presented with flank pain and hematuria. CT showed a 5-mm kidney stone and a basic metabolic panel showed no abnormalities, including normal calcium and creatinine levels. She was scheduled for a 2-week follow-up and given a urine collection container for a 24-hour calcium test and scheduled to have blood work completed. At her follow-up appointment, her 1,25-dihydroxyvitamin D level and 24-hour urine calcium level were increased. A thorough history and physical were taken, which showed no other symptoms for sarcoidosis recurrence, and she was begun on a short prednisone burst with anticipation of tapering shortly thereafter.

This patient may have recurrence of her sarcoidosis manifested by development of kidney stones. Calcium stones are common, because sarcoidosis can cause hypercalciuria and hypercalcemia. The hypercalciuria can occur without hypercalcemia. In addition, because of granulomatous inflammation, 25-hydroxyvitamin D level can be low to low-normal, whereas 1,25-dihydroxyvitamin D level can be increased. It is important to monitor the 1,25-dihydroxyvitamin D levels and not to begin patients with sarcoidosis on vitamin D or calcium supplementation because of a low 25-hydroxyvitamin D level. In the current case, this patient should receive steroid therapy and should be closely followed, because sarcoidosis can progressively affect the kidneys and because her disease pattern has changed.

Sarcoidosis can rarely affect the kidney directly, but often presents with various electrolyte and vitamin abnormalities. Hypercalcemia represents a unique challenge in sarcoidosis. The high calcium levels readily respond to corticosteroids; however, the steroid therapy itself can also cause loss of bone density, occasionally requiring treatment with bisphosphonates. Osteoporosis and fractures are common in patients with long-term sarcoidosis treated with steroids. The primary derangement in sarcoidosis is upregulation of α_1-hydroxylase in granulomas, which converts 25-hydroxyvitamin D to 1,25-dihydroxyvitamin D. Because of this factor, it is important to remember that levels of 25-hydroxyvitamin D, the typical level obtained, are inaccurate in evaluating for vitamin D levels and may be decreased by laboratory standards. The level of 1,25-dihydroxyvitamin D should be evaluated in conjunction with 25-hydroxyvitamin D. The kidneys do compensate and, therefore, hypercalciuria is a more prominent finding than hypercalcemia. This situation leads to a greatly increased risk of nephrolithiasis and long-term parenchymal damage. Hypercalcemia often responds to lower-dose oral prednisone therapy (20 mg daily with tapering to the lowest effective dose). Hydroxychloroquine can also be effective in the management of hypercalcemia. The interplay between calcium, vitamin D, osteoporosis, declining bone density, and steroid therapy makes standard recommendations uncertain, because each patient should be considered for immunosuppressive treatment, possible low-dose vitamin D replacement, and bisphosphonates on a case-by-case basis.

In addition to the manifestations of hypercalcemia and hypercalciuria, sarcoidosis can directly affect the kidneys, most commonly as granulomatous interstitial nephritis. Patients with sarcoid can also develop nongraulomatous interstitial nephritis. These are rare manifestations of sarcoidosis. A more typical disease course affecting the kidney is hypercalciuria ($\leq$50% of patients), which can lead to nephrolithiasis.

EYE INVOLVEMENT

The eye is one of the most common extrapulmonary manifestations of sarcoidosis (approximately 20%), which can lead to irreversible blindness and glaucoma.[1,19] It is more common in Japanese people and particularly in those with sarcoidosis that presents at an older age.[8] Ocular complaints include erythema, pain, photophobia, floaters, decreased vision, and sudden loss of vision or changes in color. If any clinical suspicion exists for the diagnosis of sarcoidosis, patients should be referred for appropriate ophthalmologic examination, including fundoscopic and slit-lamp evaluation. An eye examination can adequately detect anterior uveitis, posterior uveitis, and optic neuritis. Other manifestations include cataracts, vision changes, lacrimal gland swelling, and retinal periphlebitis.[19] In a patient with known sarcoidosis who presents with new eye complaints, repeat eye examination, including slit-lamp examination, is necessary to detect any abnormalities.

Eye abnormalities should always be treated. With the help of an ophthalmologist, steroid droplets can be used to treat anterior uveitis, but this route of administration does not adequately penetrate the posterior chamber or optic nerve. Patients diagnosed with posterior uveitis or optic neuritis should receive systemic corticosteroids or intraocular steroid injections. If a patient with sarcoidosis presents with rapidly changing visual symptoms, they should be admitted to the hospital for further workup as well as consideration for intravenous steroid therapy to preserve vision and eye function.

Once a patient is diagnosed with sarcoidosis, they should receive an initial eye evaluation and one annually indefinitely. They should also undergo an eye evaluation with any vision or ocular symptom changes. Hydroxychloroquine and chloroquine are commonly used to treat symptoms of sarcoidosis. All patients receiving these medications should receive annual eye examinations, because of the risk of retinal toxicity.

CUTANEOUS INVOLVEMENT

The cutaneous involvement of sarcoidosis is diverse, with several manifestations suggestive of systemic sarcoidosis (**Fig. 2**). These manifestations are described in more detail in **Table 6**. EN is the most common skin manifestation, especially in those at risk or with a family history of sarcoidosis. However, EN is a general inflammatory state and is not caused by noncaseating granulomas. A biopsy of the EN lesion does not aid in diagnosis. EN is less commonly seen in African Americans and Japanese people compared with other ethnic groups and typically represents a more acute and regressive disease course.[8] Lupus pernio or violaceous plaques may represent a more severe form of sarcoidosis and are more common in African Americans. Lupus pernio (associated with 4% to 9% of patients with sarcoidosis as a destructive and violaceous lesions of the ears and malar region) is classically associated with chronic and more severe sarcoidosis, with involvement of the upper lung, more advanced fibrosis, bone involvement, and ocular disease.[19] Other cutaneous manifestations of the disease include scar-associated or tattoo-associated lesions, alopecia, scarring, ulcers, and icthyosis.[20]

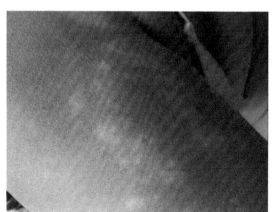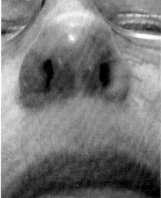

Fig. 2. Hypopigmented version of cutaneous sarcoid of upper extremity and cutaneous sarcoid presenting as thickening of alar rim and columella.

Table 6	
Cutaneous manifestations of sarcoidosis	
Skin Manifestation	**Description**
EN	Erythematous and painful subcutaneous nodules, usually located on the anterior lower legs. Often, but not necessarily, included in Löfgren syndrome
Lupus pernio	Destructive, violaceous, and nodular plaques across malar region, nose, and ears
Plaque sarcoid	Skin-colored to violaceous plaquelike lesions more commonly found on the limbs, trunk, and back
Subcutaneous sarcoid (Darier-Roussy)	Erythematous, violaceous, flesh-colored, or hyperpigmented nodules most commonly located on the upper extremities
Hypopigmented	Almost exclusively seen in dark-skinned individuals (especially African Americans). Hypopigmented skin more than plaques or nodules
Mucocutaneous	Small mucous membrane lesions
Koebner phenomenon	Lesions appearing on old scars or tattoos

There are several available options to treat cutaneous sarcoidosis, but the treatment often depends on presentation and response to therapy. If a patient is receiving oral steroids for another affected organ system, the cutaneous manifestations often respond and may be used as an indicator of response. If there are no other systemic symptoms, use of topical steroids, such as clobetasol or halobetasol, are the treatment of choice and limit systemic effects from oral steroids. A lower-potency steroid should be used if the lesions involve the face. Alternatively, intralesional steroid therapy is another option that allows targeted and direct action of corticosteroids. Triamcinolone 5 to 40 mg/mL can be injected directly into lesions every 3 to 4 weeks until the disease resolves.[20] The lesions may respond readily, or it can take up to 3 months of topical therapy to show resolving changes. Side effects of topical or intralesional steroids include atrophy, striae, telangiectasia formation, and hypopigmentation.

If cutaneous lesions become destructive with the fear of irreversible changes or are rapidly progressive, then, systemic steroid therapy is indicated (**Fig. 3**). The cutaneous manifestations of sarcoid respond well to hydroxychloroquine (or chloroquine) with or without minocycline, which may be the most effective medicine for skin disease.[5] The initial dose of hydroxychloroquine should be 200 mg twice a day. A taper can be implemented once the lesions disappear over 2 to 3 months. If cutaneous disease continues to be recalcitrant to these efforts, then, escalating to methotrexate and possibly the TNF-α inhibitors can be considered. In addition, a dermatologist with experience in treating cutaneous sarcoidosis can be helpful to optimize treatment effects.

OTHER MANIFESTATIONS

A 33-year-old man with sarcoidosis presented to his primary care physician complaining of increasing fatigue. Basic serum chemistries, CBC with differential, and chest radiograph were unchanged from baseline.

Fatigue is a common symptom in patients with sarcoidosis. Most of the time, the fatigue is not directly related to the patient's sarcoid. The first point in evaluation of

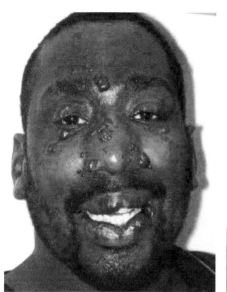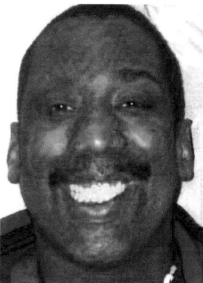

Fig. 3. Patient presenting with lupus pernio before and after treatment with prednisone and chloroquine.

fatigue is to make sure that the patient does not have a sleep disorder. Corticosteroids can cause insomnia, and chronic use can lead to weight gain, which puts patients at increased risk for the development of sleep apnea. Corticosteroid use also increases the risk of depression, which frequently manifests as fatigue. An approach to workup of fatigue in the patient with sarcoid is outlined in **Box 4**. The key approach is to focus on history to find out if there is a likely diagnosis for the patient's fatigue apart from sarcoidosis, focus on the physical examination to see if there are any signs of increased sarcoid activity, and perform judicious laboratory testing for signs of active sarcoid.

Sarcoid can affect any organ system and the disease manifestations can be varied. In addition to the issues discussed earlier, other difficult clinical characteristics include hypertension (both pulmonary and systemic; exacerbated by steroids, NSAIDs, and renal disease), as well as arthritis, generalized lymphadenopathy and involvement of the reticuloendothelial system, larynx, bone marrow, and sinuses.

LÖFGREN SYNDROME

Löfgren syndrome is characterized by fever, EN, bilateral ankle pain and swelling, and bihilar lymphadenopathy. The classic and sudden manifestation of Löfgren syndrome does not require the demonstration of granulomas on tissue histopathology for diagnosis, because it has a 95% specificity for sarcoidosis. EN is a nongranulomatous manifestation of sarcoidosis. It is more common in women than men, whereas bilateral ankle arthritis or periarticular inflammation is more common in men.[21] Some patients with Löfgren syndrome have additional findings on chest radiograph, such as pulmonary infiltrates present in about 23% of patients with Löfgren syndrome. This additional finding does not change their outcome. Löfgren syndrome is associated with a good clinical outcome, because the disease resolves in approximately 84% of patients within 2 years, although recurrence occurs in approximately 3% of patients.[21]

Box 4
Evaluation of the sarcoid patient with fatigue

History

Currently using corticosteroids?

Weight gain?

Snoring/witnessed apnea (administer Epworth sleepiness scale)?

Symptoms of depression (administer PHQ9)?

Examination

Physical examination for evidence of active sarcoid iritis?

Lymphadenopathy?

Skin lesions?

Pulmonary findings?

Hepatosplenomegaly?

Testing

CBC with differential (especially pay attention to lymphocyte count)

Erythrocyte sedimentation rate

C-reactive protein

Basic metabolic panel (focusing on calcium level and renal function)

Chest radiograph (if patient has not had one in the past 6 mo)

Löfgren syndrome is associated with HLA DRB1*0301 and DQB1*0201 alleles. In the sarcoidosis population with these HLA alleles, sarcoidosis has a high rate of resolving disease, up to 98% resolution within 2 years.

SINONASAL SARCOIDOSIS

Sinonasal sarcoidosis can sometimes be the only manifestation of sarcoidosis, but certain nasal and sinus symptoms have been associated with the disease. The most common of these symptoms are nasal obstruction, nasal crusting, anosmia, and epistaxis.[22] Nasal crusting may be the most common complaint, followed by anosmia. Polyposis is also commonly reported. The diagnosis of sarcoid rhinosinusitis is similar to that of sarcoidosis and can be determined by: (1) appropriate imaging, such as CT showing mucoperiosteal inflammation or sinus opacification, (2) evidence of granulomatous inflammation with staining to exclude fungal and mycobacterial disease, and (3) exclusion of other granulomatous inflammatory disorders, notably granulomatosis with polyangiitis (Wegener syndrome). The nasal mucosa when visualized can show discrete nodules on a background of granular mucosa, crusting and suppuration, elevated yellow lesions, atrophic mucosa, or normal appearing mucosa. Nasal steroids can be beneficial for patients and should be trailed, because they are low risk. Sarcoid rhinosinusitis is often a chronic manifestation of the disease with an unpredictable course. Long-term oral steroids are often necessary, but steroid-sparing agents and nasal steroids can help alleviate symptoms and steroid side effects. Bacterial sinusitis can be a recurrent complication and should be considered when patients have a flare in their symptoms.

BONE DISEASE

Sarcoid bone disease occurs in 5% of those with sarcoidosis (**Fig. 4**). It is often associated with cutaneous involvement, such as lupus pernio, and almost all patients also have concomitant intrathoracic disease. The manifestation most commonly involves the digits, with osteopenia, cystic lesions, or fine lattice formation found on radiograph. Joint arthralgias are also common, and bilateral ankle arthritis is included in Löfgren presentation. With severe sarcoidosis, the bone involvement is usually found as an incidental finding.

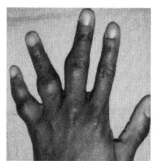 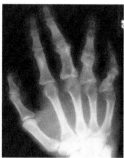 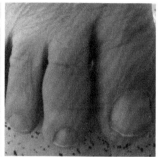

Fig. 4. Sarcoidosis-associated bone disease. Typical sausage digit seen on second toe.

MISCELLANEOUS PRESENTATIONS

Nonspecific findings, such as weight loss and fever, are common manifestations found in 30% of those with sarcoidosis.[1] These constitutional findings are usually mild, with weight loss less than 10% of total body weight and low-grade fever. High fever is uncommon, but is sometimes seen with Heerfordt and Löfgren syndrome. If a high fever is present, an alternative diagnosis should be sought. Fatigue is a common complaint in sarcoidosis, but this should be evaluated separately from the diagnosis. This separate evaluation is necessary is because patients afflicted with systemic sarcoidosis usually have a complicated clinical picture, with intricate comorbid drug side effects and other comorbidities. The high-dose steroid regimens can cause hypertension, central obesity, diabetes, glaucoma, skin thinning, and avascular necrosis of the hip, which significantly affect the patient's psychosocial mentality and can lead to depressivelike symptoms. If a patient does require therapy, there are limited data that support neurostimulants and TNF-α inhibitors.[11] In addition, dexmethylphenidate and armofafanil may also decrease subjective feelings of fatigue.

Peripheral lymph nodes are palpable in 10% to 15% of patients with sarcoidosis, but this has been reported as high as 32% to 76%.[1,5] The lymphadenopathy is typically painless and bilateral, most commonly affecting the cervical, epitrochlear, and inguinal lymph node tracts. If a patient with sarcoidosis has lymphadenopathy, these sites are readily available for biopsy. Painless hepatomegaly or splenomegaly can be seen with sarcoidosis and usually causes no associated symptoms or sequelae, although thrombocytopenia may be found on blood tests. Incidental increases in LFT results may be the first indication of sarcoidosis in some patients. Alkaline phosphatase level is most commonly increased, whereas hyperbilirubinemia suggests a more severe clinical and progressive picture. Leukopenia and anemia are found in approximately 20% of patients with sarcoid.[1] Lymphopenia is common and can correlate with disease activity.

Hepatic involvement in sarcoid is common and is seen in more than 50% of sarcoid patients on liver biopsy.[23] Abnormalities in transaminases and alkaline phosphatase are also common, occurring in 35% of patients.[24] Most patients with sarcoid liver involvement are asymptomatic and do not require treatment. Hepatic involvement with sarcoid is about 3 times more common in African Americans than in Caucasians.[25] The most common symptomatic presentations of hepatic sarcoid are pruritus and abdominal pain. Hepatomegaly (16%) and splenic abnormalities (53%) are common findings on CT scans of patients with sarcoidosis.[26] Cirrhosis is a rare complication of hepatic involvement in sarcoidosis. Symptomatic hepatic sarcoid should be initially treated with prednisone. Methotrexate can be an effective steroid-sparing agent if longer-term treatment is needed.[27]

TREATMENT

A 34-year-old woman with known sarcoidosis presented for follow-up. She was diagnosed with pulmonary sarcoidosis, complicated by lupus pernio, nasal obstruction, and bilateral ankle arthralgias, 1 year previously. This was her fourth 3-month visit and she had recently begun on a steroid regimen for dyspnea, evolving pulmonary findings on her chest radiograph, and nasal obstruction. She had felt more fatigued recently and had also been seeing an outpatient psychologist.

Close follow-up typically every 3 months in the first year of diagnosis is indicated to help establish a diagnosis, assess symptoms and effect on quality of life, and follow potential regression. This patient requires steroid treatment of her symptomatic pulmonary manifestations. The steroids will also assist with clearing her nasal obstructive symptoms. For her lupus pernio, she may need additional therapy beyond steroids, such as methotrexate and chloroquine. The steroids will undoubtedly help alleviate her joint arthralgia. It is also important to counsel her that her fatigue could be caused by several factors, although it is unlikely to be a direct effect of her sarcoidosis, such as depression, disease impact, and steroid treatment. This scenario is likely why she was referred for psychological evaluation.

As with laboratory evaluation and diagnostic testing, there are no standard protocols or guidelines for the treatment of sarcoidosis. Many patients with milder symptoms or asymptomatic findings on chest radiograph experience spontaneous regression of their disease. In a newly diagnosed patient with acute sarcoidosis and without worrisome clinical findings, treatment may be withheld to assist with establishing the diagnosis, defining the disease manifestations, and in assessing whether spontaneous regression will occur.

If treatment is required, steroids are the primary option. In general, asymptomatic patients can be observed with close follow-up, whereas more severe disease or disease that involves vital organs needs to be treated with oral steroid therapy. Symptomatic pulmonary, cardiac, ophthalmologic, and renal disease, as well as disfiguring cutaneous lesions, such as lupus pernio, require immediate treatment, because progressive inflammation in any of these systems can lead to irreversible damage or urgent clinical situations. Referral to an appropriate expert is indicated in all such cases. Cutaneous lesions other than lupus pernio can be managed effectively with topical or intralesional corticosteroids or low-dose oral corticosteroids (10–15 mg prednisone daily), whereas anterior uveitis can be treated with steroid eyedrops. Mild cases of EN and joint inflammation can be managed with NSAIDs. Corticosteroids work rapidly and are effective for more severe EN and acute arthritis caused by sarcoid.

A vigilant approach needs to be conducted for those at risk for steroid side effects, particularly osteoporosis and glaucoma. It is critical to evaluate for potential osteoporosis, because many patients are at increased risk while currently or previously on corticosteroids, particularly if the patient is older. This situation can be difficult to navigate, and a DEXA (dual-energy X-ray absorptiometry) scan and bisphosphonate therapy may be indicated. If a patient has been on steroid therapy previously, sarcoid recurrence is common in up to 80% of individuals.[1] If a patient has continued relapses, it is appropriate to consider low-dose steroids or steroid therapy on alternate days to prevent future recurrence, minimizing the steroid side effect profile.

Immunomodulatory agents, such as methotrexate, azathioprine, or hydroxychloroquine, can be considered in refractory cases or as adjunct agents. Methotrexate is the first choice of the disease-modifying antisarcoid drugs (DMASDs) among experts and has the most evidence for use. For pulmonary and extrapulmonary sarcoidosis, there is a 60% to 80% response to methotrexate in steroid-refractory cases or when adverse effects to steroids are present, although it takes approximately 6 months of treatment before it reaches maximum efficacy.[12] Methotrexate may be more effective than steroids for certain disease manifestations, such as refractory anterior uveitis or neurosarcoidosis, and can be used in combination with steroids, either initially, with treatment failure, or for a steroid-sparing effect. Patients with osteoporosis, diabetes, or those who are obese may benefit from a combination of methotrexate and low-dose steroids. World sarcoidosis experts believe that methotrexate is not used enough in general practice.[12] The recommended initial dose is 5 to 15 mg of oral methotrexate weekly along with 5 mg of folic acid once a week. Dose escalation can be considered, up to a maximum of 20 mg weekly, but requires more stringent safety monitoring and possible referral to a sarcoidosis expert or rheumatologist. Before initiation of methotrexate, basic laboratories values should be evaluated, including LFT, CBC for cell line assessment, and human immunodeficiency virus, hepatitis, and mycobacterium TB testing. Contraindications include liver disease, renal disease, bone marrow failure, chronic infection, and intent of either the man or woman for upcoming pregnancy. If a patient develops significant gastrointestinal side effects, the oral dose can be split or enteral administration can be considered.

Other steroid-sparing agents to consider, particularly in those with steroid-induced side effects or methotrexate intolerance, include azathioprine, leflunomide, hydroxychloroquine, and cyclosporine. Azathioprine has similar side effects to methotrexate but a higher infection rate. Leflunomide has a more tolerable side effect profile compared with methotrexate, but there are no comparison studies based on efficacy. Although more studies need to be conducted on DMASDs, they can be safe for use in those with more resistant sarcoidosis or in those who are unable to take or are intolerable of steroids. This situation requires more rigorous monitoring, with more cautious follow-up; evaluating new symptoms; basic laboratory tests, including CBC, basic metabolic panel, LFTs; and potentially more specialty-specific evaluations. A summary of DMASDs with side effect information is provided in **Box 4**. If a patient is nonresponsive to steroids or second-line agents, TNF-α inhibitors can be used as salvage therapy and have shown great benefit in pulmonary and extrapulmonary sarcoidosis, although they come with additional side effects. These side effects are also included in **Table 7**.

Patients with sarcoidosis are under great emotional stress. This factor, combined with lower oxygenation levels and other comorbidity, can lead to depression. Corticosteroid treatment further increases the risk of developing depression. Nonpharmacologic treatments should be considered, including patient education, exercise

Table 7
Side effect information for DMASDs

DMASDs	Indications	Side Effects
Methotrexate	First choice for second-line treatment of sarcoidosis	Bone marrow suppression, kidney failure, hepatotoxicity, pneumonitis, gastrointestinal toxicity, lymphoma
Azathioprine	Similar efficacy as methotrexate, but increased risk of infections	Malaise, gastrointestinal toxicity, bone marrow suppression, infections, hepatotoxicity
Mycophenolate mofetil	Effective for neurosarcoidosis	Hypertension, hypotension, peripheral edema, tachycardia, chest pain. Headache, insomnia, hyperglycemia, electrolyte abnormalities, bone marrow suppression, hepatotoxicity, renal failure
Leflunomide	Less effective for musculoskeletal and neurologic involvement Effective for cutaneous, ocular, and sinonasal involvement	Gastrointestinal toxicity, emaciation, severe weight loss, infections, hypertension, peripheral neuropathy, liver fibrosis, respiratory tract infections, and skin rash or hair loss
Hydroxychloroquine/ chloroquine	Most effective for cutaneous sarcoidosis	Ocular toxicity (retinal toxicity and corneal deposits), Cardiomyopathy, EKG changes, bone marrow suppression, myopathy (chloroquine), hepatitis, ototoxicity
Cyclophosphamide	Potentially effective for cardiac and neurosarcoidosis	Nausea, vomiting, hemorrhagic cystitis, recurrent pneumonia, transaminitis, gonadal suppression, alopecia, and bone marrow suppression
Apremilast, pentoxifylline (phosphodiesterase inhibitors)	Apremilast may be efficacious with cutaneous sarcoidosis	Apremilast: headache, weight loss, gastrointestinal toxicity, and upper respiratory infection Pentoxifylline: gastrointestinal toxicity, anaphylaxis, bone marrow suppression
Adalimumab, infliximab (TNF-α inhibitors)	Third-line treatment, refractory and severe disease	Injection site reactions, neutropenia, TB reactivation, infections, sarcoidlike granulomatosis, heart failure, and demyelinating disease
Rituximab	May be more effective for ocular sarcoidosis	Infusion reactions, hepatitis B virus reactivation, multifocal leukoencephalopathy, peripheral edema, rash, insomnia, angioedema, cytopenia, hepatotoxicity, neuropathy

rehabilitation, and oxygen therapy in patients who have advanced lung disease. Pneumococcal and influenza vaccination is recommended. Patients with severe cardiomyopathy or end-stage lung disease may be considered for organ transplantation.

SUMMARY

Sarcoidosis is an idiopathic, systemic granulomatous disease, which can affect any organ system, most commonly the lung. A high clinical suspicion, or at least consideration with pulmonary, cardiac, ocular, and neurologic complaints, is imperative for rapid identification and the institution of systemic steroid therapy. Patients with unexplained abnormalities on laboratory tests, such as increased LFT results, hypercalcemia, or reduced cell lines, should also be suspected of having the disease. The diagnosis is one of exclusion, which may evolve over several months. Close followup during this time, and for those on immunosuppression or those with changing clinical pictures, can offer reassurance and prevent life-threatening pathophysiologic changes. Oral steroids are the first-line treatment, but not every patient requires systemic corticosteroid therapy, although clinicians should feel comfortable offering methotrexate in those who do not respond or have a high demand for chronic immunosuppression. Inhaled, topical or intralesional, and eye droplet corticosteroid treatment can be used safely as an adjunct. If a patient presents with a changing clinical picture, the physician should reassess the diagnosis and pursue a thorough workup to exclude other granulomatous inflammatory disorders, opportunistic infections, and medication side effects. Overall, the disease most commonly remits within several years, but can be life threatening, particularly with pulmonary fibrosis, neurosarcoidosis, and cardiac sarcoidosis. Even so, a primary care physician is in an ideal position to diagnose and then manage sarcoidosis.

REFERENCES

1. O'Regan A, Berman JS. Sarcoidosis. Ann Intern Med 2012;156(9):ITC 5-1.
2. Winterbauer RH, Belic N, Moores KD. Clinical interpretation of bilateral hilar adenopathy. Ann Intern Med 1973;78:65–71.
3. Judson MA. The management of sarcoidosis by the primary care physician. Am J Med 2007;120:403–7.
4. Milman N, Soberg B, Svendsen CB, et al. Quantiferon test for tuberculosis screening in sarcoidosis patients. Scand J Infect Dis 2011;43:728–35.
5. Irwin RS, Corrao WM. Sarcoidosis. Prim Care 1978;5(3):447–64.
6. Poh SC. Bilateral hilar adenopathy: its significance. Singapore Med J 1982;23(5): 279–82.
7. Valeyre D, Bernaudin JF, Uzunhan Y, et al. Clinical presentation of sarcoidosis and diagnostic work-up. Semin Respir Crit Care Med 2014;35:336–51.
8. Kalkanis A, Judson MA. Distinguishing asthma from sarcoidosis: an approach to a problem that is not always solvable. J Asthma 2013;50(1):1–6.
9. Paramothayan S, Lasserson T. Treatment for pulmonary sarcoidosis. Respir Med 2008;102:1–9.
10. Amin EN, Closser DR, Crouser ED. Current best practice in the management of pulmonary and systemic sarcoidosis. Ther Adv Respir Dis 2014;8(4):111–32.
11. Jamilloux Y, Valeyre D, Lortholary O, et al. The spectrum of opportunistic diseases complicating sarcoidosis. Autoimmun Rev 2015;14:64–74.
12. Cremers JP, Drent M, Bast A, et al. Multinational evidence-based world association of sarcoidosis and other granulomatous disorders recommendations for the use of methotrexate in sarcoidosis: integrating systemic literature research and

expert opinion of sarcoidologists worldwide. Curr Opin Pulm Med 2013;19: 545–61.

13. Birnie DH, Sauer WH, Bogun F, et al. HRS expert consensus statement on the diagnosis and management of arrhythmias associated with cardiac sarcoidosis. Heart Rhythm 2014;11(7):1305–23.

14. Mehta D, Lubitz SA, Frankel Z, et al. Cardiac involvement in patients with sarcoidosis. Chest 2008;133(6):1426–35.

15. Segal BM. Neurosarcoidosis: diagnostic approaches and therapeutic strategies. Curr Opin Neurol 2013;26:307–13.

16. Ginat DT, Dhillon G, Almast J. Magnetic resonance imaging of neurosarcoidosis. J Clin Imaging Sci 2011;1:15.

17. Hebel R, Dubaniewicz-Wybieralska M, Dubaniewicz A. Overview of neurosarcoidosis: recent advances. J Neurol 2015;262(2):258–67.

18. Korsten P, Mirsaeidi M, Sweiss NJ. Nonsteroidal therapy for sarcoidosis. Curr Opin Pulm Med 2013;19(5):516–23.

19. Belfer MH, Stevens WR. Sarcoidosis: a primary care review. Am Fam Physician 1998;59(9):2041–50.

20. Wanat KA, Rosenbach M. A practical approach to cutaneous sarcoidosis. Am J Clin Dermatol 2014;15:283–97.

21. Grunewald J, Eklund A. Sex-specific manifestations of Löfgren syndrome. Am J Respir Crit Care Med 2007;175:40–4.

22. Reed J, deShazo RD, Houle TT, et al. Clinical features of sarcoid rhinosinusitis. Am J Med 2010;123:856–62.

23. Irani SK, Dobbins WO. Hepatic granulomas: a review of 73 patients from one hospital and a survey of the literature. J Clin Gastroenterol 1979;1:131–43.

24. Vatti R, Sharma OP. Course of asymptomatic liver involvement in sarcoidosis: the role of therapy in selected cases. Sarcoidosis Vasc Diffuse Lung Dis 1997;14:73–6.

25. Braughman RP, Tierstein AS, Judson MA, et al. Clinical characteristics of patients in a case control study of sarcoidosis. Am J Respir Crit Care Med 2001;164: 1885–9.

26. Folz SJ, Johnson CD, Swensen SJ. Abdominal manifestations of sarcoidosis in CT studies. J Comput Assist Tomogr 1995;19(4):573–9.

27. Kennedy PT, Zakaria N, Modawi SB, et al. Natural history of hepatic sarcoidosis and its response to treatment. Eur J Gastroenterol Hepatol 2006;18:721.

Index

Note: Page numbers of article titles are in **boldface** type.

A

Abdomen, radiation therapy in, late effects of, 1069
Abdominal pain
    in alcohol misuse, 998
    in inflammatory bowel disease, 973
Acamprosate, for alcohol misuse, 1006, 1029–1030
Acidosis, metabolic, in kidney disease, 947
Adalimumab
    for inflammatory bowel disease, 976, 978
    for sarcoidosis, 1137, 1146
Addiction, in homeless patients, 1028–1029
Albuminuria, in kidney disease, 944–945, 961
Albuterol, for asthma, 958, 961
Alcohol misuse, **989–1016**
    conditions associated with, 995–999
    definitions of, 990
    economic impact of, 989
    epidemiology of, 990–994
    harms of, 994
    in liver disease, 916
    in solid organ transplant recipients, 1087
    screening for, 999–1001
    terminology of, 990
    treatment of, 1001–1007
    versus alcohol benefits, 994–995
    withdrawal in, 1005
Alcohol use disorder
    asking about, 993
    definition of, 990
Alcohol Use Disorders Identification Test (AUDIT), 999–1001
Alcoholic liver disease, 915
Alcoholics Anonymous, 1001–1003
Allergic rhinitis, asthma in, 955–956
5-Aminosalicylates, for inflammatory bowel disease, 976–977
Amiodarone
    avoidance of, in liver disease, 920
    for solid organ transplant recipients, 1093
Ammonia accumulation, in liver disease, 927–929
Amnesty International Report on torture, 1047
Anemia
    in alcohol misuse, 999

Med Clin N Am 99 (2015) 1149–1165
http://dx.doi.org/10.1016/S0025-7125(15)00116-9
0025-7125/15/$ – see front matter © 2015 Elsevier Inc. All rights reserved.

medical.theclinics.com

Printed and bound by CPI Group (UK) Ltd, Croydon, CR0 4YY

03/10/2024

01040494-0011